theclinics.com

# MEDICAL CLINICS OF NORTH AMERICA

## Common Gastrointestinal Emergencies

GUEST EDITOR
Mitchell S. Cappell, MD, PhD

May 2008 • Volume 92 • Number 3

SAUNDERS

An Imprint of Elsevier, Inc.
PHILADELPHIA LONDON TORONTO MONTREAL SYDNEY TOKYO

**W.B. SAUNDERS COMPANY**
*A Division of Elsevier Inc.*

1600 John F. Kennedy Boulevard • Suite 1800 • Philadelphia, Pennsylvania 19103-2899

http://www.theclinics.com

**MEDICAL CLINICS OF NORTH AMERICA**
**May 2008**
Editor: Rachel Glover

**Volume 92, Number 3**
**ISSN 0025-7125**
**ISBN-13: 978-1-4160-5862-5**
**ISBN-10: 1-4160-5862-1**



*Medical Clinics of North America* (ISSN 0025-7125) is published bimonthly by W.B. Saunders, 360 Park Avenue South, New York, NY 10010-1710. Business and editorial offices: 1600 John F. Kennedy Boulevard, Suite 1800, Philadelphia, PA 19103-2899. Accounting and circulation offices: 6277 Sea Harbor Drive, Orlando, FL 32887-4800. Periodicals postage paid at New York, NY, and additional mailing offices. Subscription prices are USD 173 per year for US individuals, USD 306 per year for US institutions, USD 89 per year for US students, USD 220 per year for Canadian individuals, USD 389 per year for Canadian institutions, USD 131 per year for Canadian students, USD 250 per year for international individuals, USD 389 per year for international institutions and USD 131 per year for international students. To receive student/resident rate, orders must be accompanied by name of affiliated institution, date of term, and the *signature* of program/residency coordinator on institution letterhead. Orders will be billed at individual rate until proof of status is received. Foreign air speed delivery is included in all *Clinics* subscription prices. All prices are subject to change without notice. POSTMASTER: Send address changes to *Medical Clinics of North America*, Elsevier Periodicals Customer Service, 6277 Sea Harbor Drive, Orlando, FL 32887-4800. **Customer Service: 1-800-654-2452 (US). From outside the United States, call: 1-407-563-6020. Fax: 1-407-363-9661. E-mail: JournalsCustomerService-usa@elsevier.com.**

*Reprints*. For copies of 100 or more, of articles in this publication, please contact the Commercial Reprints Department, Elsevier Inc., 360 Park Avenue South, New York, New York 10010-1710. Tel.: (+1) (212) 633-3813; Fax: (+1) (212) 462-1935; E-mail: reprints@elsevier.com.

*Medical Clinics of North America* is also published in Spanish by McGraw-Hill Interamericana Editores S. A., P.O. Box 5-237, 06500 Mexico, D.F., Mexico.

*Medical Clinics of North America* is covered in *Index Medicus, Current Contents, ASCA, Excerpta Medica, Science Citation Index*, and *ISI/BIOMED.*

Printed in the United States of America.

**GOAL STATEMENT**

The goal of *Medical Clinics of North America* is to keep practicing physicians up to date with current clinical practice by providing timely articles reviewing the state of the art in patient care.

**ACCREDITATION**

The *Medical Clinics of North America* is planned and implemented in accordance with the Essential Areas and Policies of the Accreditation Council for Continuing Medical Education (ACCME) through the joint sponsorship of the University of Virginia School of Medicine and Elsevier. The University of Virginia School of Medicine is accredited by the ACCME to provide continuing medical education for physicians.

The University of Virginia School of Medicine designates this educational activity for a maximum of 90 *AMA PRA Category 1 Credits*™. Physicians should only claim credit commensurate with the extent of their participation in the activity.

The American Medical Association has determined that physicians not licensed in the US who participate in this CME activity are eligible for *AMA PRA Category 1 Credits*™.

Credit can be earned by reading the text material, taking the CME examination online at http://www.theclinics.com/home/cme, and completing the evaluation. After taking the test, you will be required to review any and all incorrect answers. Following completion of the test and evaluation, your credit will be awarded and you may print your certificate.

**FACULTY DISCLOSURE/CONFLICT OF INTEREST**

The University of Virginia School of Medicine, as an ACCME accredited provider, endorses and strives to comply with the Accreditation Council for Continuing Medical Education (ACCME) Standards of Commercial Support, Commonwealth of Virginia statutes, University of Virginia policies and procedures, and associated federal and private regulations and guidelines on the need for disclosure and monitoring of proprietary and financial interests that may affect the scientific integrity and balance of content delivered in continuing medical education activities under our auspices.

The University of Virginia School of Medicine requires that all CME activities accredited through this institution be developed independently and be scientifically rigorous, balanced and objective in the presentation/discussion of its content, theories and practices.

All authors/editors participating in an accredited CME activity are expected to disclose to the readers relevant financial relationships with commercial entities occurring within the past 12 months (such as grants or research support, employee, consultant, stock holder, member of speakers bureau, etc.). The University of Virginia School of Medicine will employ appropriate mechanisms to resolve potential conflicts of interest to maintain the standards of fair and balanced education to the reader. Questions about specific strategies can be directed to the Office of Continuing Medical Education, University of Virginia School of Medicine, Charlottesville, Virginia.

**The authors/editors listed below have identified no professional or financial affiliations for themselves or their spouse/partner:**

Mihaela Batke, MD; Mitchell S. Cappell, MD, PhD (Guest Editor); David Friedel, MD; Rachel Glover (Acquisitions Editor); John T. Langell, MD, PhD, MPH; Francisco J. Marrero, MD; Sean J. Mulvihill, MD; David M. Poppers, MD, PhD; Mohammed A. Qadeer, MD; Arun J. Sanyal, MBBS, MD; Charles J. Shanley, MD, FACS; Nagib Toubia, MD; and Jeffrey B. Weinberger, MD.

**The authors/editors listed below identified the following professional or financial affiliations for themselves or their spouse/partner:**

**Gregory B. Haber, MD, FRCPC** is a consultant, serves on the Speaker's Bureau and Advisory Committee for Boston Scientific, NDO, USGI, Olympus, Spirus, Fujinon, Pentax, Cook, Bard, ASTRA, and TAP.

**Bret A. Lashner, MD** serves on the Advisory Committee for Elan, Procter & Gamble, Shire, Abbott, UCB, and Prometheus.

*Disclosure of Discussion of non-FDA approved uses for pharmaceutical products and/or medical devices:*

**The University of Virginia School of Medicine, as an ACCME provider, requires that all faculty presenters identify and disclose any "off label" uses for pharmaceutical and medical device products. The University of Virginia School of Medicine recommends that each physician fully review all the available data on new products or procedures prior to instituting them with patients.**

**TO ENROLL**

To enroll in the Medical Clinics of North America Continuing Medical Education program, call customer service at 1-800-654-2452 or visit us online at http://www.theclinics.com/home/cme. The CME program is available to subscribers for an additional fee of USD 205.

## FORTHCOMING ISSUES

July 2008

**Common Hepatic Emergencies**
Mitchell S. Cappell, MD, PhD, *Guest Editor*

September 2008

**Women's Health**
Tony Ogburn, MD, and
Carolyn Voss, MD, *Guest Editors*

November 2008

**Emerging Infectious Diseases**
Mary Wilson, MD, *Guest Editor*

## RECENT ISSUES

March 2008

**Hospital Medicine**
Scott A. Flanders, MD, Vikas I. Parekh, MD, and
Lakshmi Halasyamani, MD, *Guest Editors*

January 2008

**Atrial Fibrillation**
Ranjan K. Thakur, MD, and
Andrea Natale, MD, FACC, FHRS, *Guest Editors*

November 2007

**Metabolic Syndrome**
Robert T. Yanagisawa, MD, and
Derek LeRoith, MD, PhD, *Guest Editors*

July 2007

**Acute Myocardial Infarction**
Mandeep Singh, MD, and
David R. Holmes, Jr., MD, *Guest Editors*

# GUEST EDITOR

**MITCHELL S. CAPPELL, MD, PhD,** Chief, Division of Gastroenterology, Department of Medicine, William Beaumont Hospital, Royal Oak, Michigan

# CONTRIBUTORS

**MIHAELA BATKE, MD,** Fellow, Division of Gastroenterology, Department of Medicine, William Beaumont Hospital, Royal Oak, Michigan

**MITCHELL S. CAPPELL, MD, PhD,** Chief, Division of Gastroenterology, Department of Medicine, William Beaumont Hospital, Royal Oak, Michigan

**DAVID FRIEDEL, MD,** Division of Gastroenterology, Department of Medicine, Winthrop Medical Center, Mineola, New York

**GREGORY B. HABER, MD, FRCPC,** Chief, Division of Gastroenterology, Center for Advanced Therapeutic Endoscopy, Lenox Hill Hospital, New York, New York

**JOHN T. LANGELL, MD, PhD, MPH,** Assistant Professor of Surgery; Director of Acute Care Surgery, Department of Surgery, University of Utah, Salt Lake City, Utah

**BRET A. LASHNER, MD,** Professor of Medicine, Department of Gastroenterology and Hepatology, Cleveland Clinic, Cleveland, Ohio

**FRANCISCO MARRERO, MD,** Fellow, Department of Gastroenterology and Hepatology, Cleveland Clinic, Cleveland, Ohio

**SEAN J. MULVIHILL, MD,** Professor of Surgery; Chairman, Department of Surgery, University of Utah; Senior Director of Clinical Affairs, Huntsman Cancer Institute, Salt Lake City, Utah

**DAVID M. POPPERS, MD, PhD,** Advanced Therapeutic Endoscopy Fellow, Division of Gastroenterology, Center for Advanced Therapeutic Endoscopy, Lenox Hill Hospital, New York, New York

**MOHAMMED A. QADEER, MD,** Fellow, Department of Gastroenterology and Hepatology, Cleveland Clinic, Cleveland, Ohio

**ARUN J. SANYAL, MBBS, MD,** Chairman, Division of Gastroenterology, Hepatology and Nutrition, Virginia Commonwealth University School of Medicine, Richmond, Virginia

**CHARLES J. SHANLEY, MD, FACS,** Senior Vice President for Surgical Services; Chairman, Department of Surgery, William Beaumont Hospital, Royal Oak, Michigan

**NAGIB TOUBIA, MD,** Division of Gastroenterology, Hepatology and Nutrition, Virginia Commonwealth University School of Medicine, Richmond, Virginia

**JEFFREY B. WEINBERGER, MD,** Chief Resident, Department of Surgery, William Beaumont Hospital, Royal Oak, Michigan

# CONTENTS

ELSEVIER
SAUNDERS

Med Clin N Am 92 (2008) xi–xiv

THE MEDICAL CLINICS OF NORTH AMERICA

# Preface

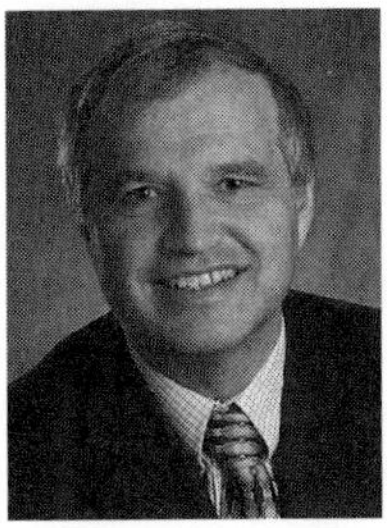

Mitchell S. Cappell, MD, PhD
*Guest Editor*

Gastrointestinal emergencies are important to clinicians and their patients. They are relatively common. Mechanical gastrointestinal obstruction and acute upper gastrointestinal bleeding, for example, are each individually responsible for more than 300,000 hospitalizations each year in the United States [1,2]. These emergencies require urgent, correct, life-or-death decisions for a successful outcome. The clinician has to recognize a true gastrointestinal emergency among the vast number of patients presenting with mostly mundane abdominal complaints. Is this mundane chronic constipation or acute gastrointestinal obstruction? Does this abdominal pain arise from the irritable bowel syndrome or from early acute mesenteric ischemia? Is this bright red blood per rectum from hemorrhoids, the most common and least significant cause of gastrointestinal bleeding, or from exsanguinating upper gastrointestinal hemorrhage, a less common but highly lethal condition? If therapy is delayed because the emergency goes unrecognized, the mortality increases dramatically, as, for example, occurs with acute mesenteric ischemia [3].

For an emergency, the physician, perforce, compresses the usual elective evaluation into a rapid diagnostic algorithm. The history, physical examination, and diagnostic tests have to be appropriate and thorough but severely compressed in time, while the therapy is emergently instituted. The penalty for delays or errors is likely death [4].

Physicians confronted by these multiple challenges generally perform admirably. But as clinicians, we can do better. The overall mortality of gastrointestinal emergencies is 10% or greater. Even a 3% decrease in


doi:10.1016/j.mcna.2008.01.008

mortality, when applied to the estimated one million or more gastrointestinal emergencies per year in America, translates into 30,000 lives saved each year! This number of saved lives is more than 10 fold greater than the annual mortality from the current American war in Iraq.

New clinical data based on clinical trials, novel diagnostic tests, and high technology therapies are increasing exponentially. For example, at least 10 different endoscopic therapies are available for hemostasis of upper gastrointestinal bleeding (see the article by Cappell and Friedel elsewhere in this issue). But which therapy is best for a given patient bleeding from a given gastrointestinal lesion?

To improve physician performance and decrease mortality, the physician has to function at an extremely high level, armed with the newest clinical studies, the most authoritative clinical algorithms, the latest consensus statements, and the best expert opinions. How is the busy practitioner—burdened by paperwork from insurance companies, mundane requirements of hospital bureaucracies, increasing governmental regulations, and increasing fiscal restraints in medical practice—expected to achieve this high level of performance? The clinician needs an up-to-date, authoritative, and concise but thorough clinical review.

The clinician employs the *Medical Clinics of North America* format of concise, up-to-date articles to try to achieve these goals. Gastrointestinal emergencies selected for this issue are relatively common, frequently life-threatening disorders that are rapidly changing in terms of diagnosis and therapy. The selected authors are practicing clinicians who are nationally recognized authorities in their fields. This issue is intended to aid the entire medical team involved in gastrointestinal emergencies: the internist requiring a sound working knowledge of the field, the gastroenterologist and other subspecialists needing an in-depth and up-to-date understanding of the field, the clinical researcher to comprehend areas of uncertainty and controversy to stimulate new clinical protocols and trials, and the medical inventor to understand the clinical needs and technical shortcomings of current devices to invent better ones.

Consider upper gastrointestinal bleeding. Despite the revolutionary development of endoscopic hemostasis, the mortality of this bleeding has stubbornly persisted at about 10% during the last 30 years [5]. Among other explanations for this phenomenon, lack of effective clinical implementation of endoscopic therapy is undoubtedly a contributing factor, as is insufficient medical resuscitation before endoscopy. The principles of rapid but thorough diagnostic evaluation as well as adequate fluid resuscitation, blood transfusion, and cardiopulmonary support are comprehensively reviewed in the first article by Drs. Cappell and Friedel. In a companion article the same authors extensively review the endoscopic diagnosis of gastrointestinal bleeding, the available endoscopic therapies, and their individual advantages, disadvantages, and indications, with a focus on novel therapies.

Variceal bleeding is highly important clinically because of its high mortality [6]. Drs. Toubia and Sanyal extensively cover the pathophysiology, diagnosis, and therapy of varcieal bleeding. Mechanical intestinal obstruction still has a 10% mortality, mostly due to delayed and ineffective therapy. This disease is reviewed from the medical perspective by two gastroenterologists, Drs. Cappell and Batke, to emphasize the importance of rapid, effective diagnosis for aggressive surgery before ischemia or necrosis supervenes. Drs. Batke and Cappell also review colonic pseudoobstruction and ileus, medical conditions that closely mimic mechanical obstruction but are treated very differently. Their article comprehensively reviews this subject. The discussion on neostigmine is particularly important because neostigmine is insufficiently, clinically applied despite manifest efficacy [7].

Drs. Langell and Mulvihill admirably review gastrointestinal perforation and the acute abdomen. Of particular interest is the discussion of the pathophysiology and the differences between gastric, small intestinal, and colonic perforations. Acute vascular emergencies are highly important due to the frequency of clinical misdiagnosis with a consequently poor outcome. I commend Drs. Shanley and Weinberger on their authoritative review of this subject. The internist, general practitioner, and gastroenterologist must be knowledgeable about complications of inflammatory bowel disease. Drs. Marrero, Qadeer, and Lashner provide a superb review of this insufficiently appreciated subject.

Finally, the article on endoscopic mucosal resection (EMR) is essential reading for any student of gastrointestinal disease. The clinical benefits of this novel therapy are realized only insofar as this technique is clinically implemented. While widely implemented in Japan and Europe, advanced EMR is still unavailable in most American hospitals! Drs. Poppers and Haber provide a unique insight into this area as practitioners and researchers.

I thank my supervisors, Drs. Ananias Diokno, Leslie Rocher, Mike Maddens, and John Musich, for their encouragement and support for this academic endeavor. I thank Rachel Glover, the editor, for her extremely helpful advice, wonderful guidance, and friendly collaboration in this project, as well as the folks at Elsevier for an ongoing relationship that has allowed me to serve as guest editor of 10 issues in the *Clinics of North America* series. I thank my secretary Mary Fronczak for help in typing. I thank the librarians at William Beaumont Hospital, including Janet Zimmerman, Andrea Rogers, Ken Nelson, Janet West, and Chris Smitacz, for their help in literature searches and procuring articles form other libraries. I thank Mike Holland, of the Continuing Medical Education Department at William Beaumont Hospital, for his generous help in setting up flow charts in this issue. Finally, I thank my wife for tolerating my absence from home during nights and weekends while working on this issue, and my kids Adina, David, Miriam, and Daniel for their support.

On a personal note, this has been an immensely satisfying experience as a practicing clinician, clinical researcher, and educator.

Mitchell S. Cappell, MD, PhD
*Division of Gastroenterology*
*Department of Medicine*
*William Beaumont Hospital*
*MOB 233*
*3601 West Thirteen Mile Road*
*Royal Oak, MI 48073, USA*

## References

[1] Ray NF, Denton WG, Thamer M, et al. Abdominal adhesiolysis: inpatient care and expenditures in the United States in 1994. J Am Coll Surg 1998;186(1):1–9.
[2] Fallah MA, Prakash C, Edmundowicsz S. Acute gastrointestinal bleeding. Med Clin North Am 2000;84(5):1183–208.
[3] Kougias P, Lau D, El Sayed HF, et al. Determinants of mortality and treatment outcome following surgical interventions for acute mesenteric ischemia. J Vasc Surg 2007;46(3):467–74.
[4] Fevang BT, Fevang J, Stangeland L, et al. Complications and death after surgical treatment of small bowel obstruction: a 35-year institutional experience. Ann Surg 2000;231(4):529–37.
[5] Palmer K. Acute upper gastrointestinal haemorrhage. Br Med Bull 2007;83:307–24.
[6] Habib A, Sanyal AJ. Acute variceal hemorrhage. Gastrointest Endosc Clin N Am 2007;17(2): 223–52.
[7] Loftus CG, Harewood GC, Baron TH. Assessment of predictors of response to neostigmine for acute colonic pseudo-obstruction. Am J Gastroenterol 2002;97(12):3118–22.

ELSEVIER
SAUNDERS

THE MEDICAL CLINICS OF NORTH AMERICA

Med Clin N Am 92 (2008) 491–509

# Initial Management of Acute Upper Gastrointestinal Bleeding: From Initial Evaluation up to Gastrointestinal Endoscopy

Mitchell S. Cappell, MD, PhD[a,*], David Friedel, MD[b]

[a]*Division of Gastroenterology, Department of Medicine, William Beaumont Hospital, MOB 233, 3601 West Thirteen Mile Road, Royal Oak, MI 48073, USA*
[b]*Division of Gastroenterology, Department of Medicine, Winthrop Medical Center, 222 Station Plaza North, Suite 428, Mineola, NY 11501, USA*

Upper gastrointestinal bleeding (UGIB) is a common, potentially life-threatening condition responsible for more than 300,000 hospital admissions and about 30,000 deaths per annum in America [1]. Treating and preventing UGIB costs many billions of dollars per annum [2]. Accurate patient evaluation and appropriate early management before esophagogastroduodenoscopy (EGD) is critical to decrease the morbidity and mortality. The early management focuses on resuscitative measures of fluid infusion or blood transfusion to reverse the direct consequences of bleeding; prevention of end-organ damage induced by the bleeding, such as hypoxia or prerenal azotemia; and general measures to promote hemostasis before EGD. Clinicians—whether internists, intensivists, gastroenterologists, or gastrointestinal surgeons—have to be familiar with the initial evaluation and therapy to form a knowledgeable and cohesive team. This article focuses on the initial assessment, early resuscitative measures, and general therapy of UGIB before EGD, with a focus on new techniques, to optimize the patient therapy and thereby decrease patient morbidity and mortality.

## Epidemiology

UGIB is defined as bleeding proximal to the ligament of Treitz, to differentiate it from lower gastrointestinal bleeding involving the colon, and middle gastrointestinal bleeding involving the small intestine distal to the

* Corresponding author.
*E-mail address:* mscappell@yahoo.com (M.S. Cappell).


doi:10.1016/j.mcna.2008.01.005 ***medical.theclinics.com***

ligament of Treitz [1]. The annual incidence of hospitalization for acute UGIB is 1 per 1000 people in America [3]. It has a mortality of 7% to 10% [4]. The mortality has decreased only minimally during the last 30 years, despite the introduction of endoscopic therapy that reduces the rate of rebleeding [4]. This phenomenon has been attributed to the increasing percentage of UGIB occurring in the elderly, who have a much worse prognosis than other patients because of their frequent use of antiplatelet medications or anticoagulants, and their frequent comorbid conditions [5,6]. About 45% of patients now hospitalized for UGIB are more than 60 years old [7]. Endoscopic therapy has, however, led to a recent decrease in the need for blood transfusions or surgery for UGIB [1]. The mortality of UGIB is much higher for patients who bleed after hospital admission than for those admitted for gastrointestinal bleeding [1,8,9].

## Etiology

Major and minor causes of UGIB are listed in Box 1, and the frequency distribution of the major causes are listed in Table 1 [3,10,11]. Peptic ulcer disease (PUD) accounts for about half of all UGIB (see Table 1) [1,7]. Major risk factors for PUD include *Helicobacter pylori* infection, use of nonsteroidal antiinflammatory drugs (NSAIDs) or aspirin, smoking, alcoholism, and prior history of PUD [9,12]. Patients who bleed after admission for another problem usually have PUD [8]. One study suggests a recent moderate decrease in PUD as a cause of UGIB, despite a marked increase in the proportion of elderly patients who have UGIB from PUD related to NSAIDs [3]. PUD surgery is performed less than previously, but increasingly bariatric surgery causes postoperative bleeding ulcers [13]. Variceal hemorrhage accounts for 10% to 25% of UGIB, depending on the catchment area [1,7]. Other relatively common causes of UGIB are inflammatory lesions of the upper gastrointestinal tract, Mallory-Weiss tears, angiodysplasia, and Dieulafoy lesions (see Table 1) [3,10,11]. Postprocedural bleeding is usually related to endoscopic biopsy or therapy [14].

## Clinical assessment

Patients who have UGIB must be promptly and accurately clinically assessed, as described in Box 2, to provide a rational basis for key early decisions on their medical management, as enumerated in Box 3. The medical history, physical examination, and initial laboratory values are important in assessing resuscitation requirements, triage, endoscopy timing, consultation requirements, and prognostication [15].

### *Medical history*

Although a complete medical history is obtained, it should be focused on the gastrointestinal tract, other highly relevant history, and significant

**Box 1. Causes of upper gastrointestinal hemorrhage**

*Major causes*
Peptic ulcer disease
Esophageal and gastric varices
Hemorrhagic gastritis
Esophagitis
Duodenitis
Mallory-Weiss tear
Angiodysplasia
Upper gastrointestinal malignancy
Anastomotic ulcers (after PUD surgery or bariatric surgery)
Dieulafoy lesion

*Minor causes*
Cameron lesion
Gastric antral vascular ectasia (watermelon stomach)
Portal hypertensive gastropathy
Post chemotherapy or radiation sequelae
Gastric polyps
Aortoenteric fistula
Submucosal lesion/mass (eg, leiomyoma)
Connective tissue disease
Hemobilia
Hemosuccus pancreaticus
Kaposi sarcoma
Foreign bodies
Postprocedural: nasogastric tube erosions, endoscopic biopsy, endoscopic polypectomy, EMR, endoscopic sphincterotomy

*Abbreviations:* EMR, endoscopic mucosal resection; PUD, peptic ulcer disease.

comorbid conditions (Box 4). In a patient in hypovolemic shock or otherwise in extremis, the medical history is initially obtained rapidly in summary form because of the need for emergency resuscitation, but a complete history is obtained after patient stabilization. The medical history includes past episodes of gastrointestinal bleeding and their causes, because up to 60% of UGIB is from the same gastrointestinal lesion that previously bled [16]; prior use of gastrotoxic drugs, such as NSAIDs or aspirin; and prior use of drugs that promote bleeding, such as antiplatelet agents or anticoagulants. The risk of bleeding from PUD is increased up to fivefold with administration of nonselective NSAIDs or higher doses ($\geq$325 mg/d) of aspirin [17,18]. Administration of anticoagulants in the therapeutic range, low-dose aspirin (<100 mg/d), or the antiplatelet drugs clopidogrel and

Table 1
Endoscopic diagnoses in patients who have overt upper gastrointestinal bleeding

| | Incidence (%) | | |
|---|---|---|---|
| Diagnosis | Silverstein et al [11][a] | Jutabha and Jensen [10] | Boonpongmanee et al [3][b] |
| Peptic ulcers | — | 55 | — |
| Duodenal ulcer | 24.3 | — | 13.9 |
| Gastric ulcer | 21.3 | — | 23.1 |
| Erosive disease | | | |
| Esophagitis | 6.3 | 6 | 3.7 |
| Gastric erosions/gastritis | 23.4 | — | 4.7 |
| Duodenitis | 5.8 | — | 3.7 |
| Esophageal varices | 10.3 | 14 | 23.1 |
| Mallory-Weiss tear | 7.2 | 5 | 10.2 |
| Neoplasm | 2.9 | 4 | — |
| Stomal (marginal) ulcer | 1.8 | — | — |
| Esophageal ulcer | 1.7 | — | — |
| Angiodysplasia | — | 6 | — |
| Dieulafoy lesion | — | 1 | — |
| Other/miscellaneous | 6.8 | 11 | 17.6 |

[a] Results total more than 100% because of inclusion of multiple endoscopic diagnoses in some individual patients.

[b] Patients who had a nondiagnostic esophagogastroduodenoscopy excluded.

ticlopidine increase the risk of UGIB by threefold, whereas the selective COX-II (cyclooxygenase-II) inhibitor celecoxib only modestly increases the risk [18,19].

The medical history provides clues to the cause of the UGIB, as summarized in Table 2. A history of alcoholism increases the risk for cirrhosis, portal hypertension, and bleeding from esophageal varices. In cirrhotics, about 60% of an initial UGIB is from esophageal varices [20]. Alcoholism also increases the incidence of PUD [21]. A history of smoking cigarettes is relevant. Duodenal ulcers heal more slowly and recur more frequently with therapy in smokers than in nonsmokers [22]. Smoking and alcoholism are also associated with gastrointestinal malignancy. The patient should be asked about prior *H pylori* infection and therapy. *H pylori* most commonly produces

**Box 2. Key aspects in the initial assessment of the patient who has acute gastrointestinal bleeding**

Bleeding severity
Bleeding acuity
Bleeding activity
Bleeding location: upper versus lower gastrointestinal bleeding
Variceal versus nonvariceal upper gastrointestinal bleeding
Associated coagulopathy

**Box 3. Key early decisions in the medical management of acute upper gastrointestinal bleeding**

*Triage*

Admit to hospital versus discharge from emergency room
Admit to ICU versus monitored bed versus unmonitored hospital bed
Emergency versus routine gastroenterology consult
Surgical consult or not

*Intensive monitoring*

Nasogastric tube insertion or not
Central venous line or Swann-Ganz catheter or not
Foley insertion or not

*General supportive therapy*

Endotracheal intubation or not
Transfuse packed erythrocytes or not
Transfuse other blood products or not
PPI therapy or not
Octreotide therapy or not

*Endoscopy*

Emergency versus elective endoscopy
EGD versus colonoscopy
Endoscopic therapy or not
Specific modality of endoscopic therapy

*Abbreviations:* EGD, esophagogastroduodenoscopy; PPI, proton pump inhibitor.

**Box 4. Key aspects in the medical history of patients who have significant acute upper gastrointestinal bleeding**

Prior history of GI bleeding
GI symptoms
Character of GI bleeding
GI medications
Gastrotoxic medications
Anticoagulants
Social habits
Medical comorbidities
Other relevant history

*Abbreviation:* GI, gastrointestinal.

Table 2
Clues provided by the medical history regarding the cause of acute upper gastrointestinal bleeding

| Bleeding etiology | Historical clues |
|---|---|
| Mallory-Weiss tear | Emesis before hematemesis, alcoholism |
| Esophageal ulcer | Odynophagia, GERD, esophagotoxic pill ingestion |
| Peptic ulcer | Epigastric/RUQ pain, NSAID or aspirin use |
| Stress gastritis | Patient in an ICU, gastrointestinal bleeding occurring after admission, respiratory failure, multiorgan failure |
| Varices, portal gastropathy | Alcoholism, cirrhosis |
| Gastric antral vascular ectasia | Renal failure, cirrhosis |
| Malignancy | Recent involuntary weight loss, dysphagia, cachexia, early satiety |
| Angiodysplasia | Chronic renal failure, hereditary hemorrhagic telangiectasia |
| Aortoenteric fistula | Known aortic aneurysm, prior abdominal aortic aneurysm repair |

*Abbreviations:* GERD, gastroesophageal reflux disease; NSAID, nonsteroidal anti-inflammatory drug; RUQ, right upper quadrant.

PUD when contracted at a young age, a phenomenon more frequent in immigrants to America [23]. Aortoenteric fistula is strongly associated with prior aortic surgery, aortic aneurysms, and severe atherosclerosis [24].

Gastrointestinal symptoms are highly relevant. Patients who have PUD often have chronic epigastric pain. A duodenal ulcer typically causes abdominal pain that is initially relieved by eating, but recurs 1 to 2 hours postprandially. Mesenteric ischemia often presents with self-limited gastrointestinal bleeding associated with severe abdominal pain. Reflux esophagitis typically causes pyrosis. Other forms of gastrointestinal bleeding are typically painless. Vomiting, coughing, or retching before bleeding suggests a Mallory-Weiss tear [25]. Involuntary weight loss suggests chronic disease, particularly gastrointestinal malignancy. Regurgitation, water brash, or dysphagia suggests possible gastroesophageal reflux disease (GERD). The differential of dysphagia with UGIB includes reflux esophagitis, esophageal infections, esophageal malignancy, benign peptic stricture, pill esophagitis, and esophageal ulcers.

The presentation and appearance of the blood helps to localize the site of bleeding and to evaluate its acuity and severity. Melena is recognized as black and tarry stools. It should be differentiated from black stools secondary to iron or bismuth ingestion. Patients who have gross UGIB present with melena in about 75% of cases and with hematemesis in about 50% [6]. Hematemesis indicates bleeding proximal to the ligament of Treitz. Moderate amounts of "coffee-ground" or altered blood emesis suggest more limited bleeding than does hematemesis. About 90% of melena arises from bleeding proximal to the ligament of Treitz because of degradation of blood during gastrointestinal transit, whereas 10% of melena arises from the small bowel or right colon. Bright red blood per rectum usually arises from a lower gastrointestinal source, most commonly from hemorrhoids. Hemorrhoidal bleeding classically presents with a clinical triad of bright red blood per rectum attributable to the presence of arterialized blood in the hemorrhoidal plexus; blood coating the stools attributable to insufficient time for admixture; and postdefecatory bleeding attributable to hemorrhoidal trauma during stool evacuation. Bright red blood per rectum occasionally arises from a massive UGIB [26]. A UGIB must be excluded when fresh rectal bleeding is accompanied by signs of hypovolemia or hypoperfusion.

The patient's evaluation of the severity of gastrointestinal bleeding is generally not quantitative and often inaccurate [27]. Orthostatic dizziness, mental confusion, cold clammy extremities, angina, or severe palpitations suggest hemodynamic compromise from massive bleeding. Symptoms of excessive bleeding when brushing the teeth, hematuria, or easy bruisability suggest a coagulopathy that can contribute to the bleeding. Jaundice, weakness, fatigue, anorexia, and abdominal distention from ascites are consistent with chronic liver disease.

*Physical examination*

The physical examination, while complete, is directed at findings relevant to gastrointestinal bleeding (Box 5). The severity of blood loss is roughly estimated by the hemodynamic status and other key signs (Table 3). Resting tachycardia, in the absence of another cause, suggests mild to moderate hypovolemia. Orthostatic hypotension is defined as a decrease in the systolic blood pressure of more than 20 mm Hg or an increase in the pulse of more than 20 beats/min from recumbency to standing. Orthostatic hypotension suggests loss of 15% or more of the blood volume. Hypotension is associated with a 40% loss of blood volume [28]. Patients in shock typically have a thready, weak pulse and cold, clammy extremities. Stigmata of chronic liver disease, such as jaundice, spider angiomata, palmar erythema, hepatomegaly, ascites, and caput medusa suggest UGIB from esophageal varices. Ecchymoses or petechiae are signs of a coagulopathy.

The abdomen is carefully examined. Hyperactive bowel sounds are consistent with a UGIB because blood in the proximal gut is an irritant that stimulates peristalsis, whereas normoactive bowel sounds are more consistent with lower gastrointestinal bleeding. Hypoactive bowel sounds suggest bowel ischemia, an ileus, or mechanical obstruction. Abdominal tenderness is uncommon with uncomplicated UGIB, except occasionally for PUD. Severe abdominal tenderness suggests gastrointestinal bleeding associated with bowel ischemia, gastrointestinal obstruction, or gastrointestinal perforation. Severe direct abdominal tenderness, rebound tenderness, or involuntary guarding suggests a possible acute abdomen that requires exclusion of gastrointestinal perforation before performing EGD. A careful rectal examination should be performed, including determination of the type of bleeding, whether hematochezia, maroon stools, or melena; testing for fecal occult blood; and inspection for external hemorrhoids or anal fissures.

**Box 5. Critical aspects of the physical examination in patients who have acute gastrointestinal bleeding**

*Hemodynamic stability*
Tachycardia, thready pulse
Hypotension
Orthostatic hypotension
Hypoxia

*Careful abdominal examination*
Bowel sounds
Abdominal tenderness
Ascites—shifting dullness

*Signs of chronic liver disease or portal hypertension*
Hepatomegaly
Splenomegaly
Palmar erythema
Caput medusa
Spider angiomata
Peripheral edema

*Signs of shock*
Cold clammy extremities
Poor mentation
(Also see vital signs listed above)

*Rectal examination*
Occult blood
Gross blood
- Bright red blood per rectum
- Melena
- Burgundy stools
- Blood coating stools versus within stools
- Bloody diarrhea

*Laboratory data*

The decline in hematocrit reflects the degree of blood loss after a delay of 24 hours or more from an acute UGIB. The hematocrit does not immediately decline during bleeding because whole blood, containing a proportionate amount of plasma and erythrocytes, is initially lost. The hematocrit subsequently declines because of dilution from influx of extravascular fluid into the vascular space. This dilution is augmented by intravenous hydration. The initial hematocrit on admission is best interpreted when a recent

Table 3
Correlation between physical signs and the severity of upper gastrointestinal bleeding

| Physical signs or degree of blood loss | Bleeding severity: Mild | Moderate | Severe |
|---|---|---|---|
| Blood loss | <1 L | 1–2 L | ≥2 L |
| Blood pressure | Normal | Normal–borderline low | Hypotensive |
| Orthostasis | No | Possible | Likely |
| Tachycardia | None–mild | Moderate | Severe |
| Skin | Warm, well perfused | Diaphoretic | Cool–cold, clammy |
| Respiratory rate | Normal | Normal–slightly decreased | Irregular |
| Urine output | Normal | Diminished | Poor |
| Sensorium | Alert/anxious | Anxious | Confused/drowsy |

prior baseline hematocrit is available for comparison. Serial hematocrits are helpful to assess the severity of a UGIB but should be integrated with the hemodynamic assessment because overhydration falsely depresses the hematocrit. A central venous pressure or Swann-Ganz catheter more accurately reflects the volume status than the physical examination or serial hematocrit levels [29,30]. These catheters are indicated when such information is essential for proper fluid management.

Other important laboratory parameters include the coagulation profile; routine serum chemistries, especially the blood urea nitrogen (BUN) and creatinine levels; and serum biochemical parameters of liver function. Patients who have UGIB typically have an elevated BUN level because of absorption of degraded blood during intestinal transit and prerenal azotemia from hypovolemia [31], and have a BUN/creatinine ratio greater than 20:1 [32]. The erythrocytes are typically normocytic with an acute UGIB and are typically microcytic with a chronic UGIB. Iron deficiency anemia is consistent with chronic blood loss. Although leukocytosis may be secondary to the stress of acute bleeding, leukocytosis requires exclusion of underlying infection by appropriate cultures and analyses of blood, sputum, urine, or ascitic fluid as necessary.

Myocardial infarction should be excluded by serial electrocardiography and serum cardiac enzymes in elderly patients who have hypotension and in all patients who have massive bleeding because of a significant risk for myocardial infarction from coronary artery hypoperfusion from hypovolemia. For example, in a study of 113 patients who had severe gastrointestinal bleeding undergoing serial serum cardiac enzyme determinations, 16 (12.3%) patients had myocardial infarction [33]. Patients who have myocardial infarction consequent to massive bleeding often do not experience chest pain, or the chest pain may be misinterpreted as epigastric pain. For example, in a study of 36 patients who had gastrointestinal bleeding complicated by simultaneous myocardial infarction only half of the patients had chest pain [34].

*Nasogastric aspiration*

Nasogastric aspiration with saline lavage is beneficial to detect the presence of intragastric blood, to determine the type of gross bleeding, to clear the gastric field for endoscopic visualization, and to prevent aspiration of gastric contents. A grossly bloody aspirate in the absence of traumatic intubation confirms a UGIB. Red blood suggests currently active bleeding, whereas coffee grounds suggest recently active bleeding. Continued aspiration of red blood suggests severe, active hemorrhage [35]. Nasogastric aspiration of red blood is associated with a significantly higher rate of active bleeding or other endoscopic stigmata of recent hemorrhage (SRH) at emergency EGD, as compared with a nasogastric aspirate of coffee grounds or nonbloody material [36].

A nonbloody nasogastric aspirate does not preclude a recent gastric bleed that ceased several hours earlier because of evacuation of gastric contents during the interim, and does not preclude a duodenal bleed because duodenal contents may not have been sampled because of pylorospasm [37,38]. A bilious, nonbloody aspirate virtually excludes these alternatives, however, and strongly suggests that the bleeding is distal to the ligament of Treitz or stopped many hours earlier.

Nasogastric tube insertion is uncomfortable, but rarely causes complications. The main complications are epistaxis from traumatic tube insertion and gastric erosions from nasogastric suctioning. Nasogastric tube erosions are recognized as multiple, collinear, equidistant, round, and relatively uniform erythematous erosions that are in register with the apertures of the nasogastric tube and that are at the same stage of evolution because of their simultaneous creation [24,39]. In a review of 152 nasogastric tube insertions for gastrointestinal bleeding within 30 days of myocardial infarction among 125 patients, only 2 (1.3% rate) cases of clinically significant complications occurred, including epistaxis in 1 patient and nasogastric tube–induced gastric erosions in 1 patient [36]. Both complications were easily managed without clinical sequelae by transfusions of packed erythrocytes. The risk of epistaxis is greatly decreased by gentle insertion technique, lubrication of the tip of the tube, patient cooperation during insertion, discontinuation of intravenous heparin therapy more than 4 hours before insertion, and avoidance of insertion in the presence of a coagulopathy. The risk of inducing gastric erosions is decreased by applying nasogastric suction only intermittently, by using low-pressure negative suction, by early tube removal after the bleeding ceases, and by use of modern, flexible nasogastric tubes with multiple apertures.

Failure to clear the fundus of blood before EGD can result in missed pathology at EGD because of poor endoscopic visibility and can necessitate repeat EGD [40]. If the stomach is not cleared by nasogastric aspiration and lavage, parenteral erythromycin promotes evacuation of intragastric blood and improves endoscopic visualization [41].

## General therapy

Patient resuscitation includes fluid administration, blood transfusion, cardiorespiratory support, and treatment of significant comorbid diseases, such as sepsis or coronary artery disease. In patients who have severe hemodynamic or pulmonary instability, EGD should be delayed until the patient is adequately resuscitated and stabilized.

### *General supportive measures*

Patients generally receive supplemental oxygen by nasal cannula to counteract the loss of oxygen carrying capacity from loss of erythrocytes. Patients who have massive bleeding, active hematemesis, hypoxia, severe tachypnea, or altered mental status should be evaluated for endotracheal intubation to protect the airway and to supplement tissue oxygenation [42]. Patients who have acute UGIB should receive nothing per os because of the urgent need for EGD and the potential need for abdominal surgery. A Foley catheter is inserted in patients in shock or in those who have massive bleeding to monitor the urine output [43]. Cardiac telemetry and pulse oximetry are generally recommended.

### *Fluid resuscitation*

Patients are assessed for hypovolemia and shock to determine requirements for fluid infusion and transfusion of packed erythrocytes, and are assessed for comorbid diseases, especially cardiovascular disease. Intravenous access is secured at two or more sites using 18-gauge or larger catheters. Patients who have active bleeding receive at least 500 mL of saline, or another crystalloid solution, during the first 30 minutes to maintain the blood pressure, while several units of packed erythrocytes are typed and crossed [27,44]. Fluid infusion is increased if the blood pressure fails to increase or declines.

### *Blood transfusions*

Packed erythrocytes are transfused to improve tissue oxygenation and prevent end-organ damage. The need for blood transfusions is individualized. No absolute hematocrit level is required to preserve life and organ function, and blood is not transfused according to rigid, arbitrary, minimum hematocrit levels. Transfusion requirements are determined by multiple factors, including patient age, presence of comorbidities, cardiovascular status, baseline hematocrit, and tempo of the bleeding, along with the current hematocrit level. Packed erythrocytes are transfused in patients who have significant blood loss, continuing active bleeding, and those who manifest cardiac, renal, or cerebral ischemia. The rate of blood transfusion is determined by the severity of the hypovolemia, by the tempo of the bleeding, and by the presence of cardiac, renal, or cerebrovascular comorbidities. Patients who have severe ongoing bleeding, with hemodynamic instability associated with the bleeding and with recent angina are aggressively transfused. Patients who have variceal bleeding are conservatively transfused to a hematocrit of only 27 to avoid exacerbating the bleeding by increasing the portal pressure. Overtransfusion in cirrhotic laboratory animals produces a rebound in portal pressure that can precipitate variceal bleeding [45]. Similarly, in a small, randomized, controlled study, 25 cirrhotic patients who were transfused aggressively, with transfusion of at least 2 units of packed erythrocytes, had a significantly higher risk for rebleeding than 25 similar cirrhotic patients who were transfused conservatively with transfusion only for shock or a hemoglobin less than 8 [46]. A hematocrit of 25 to 27 is, likewise, generally adequate to maintain tissue oxygenation in young healthy patients who do not have comorbid disorders [47]. Elderly patients, however, have less cardiopulmonary reserve and may not tolerate mild anemia. For example, a hematocrit less than 28 was associated with myocardial ischemia in elderly men undergoing medical prostatectomy [48].

Severe coagulopathy can exacerbate the bleeding and must be treated by transfusion of fresh frozen plasma or platelets, as appropriate. A useful guideline is to transfuse 1 unit of fresh frozen plasma for every 4 units of packed erythrocytes transfused to replace lost coagulation factors [49]. An international normalized ratio (INR) of less than 1.5 does not require therapy. Mild thrombocytopenia (50,000–90,000 platelets/μL) usually does not contribute to UGIB and does not require platelet transfusion. Platelet counts less than 50,000/μL in the presence of active bleeding may require platelet transfusion [10,50]. This general rule is individualized according to multiple factors, including bleeding severity, bleeding rate, presence of other coagulopathies, and presence of qualitative platelet defects, such as those induced by NSAIDs [51]. Coagulopathies are aggressively corrected before surgery for gastrointestinal bleeding [52].

Blood transfusions have rare but serious side effects. Despite screening of blood donors, HIV, human T-cell lymphotrophic virus types 1 and 2, hepatitis B, hepatitis C, and parvovirus are still very rarely transmitted by blood transfusions. Bacterial infections are also rarely transmitted by blood transfusions, particularly *Yersinia enterocolitica* with erythrocyte transfusions and *Staphylococcus aureus* with platelet transfusions [49]. Hemolytic reactions from ABO-incompatible blood rarely occur because of human error. Blood transfusion can cause fever and transfusion-associated graft-versus-host disease. Too rapid transfusion can induce congestive heart failure and pulmonary edema in patients who have prior congestive heart failure or other cardiac diseases [53]. Such patients are transfused cautiously and slowly. Diuretics may be administered before or during transfusion in such patients [28].

## *Empiric pharmacotherapy before endoscopy*

Proton pump inhibitor (PPI) therapy is recommended before EGD [54,55]. This therapy reduces the severity of SRH at endoscopy and reduces the need for endoscopic therapy as compared with no treatment or histamine-2 antagonist therapy [56,57]. PPI therapy, however, only modestly reduces the risk for rebleeding, need for surgery, and blood transfusions, and has so far not been shown to reduce mortality [58]. The benefit is greatest in patients who have high-risk SRH, such as a visible vessel. Although intravenous infusion is ideal, oral PPI therapy provides much of the benefit [59]. For example, a randomized, controlled trial from India of 220 patients showed that early oral therapy with high-dose omeprazole, a PPI, significantly reduced the rate of rebleeding and of surgery in patients who had bleeding PUD [59]. The rationale for PPI therapy is that most common causes of UGIB, including ulcers, gastritis, duodenitis, and hemorrhagic reflux esophagitis, are medically treated with acid-suppressive therapy. PPI therapy is also useful, however, for hemostasis of lesions that are not caused by acid and are not in other circumstances treated by PPI therapy, probably because neutralization of intraluminal gastric acid promotes hemostasis by stabilizing blood clots [60].

Octreotide, a somatostatin analog, is standardly used to reduce the risk of bleeding from esophageal varices because it inhibits mesenteric vasodilatation induced by glucagon [61]. Our practice is to initiate octreotide therapy in patients who have UGIB who have significant liver disease, a history of variceal bleeding, a history of alcoholism, or highly abnormal biochemical parameters of liver function because of the established benefits of this therapy for variceal bleeding [62].

## Consultation and triage

All patients who have acute UGIB require gastroenterology consultation [63]. Surgical consultation is recommended for patients who have ongoing active bleeding, massive bleeding, recurrent bleeding, bleeding associated with significant abdominal pain, acute lower gastrointestinal bleeding, variceal bleeding, and abdominal findings suggestive of an acute abdomen. Cardiology consultation is recommended in patients who have chest pain, prior severe coronary artery disease, hemodynamic instability, suspected myocardial infarction, or significant cardiac arrhythmias. Intensivist consultation is recommended for severe gastrointestinal bleeding [28]. Patients who have severe manifestations of bleeding, such as shock or continuing hematochezia, or significant comorbidities should be triaged to an ICU for monitoring by continuous electrocardiography and pulse oximetry, and by intermittent sphygmomanometry [64,65].

## Endoscopy

EGD is the prime diagnostic and therapeutic tool for UGIB. It is the procedure of choice. It accurately delineates the bleeding site and determines the specific cause, it provides a rational basis for triage of patients for routine hospital admission versus ICU admission, it helps assess the need for surgery, it provides valuable prognostic information, and it can be used to apply the recently greatly expanded armamentarium of endoscopic therapy (see the article by Cappell and Friedel elsewhere in this issue).

Therapeutic endoscopy generally produces hemostasis and prevents rebleeding [66,67]. The available therapies include injection therapy, such as injection of epinephrine; ablative therapy, such as electrocautery or argon plasma coagulation; and mechanical therapy, such as endoclips or banding. EGD rarely causes serious complications, such as gastrointestinal perforation, precipitation of bleeding, missed pathology, and anesthesia complications [14,68]. The benefit of EGD has to be weighed against the risks in high-risk patients, such as those who have acute myocardial infarction [69,70].

## Clinical parameters to assess bleeding severity and efficacy of therapies

Endoscopic findings, particularly SRH, help predict the risk for rebleeding in patients who have PUD, the need for blood transfusions, the length of hospital stay, and the mortality [71,72]. The endoscopic findings are combined with the clinical presentation and initial laboratory data in clinical scoring systems for risk stratification, triage, and prognostication [73–75]. Patient evaluation and assessment with simultaneous resuscitative measures and prompt EGD optimizes UGIB outcome (Fig. 1) [76].

Clinical parameters to assess the efficacy of pharmacologic or endoscopic therapies for UGIB include rebleeding rate, need for repeat EGD, need for surgery or angiography, blood transfusion requirements, length of hospital stay, medical costs, and mortality, including in-hospital mortality, 30-day mortality, and bleeding-associated mortality. Endoscopic parameters are used to evaluate the efficacy of pharmacotherapy.

## Challenges and prospects

Mortality has stubbornly persisted at 7% to 10% for nonvariceal UGIB (NVUGIB), perhaps because patients are older, sicker, and on an ever-increasing regimen of drugs that affect hemostasis. PPI use has been validated in patients bleeding from high-risk PUD, but guidelines still need clarification regarding patient stratification, medication formulation, and timing of administration [56,57]. The role of octreotide for NVUGIB requires further study. The clinical evaluation, diagnosis, and management of UGIB will become increasingly standardized, based on validated clinical scoring systems and management algorithms, to optimize patient care and minimize medical costs [77]. Artificial blood, such as treated bovine hemoglobin or perfluorocarbons, requires further clinical trials regarding safety and efficacy before achieving widespread clinical application [78].

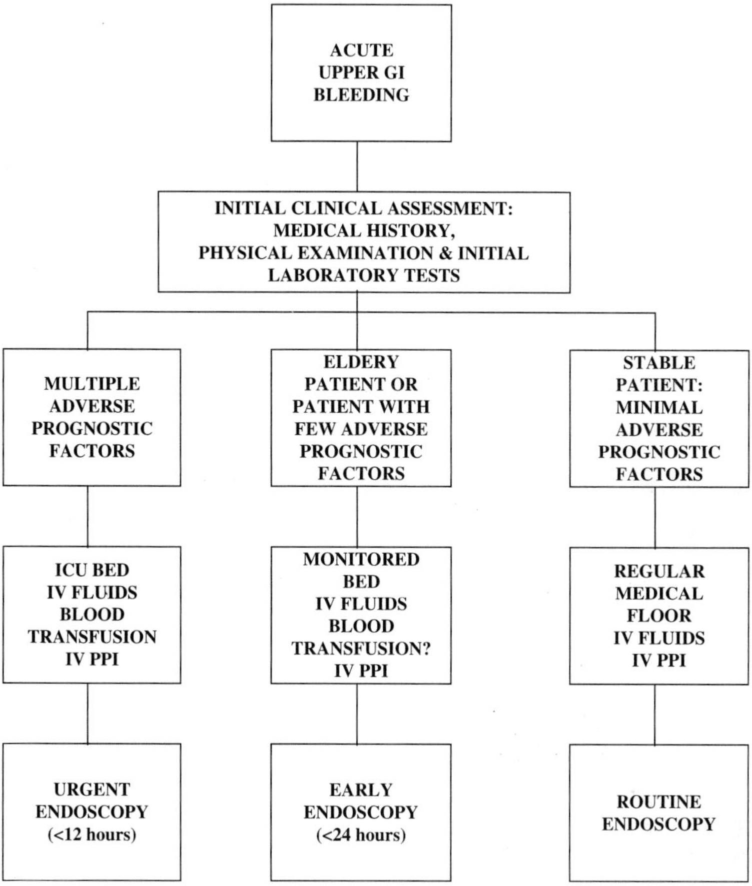


Fig. 1. An algorithm for the initial management and triage of a patient who has acute upper gastrointestinal bleeding. GI, gastrointestinal; IV, intravenous; PPI, proton pump inhibitor.

## Summary

UGIB is a relatively common, potentially life-threatening condition that requires rapid assessment of clinical presentation, rapid resuscitative measures, and appropriate medical triage. Administration of PPIs is an important adjunctive measure for NVUGIB. EGD remains the principal diagnostic, therapeutic, and prognostic modality for NVUGIB. The article by Cappell and Friedel elsewhere in this issue reviews the diagnostic and therapeutic role of EGD for NVUGIB.

## References

[1] Fallah MA, Prakash C, Edmundowicz S. Acute gastrointestinal bleeding. Med Clin North Am 2000;84(5):1183–208.

[2] Jiranek JC, Kozarek RA. A cost-effective approach to the patient with peptic ulcer bleeding. Surg Clin North Am 1996;76(1):83–103.

[3] Boonpongmanee S, Fleischer DE, Pezzulo JC, et al. The frequency of peptic ulcer disease as a cause of upper-GI bleeding is exaggerated. Gastrointest Endosc 2004;59(7):788–94.

[4] Palmer K. Acute upper gastrointestinal haemorrhage. Br Med Bull 2007;83:307–24.

[5] Kaplan RC, Heckbert SR, Koepsell TD, et al. Risk factors for gastrointestinal bleeding among older patients. Cardiovascular Health Study Investigators. J Am Geriatr Soc 2001; 49(2):126–33.

[6] Peter DJ, Doughtery JM. Evaluation of the patient with gastrointestinal bleeding: an evidence based approach. Emerg Med Clin North Am 1999;17(1):239–61.

[7] Yavorski RT, Wong RK, Maydonovitch C, et al. Analysis of 3,294 cases of upper gastrointestinal bleeding in military medical facilities. Am J Gastroenterol 1995;90(4):568–73.

[8] Lewis JD, Shin EJ, Metz DC. Characterization of gastrointestinal bleeding in severely ill hospitalized patients. Crit Care Med 2000;28(1):261–2.

[9] Longstrech GF. Epidemiology of hospitalization for acute upper gastrointestinal hemorrhage: a population based study. Am J Gastroenterol 1995;90(2):206–10.

[10] Jutabha R, Jensen DM. Management of upper gastrointestinal bleeding in the patient with chronic liver disease. Med Clin North Am 1996;80(5):1035–68.

[11] Silverstein FE, Gilbert DA, Tedesco FJ, et al. The National ASGE survey on upper gastrointestinal bleeding: 1. Study design and baseline data. Gastrointest Endosc 1981; 27(2):73–9.

[12] Bayyurt N, Abasiyanik MF, Sander E, et al. Canonical analysis of factors involved in the occurrence of peptic ulcers. Dig Dis Sci 2007;52(1):140–6.

[13] Yang CS, Lee WJ, Wang HH, et al. Spectrum of endoscopic findings in patients with upper gastrointestinal symptoms after laparoscopic bariatric surgery. Obes Surg 2006;16(9): 1232–7.

[14] Cappell MS, Abdullah M. Management of gastrointestinal bleeding induced by gastrointestinal endoscopy. Gastroenterol Clin North Am 2000;29(1):125–67.

[15] Kollef MH, O'Brien JD, Zuckerman GR, et al. BLEED: a classification to predict outcome in patients with acute upper and lower gastrointestinal hemorrhage. Crit Care Med 1997; 25(7):1101–2.

[16] McGuirk TD, Coyle WJ. Upper gastrointestinal tract bleeding. Emerg Med Clin North Am 1996;14(3):523–45.

[17] Dubois RW, Melmed GY, Henning JM, et al. Risk of upper gastrointestinal injury and events in patients treated with cyclo-oxygenase COX-1/COX-2 nonsteroidal anti-inflammatory drugs (NSAIDs), COX-2 selective NSAIDs and gastroprotective cotherapy: an appraisal of the literature. J Clin Rheumatol 2004;10(4):178–89.

[18] Lana A, Garcia-Rodriguez LA, Arroyo MT, et al. Risk of upper gastrointestinal ulcer bleeding with selective cyclo-oxygenase-2 inhibitors, traditional non-aspirin non-steroidal anti-inflammatory drugs, aspirin and combinations. Gut 2006;55(12):1731–8.

[19] Cryer B. The role of cyclooxygenase inhibitors in the gastrointestinal tract. Curr Gastroenterol Rep 2003;5(6):453–8.

[20] Sutton FM. Upper gastrointestinal bleeding in patients with esophageal varices: what is the most common source? Am J Med 1987;83(2):273–5.

[21] Andersen IB, Jorgensen T, Bonnevie O, et al. Smoking and alcohol intake as risk factors for bleeding and perforated peptic ulcers: a population-based cohort study. Epidemiology 2000; 11(4):434–49.

[22] Chiverton SG, Hunt RH. Smoking and duodenal ulcer disease. J Clin Gastroenterol 1989; 11(Suppl):s29–33.

[23] Smith BR, Stabile BE. Emerging trends in peptic ulcer disease and damage control surgery in the *H. pylori* era. Am Surg 2005;71(9):797–801.

[24] Cappell MS, Friedel D. The role of esophagogastroduodenoscopy in the diagnosis and management of upper gastrointestinal disorders. Med Clin North Am 2002;86(6):1165–216.

[25] Sugawa C, Benishek D, Walt AJ. Mallory-Weiss syndrome: a study of 224 patients. Am J Surg 1983;145(1):30–3.
[26] Jensen DM, Machicado GA. Diagnosis and treatment of severe hematochezia: the role of urgent colonoscopy after purge. Gastroenterology 1988;95(6):1569–74.
[27] Steele R. The preprocedure care of the patient with gastrointestinal bleeding. Gastrointest Endosc Clin N Am 1997;7(4):551–60.
[28] Kupfer Y, Cappell MS, Tessler S. Acute gastrointestinal bleeding in the intensive care unit. The intensivist's perspective. Gastroenterol Clin North Am 2000;29(2):275–307.
[29] Sorensen MB, Christiansen LA, Malmstrom J, et al. Central hemodynamics in acute gastrointestinal bleeding. Surg Gynecol Obstet 1977;145(5):685–90.
[30] Kwan V, Norton ID. Endoscopic management of non-variceal upper gastrointestinal haemorrhage. ANZ J Surg 2007;77(4):222–30.
[31] Stellato T, Rhodes RS, McDouglas WS. Azotemia in upper gastrointestinal hemorrhage. Am J Gastroenterol 1980;73:486–9.
[32] Richards RJ, Donica MB, Grayer D. Can the blood urea nitrogen/creatinine ratio distinguish upper from lower gastrointestinal bleeding? J Clin Gastroenterol 1990;12(5):500–4.
[33] Bhatti N, Amoateng-Adjepong Y, Qamar A, et al. Myocardial infarction in critically ill patients presenting with gastrointestinal hemorrhage: retrospective analysis of risks and outcomes. Chest 1998;114(4):1137–42.
[34] Cappell MS. A study of the syndrome of simultaneous acute upper gastrointestinal bleeding and myocardial infarction in 36 patients. Am J Gastroenterol 1995;90(9):1444–9.
[35] DiMaio CJ, Stevens PD. Nonvariceal upper gastrointestinal bleeding. Gastrointest Endosc Clin N Am 2007;17(2):253–72.
[36] Cappell MS. Safety and efficacy of nasogastric intubation for gastrointestinal bleeding after myocardial infarction: an analysis of 125 patients at two tertiary cardiac referral hospitals. Dig Dis Sci 2005;50(11):2063–70.
[37] Witting MD, Magder L, Heins AE, et al. Usefulness and validity of diagnostic nasogastric tube aspiration in patients without hematemesis. Ann Emerg Med 2004;43(4):525–32.
[38] Cuellar RE, Gavaler JS, Alexander JA, et al. Gastrointestinal tract hemorrhage: the value of a nasogastric aspirate. Arch Intern Med 1990;150(7):1381–4.
[39] Greene JF Jr, Sawicki JE, Doyle WF. Gastric ulceration: a complication of double-lumen nasogastric tubes. JAMA 1973;224(3):338–9.
[40] Stollman NH, Putcha RV, Neustater BR, et al. The uncleared fundal pool in acute upper gastrointestinal bleeding: implications and outcomes. Gastrointest Endosc 1997;46(4):324–7.
[41] Carbonell N, Pauwels A, Serfaty L, et al. Erythromycin infusion prior to endoscopy for acute upper gastrointestinal bleeding: a randomized, controlled double-blind trial. Am J Gastroenterol 2006;101(6):1211–5.
[42] Rudolph SJ, Landsverk BK, Freeman ML. Endotracheal intubation for airway protection during endoscopy for severe upper GI hemorrhage. Gastrointest Endosc 2003;57(1):58–61.
[43] McIntyre LA, Hebert PC, Fergusson D, et al. A survey of Canadian intensivists' resuscitation practices in early septic shock. Crit Care 2007;11(4):R74.
[44] Duggan JM. Personal view: crystalloid transfusion in acute gastrointestinal haemorrhage: is it beneficial? An historical perspective. Aliment Pharmacol Ther 2006;24(3):493–6.
[45] Kravetz D, Bosch J, Arderiu M, et al. Hemodynamic effects of blood volume restitution following a hemorrhage in rats with portal hypertension due to cirrhosis of the liver: influence of the extent of portal-systemic shunting. Hepatology 1989;9(6):808–14.
[46] Blair SD, Janvrin SB, McCollum CN, et al. Effect of early blood transfusion on gastrointestinal haemorrhage. Br J Surg 1986;73(10):783–5.
[47] Klein HG, Spahn DR, Carson JL. Red blood cell transfusion in clinical practice. Lancet 2007;370(9585):415–26.
[48] Hogue CW Jr, Goodnough LT, Monk TG. Preoperative myocardial ischemic episodes are related to hematocrit levels in patients undergoing radical prostatectomy. Transfusion 1998;38(10):924–31.

[49] Maltz GS, Siegel JE, Carson JL. Hematologic management of gastrointestinal bleeding. Gastroenterol Clin North Am 2000;29(1):169–87.
[50] Conteras M. Final statement from the consensus conference on platelet transfusion. Transfusion 1998;38:796–7.
[51] Cairns JA, Gent M, Singer J, et al. Aspirin, sulfinpyrazone, or both in unstable angina: results of a Canadian multicenter trial. N Engl J Med 1985;313(22):1369–75.
[52] Samama CM, Djoudi R, Lecompte T, et al. Perioperative platelet transfusion: recommendations of the Agence Française de Sécurité Sanitaire des Produits de Santé (AFSSaPS) 2003. Can J Anaesth 2005;52(1):30–7 [in French].
[53] Allen JB, Allen FB. The minimum acceptable level of hemoglobin. Int Anesthesiol Clin 1982; 20(4):1–22.
[54] Eisen GM, Dominitz JA, Faigel DO, et al. An annotated algorithmic approach to upper gastrointestinal bleeding. Standards of Practice Committee. Gastrointest Endosc 2001; 53(7):853–8.
[55] Barkun A, Bardou M, Marshall JK, et al, and the Nonvariceal Upper GI Bleeding Consensus Group. Consensus recommendations for managing patients with nonvariceal upper gastrointestinal bleeding. Ann Intern Med 2003;139(10):843–57.
[56] Andrews CN, Levy A, Fishman M, et al. Intravenous proton pump inhibitors in bleeding peptic ulcer disease with high-risk stigmata: a multicenter comparative study. Can J Gastroenterol 2005;19(11):667–71.
[57] Jensen DM, Pace SC, Soffer E, et al. 315 study Group. Continuous infusion of pantoprazole versus ranitidine for prevention of ulcer rebleeding: a US multicenter randomized double-blind study. Am J Gastroenterol 2006;101(9):1991–9.
[58] Leontiadis GI, Sharma VK, Howden CW. Systematic review and meta-analysis: proton-pump inhibitor treatment for ulcer bleeding reduces transfusion requirements and hospital stay-results from the Cochrane Collaboration. Aliment Pharmacol Ther 2005;22(3): 169–74.
[59] Khuroo MS, Yattoo GN, Javid G, et al. A comparison of omeprazole and placebo for bleeding peptic ulcer disease. N Engl J Med 1997;336(15):1054–8.
[60] Green FW Jr, Kaplan MM, Curtis LE, et al. Effect of acid and pepsin on blood coagulation and platelet aggregation: a possible contributor prolonged gastroduodenal mucosal hemorrhage. Gastroenterology 1978;74(1):38–43.
[61] Imperiale TF, Birgisson S. Somatostatin or octreotide compared to H2 antagonist and placebo in the management of acute nonvariceal upper gastrointestinal hemorrhage: a meta-analysis. Ann Intern Med 1997;127(12):1062–71.
[62] Thabut D, Bernard-Chabert B. Management of acute bleeding from portal hypertension. Best Pract Res Clin Gastroenterol 2007;21(1):19–29.
[63] Kolkman JJ, Meuwissen SG. A review of bleeding peptic ulcer: a collaborative task of gastroenterologist and surgeon. Scand J Gastroenterol Suppl 1996;218:16–25.
[64] Romagnuolo J, Barkun AN, Enns R, et al. Simple clinical predictors may obviate urgent endoscopy in patients with nonvariceal upper gastrointestinal bleeding. Arch Intern Med 2007;167(3):265–70.
[65] Tham TC, James C, Kelly M. Predicting outcome of acute non-variceal upper haemorrhage without endoscopy using the clinical Rockall Score. Postgrad Med J 2006;82(973):757–9.
[66] Adler DG, Leighton JA, Davila RE, et al. ASGE guideline: the role of endoscopy in acute non-variceal upper-GI hemorrhage. Gastrointest Endosc 2004;60(4):497–504.
[67] Rolhauser C, Fleischer DE. Nonvariceal upper gastrointestinal bleeding. Endoscopy 2002; 34(2):111–8.
[68] Reiertsen O, Skjoto J, Jacobsen CD, et al. Complications of fiberoptic gastrointestinal endoscopy: five years' experience in a central hospital. Endoscopy 1987;19(1):1–6.
[69] Lin S, Konstance R, Jollis J, et al. The utility of upper endoscopy in patients with upper gastrointestinal bleeding and acute myocardial infarction. Dig Dis Sci 2006;51(12):2377–83.

[70] Cappell MS, Iacovone FM Jr. Safety and efficacy of esophagogastroduodenoscopy after myocardial infarction. Am J Med 1999;106(1):29–35.
[71] Lau JY, Chung SC, Leung JW, et al. The evolution of stigmata of hemorrhage in bleeding peptic ulcer ulcers: a sequential endoscopic study. Endoscopy 1998;30(6):513–8.
[72] Cooper GS, Chak A, Way L, et al. Early endoscopy in upper gastrointestinal hemorrhage: association with recurrent bleeding, surgery and length of hospital stay. Gastrointest Endosc 1999;49(1):145–52.
[73] Rockall TA, Logan RF, Devlin HB, et al. Risk assessment after acute upper gastrointestinal hemorrhage. Gut 1996;38(3):316–21.
[74] Saeed ZA, Winchester CB, Michaletz PA, et al. A scoring system to predict rebleeding after endoscopic therapy of nonvariceal upper gastrointestinal hemorrhage, with a comparison of heat probe and ethanol injection. Am J Gastroenterol 1993;88(11):1842–9.
[75] Hussain H, Lapin S, Cappell MS. Clinical scoring systems for determining the prognosis of gastrointestinal bleeding. Gastroenterol Clin North Am 2000;29(2):445–64.
[76] Spiegel BM, Vakil NB, Ofman JJ. Endoscopy for acute nonvariceal upper–gastrointestinal hemorrhage: is sooner better?: a systematic review. Arch Intern Med 2001;161(11):1393–404.
[77] Podila PV, Ben-Manachem T, Batra SK, et al. Managing patients with acute nonvariceal upper gastrointestinal hemorrhage: development and effectiveness of a clinical care pathway. Am J Gastroenterol 2001;96(1):208–19.
[78] Spahn DR, Kocian R. Artificial O2 carriers: status in 2005. Curr Pharm Des 2005;11(31): 4099–114.

ELSEVIER
SAUNDERS

THE MEDICAL CLINICS OF NORTH AMERICA

Med Clin N Am 92 (2008) 511–550

# Acute Nonvariceal Upper Gastrointestinal Bleeding: Endoscopic Diagnosis and Therapy

Mitchell S. Cappell, MD, PhD[a,*], David Friedel, MD[b]

[a]*Division of Gastroenterology, Department of Medicine, William Beaumont Hospital, MOB 233, 3601 West Thirteen Mile Road, Royal Oak, MI 48073, USA*

[b]*Division of Gastroenterology, Department of Medicine, Winthrop Medical Center, 222 Station Plaza North, Suite 428, Mineola, NY 11501, USA*

Upper gastrointestinal bleeding (UGIB) is a relatively common, potentially life-threatening condition that causes more than 300,000 hospital admissions and about 30,000 deaths per annum in America [1]. Treating and preventing UGIB costs many billions of dollars per annum [2]. Endoscopic therapy has revolutionalized the treatment of UGIB, with a recently greatly expanded therapeutic armamentarium (Box 1). Clinicians—whether internists, gastroenterologists, intensivists, or gastrointestinal surgeons—have to become generally familiar with the new endoscopic therapies and their indications to form a knowledgeable and cohesive team to optimize patient care. This review of diagnostic and therapeutic esophagogastroduodenoscopy (EGD) for nonvariceal UGIB (NVUGIB) focuses on novel therapies and their indications, to optimize patient therapy and thereby decrease patient morbidity and mortality. The preceding article in this issue by the same authors discusses the initial management of acute UGIB before EGD, whereas the following article by Drs. Toubia and Sanyal reviews variceal UGIB.

## Epidemiology

UGIB is defined as bleeding proximal to the ligament of Treitz, to differentiate it from lower gastrointestinal bleeding involving the colon, and middle gastrointestinal bleeding involving the small intestine distal to the ligament of Treitz [1]. The annual incidence of hospitalization for acute UGIB is 1 per 1000 people in America [3]. UGIB has a mortality of 7%

* Corresponding author.
*E-mail address:* mscappell@yahoo.com (M.S. Cappell).


doi:10.1016/j.mcna.2008.01.001
*medical.theclinics.com*

**Box 1. Endoscopic therapies**

*Injection therapy*
Epinephrine with normal saline
Sclerotherapy
Thrombin
Fibrin sealant
Cyanoacrylate glue

*Ablative therapy*
Contact methods
- Thermocoagulation—heater probe
- Electrocoagulation—BICAP, traditional Gold probe, ERBE*
- Cryotherapy

Noncontact methods
- Photocoagulation—Nd:YAG laser
- Argon plasma coagulation (APC)

*Mechanical therapy*
Endoclips
Detachable snare—endoloop
Bands
Suturing device

*Combined therapy devices*
Probe combining electrocautery with needle injection
Device combining electrocautery with mechanical therapy

* ERBE Elektromedizin, Tubingen, Germany.
*Abbreviations:* BICAP, bipolar electrocoagulation probe; Nd:YAG, neodymium-doped yttrium aluminum garnet.

to 10% [4]. The mortality has decreased only minimally during the last 30 years, despite the introduction of endoscopic therapy that reduces the rebleeding rate. This phenomenon is attributed to the increasing percentage of UGIB occurring in the elderly, a group with a worse prognosis than other patients because of their increased use of antiplatelet medications or anticoagulants, and their frequent comorbid conditions [5,6]. Endoscopic therapy has, however, been shown to reduce the rate of rebleeding, the need for blood transfusions, and the need for surgery [1].

## Endoscopy

EGD is the prime diagnostic and therapeutic tool for UGIB [7]. It accurately delineates the bleeding site and determines the specific cause. EGD is 90% to 95% diagnostic for acute UGIB [8]. Multiple clinical scoring systems incorporate the endoscopic findings with clinical parameters on admission, including time from onset of bleeding to hospitalization, hemodynamic status, bleeding presentation, hematocrit, nasogastric tube aspirate findings, and patient comorbidities [9–11]. These scoring systems are valuable for prognostication and triage of patients who have NVUGIB [9,10]. Older age, hematochezia, shock, and a spurting artery or visible vessel at EGD are consistently negative prognostic factors, as is UGIB in patients already hospitalized for another cause [9,12]. For UGIB from peptic ulcer disease (PUD), the endoscopic findings by themselves are valuable predictors of the risk for rebleeding, need for blood transfusions, need for surgery, length of hospital stay, and mortality (Box 2) [13,14]. These prognostic data provide a rational basis for triage of patients to an unmonitored bed versus the ICU. Endoscopic parameters are also used in clinical trials to evaluate the efficacy of pharmacotherapy.

A multidisciplinary team approach, in conjunction with scoring systems that incorporate the endoscopic findings, reduces the hospital length of stay and thereby reduces hospital costs without adversely affecting patient outcome [13,15,16]. Patients who have a low clinical score, indicating a low risk for rebleeding, might conceivably be discharged immediately after EGD, but this strategy is generally not practiced [17,18]. Our practice is to perform EGD before discharge on all patients who have acute UGIB, and to admit all such patients if the EGD confirms a UGIB. Likewise, patients in the ICU who have low-risk endoscopic findings or successful endoscopic hemostasis may be triaged to a regular hospital bed [8].

The efficacy of endoscopic therapies for UGIB is assessed in clinical trials by the rebleeding rate, blood transfusion requirements, need for repeat EGD, need for surgery or angiography, length of hospital stay, medical costs, and mortality, including 30 day mortality, in-hospital mortality, or UGIB-related mortality.

### *Consent*

The endoscopist should briefly describe to the patient the procedure technique, risks, benefits, and alternatives and obtain written, signed,

**Box 2. Endoscopic findings in peptic ulcer disease as predictors of rebleeding**

*Endoscopic finding and rebleeding rate within 72 hours*
Spurting artery, 90%–100%
Actively oozing blood, 80%
Visible vessel, 40%–60%
Adherent clot, 20%–25%
Flat pigmented spots on ulcer, 13%
Clean ulcer base, 5%

and witnessed informed consent. The consent should include contemplated endoscopic therapies. If the patient is obtunded or mentally incompetent, consent is obtained from the next of kin or legal guardian. Emergency administrative consent is obtained, as per written hospital protocols, when EGD is emergently required and the next of kin is unavailable. Patients who refuse cardiac resuscitation or endotracheal intubation ("do not resuscitate" status) can still undergo EGD if appropriate consent is obtained. Our policy is to require the patient or the next of kin to waive these treatment restrictions during the EGD to handle endoscopic emergencies.

*Anesthesia*

Attendance of an anesthesiologist at EGD is currently decided arbitrarily by the endoscopist's preference, anesthesiologist's availability, and patient's wishes. Use of an anesthesiologist, a costly resource, should be allocated according to rational criteria, as proposed in Box 3. A separate consent for anesthesiology is obtained if an anesthesiologist attends the EGD. The patient should be informed of the potentially greater medical costs if an anesthesiologist is used.

EGD is generally performed with a combination of a narcotic, either fentanyl or meperidine, and a benzodiazepine, either midazolam or diazepam, administered by the gastroenterologist. EGD is increasingly performed using propofol for deeper sedation and faster recovery. The deeper sedation is advantageous in highly anxious patients, patients who have psychiatric disorders, patients who have previously not tolerated EGD, and intravenous

**Box 3. Reasonable indications for an anesthesiologist at esophagogastroduodenoscopy**

- Patient highly unstable from severe acute gastrointestinal bleeding
- American Society of Anesthesiologists class III or IV patient: mild-moderate gastrointestinal bleeding in a patient who has comorbid conditions
- Patient receiving mechanically assisted ventilation
- Severely unstable vital signs (regardless of cause)
- Highly uncooperative patient
- Active recent substance or alcohol abuse
- Advanced cirrhosis/liver failure
- Planned sclerotherapy or banding from gastroesophageal varices
- History of failed attempts at esophagogastroduodenoscopy (EGD) without anesthesiology assistance

drug abusers or alcoholics who tend to be difficult to sedate; it is advantageous in complex, prolonged procedures, such as banding of bleeding esophageal varices. The faster recovery streamlines turnover of outpatients because of shorter postprocedural monitoring.

Although traditionally administered by anesthesiologists because of the risk of respiratory depression, propofol is increasingly being administered by gastroenterologists and nurses, without anesthesiologists, with high efficacy and safety [19,20]. Nurses, under the supervision of a gastroenterologist, safely administered propofol in 36,743 endoscopic procedures with no cases requiring endotracheal intubation or resulting in death, neurologic sequelae, or other permanent injury [21]. For patient safety, the propofol dosage is titrated at EGD to a moderate level of sedation and the patient is carefully monitored for respiratory depression [22].

### *Endoscopy equipment and setting*

A large-caliber, dual-channel, therapeutic endoscope, with one channel for water lavage or suction and a second channel for insertion of therapeutic catheters, is preferred for acute UGIB. A water pump is useful to vigorously and extensively lavage blood and clots to visualize underlying lesions. At a minimum, a sclerotherapy needle for epinephrine injection and another means of therapeutic endoscopy should be available at the bedside for NVUGIB, and esophageal banding should be available for variceal UGIB. The endoscopist should test all ports, buttons, and dials on the endoscope head before the EGD to verify that they function properly. A trained assistant should be in attendance at EGD to monitor the patient's vital signs and level of consciousness and to assist in therapeutic endoscopy. For the convenience of endoscopy staff, Boxes 4 and 5 provide checklists for the patient and equipment conditions necessary for EGD.

EGD for acute UGIB should be performed in a hospital, not a freestanding ambulatory surgical center. EGD is best performed in the hospital endoscopy suite, where the required equipment and trained staff are available. Patients who have exsanguinating hemorrhage, highly unstable vital signs, or severe comorbidities may be too unstable to be transported to the endoscopy suite. In such cases, emergency EGD is performed at the bedside in a monitored unit, such as the emergency room, operating room, or ICU.

### *Esophagogastroduodenoscopy risks*

EGD rarely causes serious complications, such as gastrointestinal perforation, precipitation of gastrointestinal bleeding, aspiration pneumonia, respiratory arrest, cardiovascular complications, and missed lesions [23]. The benefit of EGD must be weighed against these risks in high-risk patients, such as those who have acute myocardial infarction [24–26].

**Box 4. Checklist for esophagogastroduodenoscopy for acute upper gastrointestinal bleeding: patient status**

- Valid EGD consent
  - Type of consent
    - Written
    - Informed
    - Includes contemplated endoscopic therapies
  - Conscious patient
    - From patient
  - Unconscious patient
    - Closest relative
    - Legal guardian
  - Administrative consent in emergency
  - Separate consent for anesthesiology if anesthesiologist in attendance
- Patient stability
  - Vital signs stabilized if possible with patient resuscitation
    - If cannot stabilize vital signs, consider EGD only if emergently indicated
  - Severe coagulopathy corrected
  - Severe electrolyte disorders corrected
  - Adequate volume resuscitation
  - Respiratory status stabilized
    - May require supplemental oxygenation
    - May require endotracheal intubation
- Secure, well-functioning, wide-bore intravenous lines in place
- Nothing per os
- Allergies checked—not allergic to contemplated endoscopic medications
- Stomach cleared
  - Nasogastric aspiration
  - Or intravenous erythromycin

*Urgent esophagogastroduodenoscopy*

Urgent EGD for NVUGIB is ideal, but significantly improves the clinical outcome over routine EGD only in special circumstances requiring urgent endoscopic hemostasis, such as severe, ongoing hemorrhage or esophageal variceal hemorrhage [27]. Early EGD may not diminish the mortality in other circumstances [28]. Early EGD helps identify stigmata of recent hemorrhage (SRH), which often disappear quickly after bleeding cessation [29]. Identification of SRH helps to determine which lesion bled when more than one lesion is identified at EGD. For example, a patient who has

**Box 5. Checklist for esophagogastroduodenoscopy for acute upper gastrointestinal bleeding: equipment status**

*Endoscopic equipment*

Double-channel therapeutic esophagogastroduodenoscope
Endoscope tested: all ports and buttons properly functioning
Endoscopic therapy
- Heater probe, BICAP, Gold probe, or APC available
- Dilute epinephrine available
- Sclerotherapy needles available
- Banding equipment or sclerosant available to treat esophageal varices
- Adequate water pump available
  - Trained endoscopy nurse available for assistance

*Other equipment*

Emergency (crash) cart
- Fully equipped with medications for cardiac resuscitation
- Electrical cardiac defibrillator machine
- Equipment for endotracheal intubation and for manual mechanical respiration

*Abbreviations:* BICAP, bipolar electrocoagulation probe; APC, argon plasma coagulation.

two ulcers of equal size likely bled from the ulcer exhibiting more severe SRH. Identification of high-risk SRH permits early endoscopic intervention to reduce the risk for rebleeding.

Prompt EGD is often unattainable [30,31]. A large multicenter study reported a mean time of 12 hours from presentation with UGIB to EGD because of obstacles, including patient presentation during off-hours, lack of on-call nurses, or patient comorbidities, such as chest pain, that required evaluation before EGD [32]. Inpatients have worse clinical outcomes than outpatients who have acute UGIB despite a shorter mean endoscopy waiting time. Greater endoscopist experience is an independent factor that improves the outcome for NVUGIB [33].

## Peptic ulcer disease

At EGD, ulcers appear as depressed craters, in contrast to erosions that lack depth. Pathologically, an ulcer penetrates through the muscularis mucosa into the submucosa. At EGD, ulcers are characterized by size, number, location, acuity, and SRH. Acute ulcers exhibit fibrinopurulent exudation, erythema, an inhomogeneous base, and edema, whereas chronic ulcers exhibit fibrosis, scarring, a homogeneous base, and partial healing.

Duodenal ulcers are rarely malignant, whereas 5% of gastric ulcers are malignant [34]. Gastric ulcers are classified at EGD as likely benign as evidenced by a round margin, smooth border, antral or prepyloric location, small size, radiating folds, and lack of an associated mass. Gastric ulcers are classified as likely malignant as evidenced by an irregular and indurated border, heaped-up margins, proximal gastric location, large size, absence of gastric folds near the ulcer, and an associated mass. Gastric ulcers are classified as indeterminate if they have ambiguous features. At EGD numerous biopsies should be taken at the margin of a gastric ulcer to exclude malignancy. Performance of at least seven biopsies from the ulcer margin and base, together with the endoscopic appearance, is 98% sensitive at diagnosing malignancy [35]. These biopsies may be deferred at an initial EGD when the ulcer is actively bleeding or has recently bled to avoid exacerbating or inducing bleeding. Gastric ulcers are generally followed by repeat EGD to document healing to exclude a nonhealing malignant ulcer [36].

Up to 80% of duodenal ulcers are caused by *Helicobacter pylori* infection, whereas about 50% of gastric ulcers are associated with this infection [37]. The prevalence of *H pylori* infection in duodenal ulcers has, however, been recently decreasing in America because of increasing administration of antibiotics in general or as specific therapy for chronic *H pylori* infection [38]. About 15% of patients who have *H pylori* infection develop duodenal ulcers. The virulent bacterial strain that contains the *cagA* gene is strongly associated with duodenal ulcers [39]. Patients who have PUD should undergo endoscopic biopsies of the antrum to test for this infection. Patients who have PUD and documented infection should receive triple therapy, including antibiotics and acid suppressive therapy, to eradicate this infection. Eradication induces ulcer healing and helps prevent ulcer recurrence [40].

Nonsteroidal anti-inflammatory drugs (NSAIDs) constitute the most important cause of PUD after *H pylori* infection. All patients who have PUD should be carefully questioned about NSAID use. Patients frequently do not report NSAID use because NSAIDs are perceived as minor painkillers and are often taken without a prescription [41]. Wilcox and colleagues [42] reported that 65% of patients who had UGIB were taking aspirin or other NSAIDs, often administered without a prescription. Although NSAIDs can cause duodenal ulcers, they most commonly produce antral ulcers [43]. They are an especially common cause of PUD in the elderly [41].

About half of NSAID-induced ulcers are painless because of the analgesic properties of NSAIDs that can mask the pain of ulcers and the early discontinuation of NSAID therapy (before developing PUD) in patients who experience abdominal pain [41]. Endoscopic biopsies are safe in patients taking aspirin or other NSAIDs, with a small increased risk of minor, clinically insignificant bleeding [44]. NSAID-induced ulcers often lack inflammation beyond the ulcer margin, whereas *H pylori*–induced ulcers usually occur in a background of chronic active gastritis [43]. NSAID-induced ulcers are treated by NSAID discontinuation or substitution of a less gastrotoxic alternative medication, discontinuation of other gastrotoxic medications, treatment of concomitant *H pylori* infection if present, and proton pump inhibitor (PPI) therapy.

The Zollinger-Ellison syndrome (gastrinoma) should be considered in the differential whenever ulcers are multiple, refractory to conventional therapy, located in otherwise unusual places (such as the second portion of the duodenum or the esophagus), associated with thickened gastric folds, associated with an acidic diarrhea, or associated with gastric hypersecretion and hyperchlorhydria [45]. The Zollinger-Ellison syndrome is diagnosed by a highly elevated fasting serum gastrin level, in the absence of pernicious anemia, atrophic gastritis, histamine-2 receptor antagonist therapy, or PPI therapy [46]. A secretin test is useful when the gastrin level is only moderately elevated. In the Zollinger-Ellison syndrome, the serum gastrin level pathologically increases by at least 200 units after secretin administration [47].

## Endoscopic therapy

About 25% of EGDs performed for UGIB incorporate endoscopic therapy [48]. UGIB usually ceases with conservative measures, but severe cases, with endoscopic SRH, require endoscopic therapy to achieve hemostasis and prevent rebleeding [49]. Without endoscopic therapy, PUD with SRH has a high incidence of rebleeding or continued bleeding (see Box 2). SRHs that require endoscopic therapy include active bleeding from an ulcer, whether severe or oozing, and a visible vessel, which refers to an elevated pigmented spot within an ulcer crater that may be red, purple, black, or gray (Fig. 1). An ulcer with a visible vessel has a high risk of rebleeding. Visible vessels that are prominently elevated or peripherally located within an ulcer base have a particularly high risk for rebleeding without endoscopic therapy [50]. Ulcers with a clean base or with a flat pigmented spot have a low risk of rebleeding and do not require endoscopic therapy. An algorithm describing which ulcers require endoscopic therapy is provided in Fig. 2.

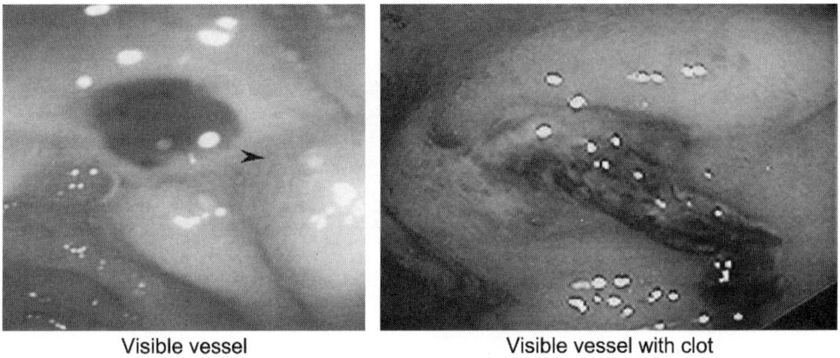


Fig. 1. (*Left*) Endoscopic videophotograph of a prominent red elevation within an ulcer that represents a visible vessel. (*Right*) Endoscopic videophotograph of an ulcer that contains a prominent dark red elevation, representing a visible vessel, with an attached clot.

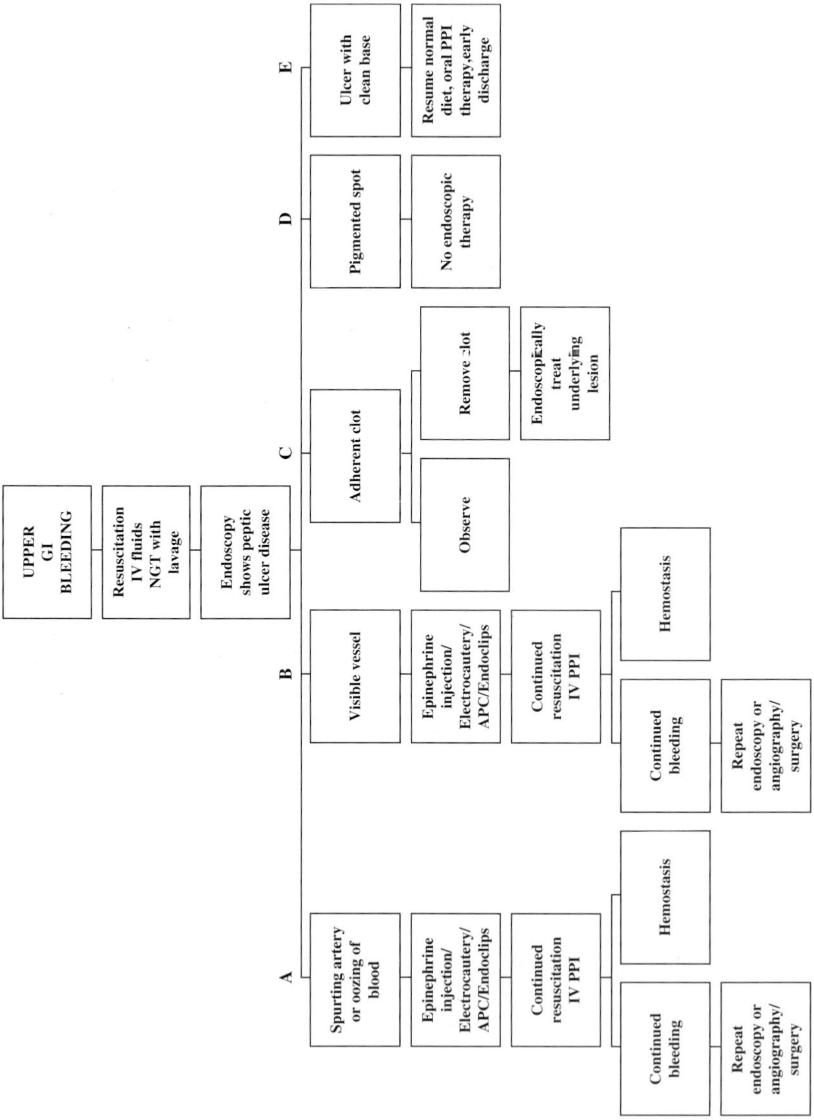
UPPER GI BLEEDING
Resuscitation IV fluids NGT with lavage
Endoscopy shows peptic ulcer disease
A
B
C
D
E
Spurting artery or oozing of blood
Epinephrine injection/ Electrocautery/ APC/Endoclips
Continued resuscitation IV PPI
Continued bleeding
Hemostasis
Repeat endoscopy or angiography/ surgery
Visible vessel
Epinephrine injection/ Electrocautery/ APC/Endoclips
Continued resuscitation IV PPI
Continued bleeding
Hemostasis
Repeat endoscopy or angiography/ surgery
Adherent clot
Observe
Remove clot
Endoscopically treat underlying lesion
Pigmented spot
No endoscopic therapy
Ulcer with clean base
Resume normal diet, oral PPI therapy,early discharge

Pooled blood partly obscuring gastrointestinal lesions should be lavaged to avoid missing high-risk SRH. It is controversial, however, whether to remove a clot attached to an ulcer with vigorous lavage or cold guillotine by way of a snare for immediate endoscopic therapy if SRH are thereby exposed. Recent data suggest such aggressive therapy can diminish the risk for rebleeding [51,52], but does not diminish the need for surgery or reduce the mortality [53]. Many endoscopists avoid clot manipulation and medically treat such an ulcer with PPI therapy to stabilize the clot and promote hemostasis [54,55].

Unfavorable peptic ulcer locations increase the risk of rebleeding because of proximity to major vessels and reduce the efficacy of endoscopic therapy because of difficult endoscopic access [56]. Unfavorable locations include the proximal lesser curvature that overlies the lesser gastric artery, and the posterior duodenal bulb that overlies the gastroduodenal artery. Large (>2 cm wide) and deep ulcers also pose a greater risk of rebleeding [57]. The requirement for endoscopic therapy is, however, determined by endoscopic SRH rather than ulcer location or size.

Endoscopic therapies include injection, ablation, and mechanical therapy (see Box 1). All three therapies are effective as monotherapies, but combined therapies increase the efficacy. Treatment of UGIB has shifted from the operating room to the endoscopy suite. Ulcers with a visible vessel have a 40% to 60% rate of rebleeding and a 35% rate of requiring surgery without endoscopic therapy that is reduced to a 5% to 15% rate of rebleeding and a 5% to 10% rate of requiring surgery after endoscopic therapy [58]. Likewise, actively bleeding ulcers have about a 90% rate of continued or subsequent bleeding if untreated, which is reduced to a 10% to 15% risk of rebleeding after endoscopic therapy (see Box 2).

### *Injection therapy*

Injection therapy for hemostasis is used for bleeding from PUD, Mallory-Weiss tears, and Dieulafoy lesions, and for bleeding after endoscopic

Fig. 2. Algorithm for endoscopic therapy of peptic ulcer disease. At endoscopy, the following ulcer characteristics determine the endoscopic therapy: (*A*) Spurting or oozing artery requires endoscopic therapy, such as epinephrine injection, thermocoagulation, APC, or endoclips, to promote hemostasis. If the attempted endoscopic hemostasis fails, the endoscopy is repeated to reapply the endoscopic therapy or the patient undergoes angiography or surgery for hemostasis. (*B*) A visible vessel within an ulcer is treated at endoscopy just like a spurting artery because of a high risk for rebleeding without therapy. (*C*) An adherent clot may be treated conservatively with PPI therapy without disrupting the clot, or may be treated aggressively by deliberate clot removal (either by vigorous lavage or guillotining the clot using a snare) followed by endoscopic therapy of the underlying lesion. Both approaches are currently considered the standard of care for an adherent clot. (*D*) Pigmented (flat) spot within an ulcer should not receive endoscopic therapy because of a low risk of rebleeding. (*E*) An ulcer with a clean base should also not receive endoscopic therapy because of a very low risk of rebleeding. A patient who has this finding can quickly resume a normal diet and be considered for early discharge. APC, argon plasma coagulation; GI, gastrointestinal; IV, intravenous; NGT, nasogastric tube; PPI, proton pump inhibitor.

polypectomy, endoscopic mucosal resection (EMR), or sphincterotomy. The assistant projects the needle, originally designed for variceal sclerotherapy, about 5 mm beyond the plastic sheath, injects the solution, and provides feedback regarding resistance during injection. No resistance suggests off-target injection. Multiple injections are applied around an ulcer and then directly at the bleeding point or visible vessel within the ulcer. Alternatively, some endoscopists initially target the bleeding site [59].

Epinephrine, at a concentration of 1:10,000, is the injection agent of choice in the United States. It is effective for hemostasis [60,61]. Epinephrine injection induces hemostasis by vasoconstriction, tamponade, and platelet aggregation [62]. Large volumes (>12 mL) are more effective than small volumes, but they might theoretically produce cardiovascular toxicity because of elevated serum epinephrine levels that last for 20 minutes after injection [63–65]. Epinephrine is not recommended as monotherapy because about 20% of patients rebleed after epinephrine injection alone [48,49]. It is often used to clear the endoscopic field before ablative or mechanical therapy. Risk factors for failure of this therapy include active bleeding, large ulcers, proximal gastric ulcers, posterior duodenal bulb ulcers, or significant coagulopathy [57,66].

Some endoscopists inject sclerosants, including sodium tetradecyl sulfate, polidocanol, or ethanol. Sclerosants cause greater vascular thrombosis than epinephrine, but induce greater tissue inflammation and injury that can cause iatrogenic ulcers or strictures. This potential for injury limits the amount of sclerosant that can be injected. Sclerosants are not combined with epinephrine injection because of an increased risk of tissue injury, without improved hemostatic efficacy [67].

Biologic glues are rarely used as injection therapy because of limited efficacy, cost, cumbersomeness, and potential toxicity. Thrombin initiates the clotting sequence and may promote ulcer healing. It is primarily an adjunctive agent. There are few clinical trials of thrombin for NVUGIB [68,69]. Fibrin sealant consists of thrombin and fibrinogen, which are combined at the needle tip in a dual-channel injection apparatus. Use of fibrin sealant does not add efficacy to the use of epinephrine alone [70]. There are numerous case reports of cyanoacrylate glue injection for gastric varices, and this glue has been used as salvage therapy after failure of traditional hemostasis. It can, however, cause pulmonary emboli [71,72].

### *Ablative therapy*

Ablative therapy includes contact methods, such as the heater probe and electrocautery with the BICAP (bipolar electrocoagulation probe) or Gold probe, and noncontact methods (Fig. 3) [48,56]. Electrocautery devices are standardly bipolar to produce focal injury from a well-localized electrical circuit. Monopolar electrocautery is used only as salvage therapy if standard endoscopic therapies fail because it produces more diffuse injury from

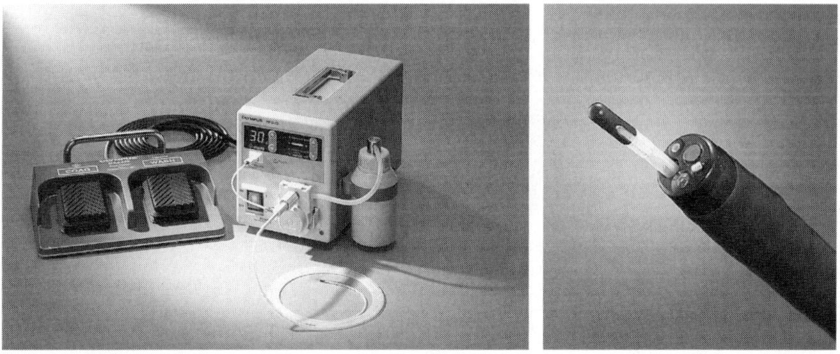

Fig. 3. Heater probe. Left photograph shows the entire heater probe apparatus, including the machine, attached water bottle for vigorous irrigation of lesions, foot pads for controlling the water irrigation, catheter (coiled plastic tube attached to the front of the machine), and wound up electrical cord. Right photograph shows a close-up view of the heater probe catheter tip extending 2 cm beyond the therapeutic channel of an endoscope. (*Courtesy of* Olympus America, Inc., Center Valley, PA; with permission.)

a poorly localized electrical circuit [73]. Bipolar electrodes complete the electrical circuit when the probe contacts the tissue [74]. The Gold probe (Microvasive Corporation, Milford, Massachusetts) has alternating spiral electrodes that form a bipolar electrode. Contact methods use coaptive coagulation, wherein the endoscopist forcefully presses the probe on the lesion while delivering electrical current and generating heat to compress, fuse, and seal the open wall of a bleeding vessel, much like a welder who applies pressure to fuse two pieces of metal together (Fig. 4). A large (3.2 mm wide) probe is applied at a low power setting for several seconds, with multiple applications, as necessary [74].

Argon plasma coagulation (APC) has supplanted the Nd:YAG laser as the noncontact ablative modality of choice for NVUGIB because of superior efficacy, greater portability, easier application, and lower cost [58,75,76]. APC produces more superficial tissue injury than the Nd:YAG laser and causes less frequent complications from deep tissue injury, such as a transmural burn or gastrointestinal perforation. APC can be used to treat ("paint") diffuse, extensive lesions, such as the watermelon stomach (Fig. 5), whereas contact therapies are designed to treat point sources of bleeding [48,76].

APC, heater probe, and BICAP electrocautery have comparable efficacy for NVUGIB [48,58,77]. Use is dictated by personal experience, training, preference, cost, and availability. Ablative therapy diminishes the need for blood transfusions, decreases the need for surgery, and decreases morbidity, but has not been demonstrated to decrease mortality [56,74]. There is a low ($<1\%$) complication rate of iatrogenically induced ulcer bleeding or gastrointestinal perforation [74]. Ablative therapy is about as effective as epinephrine injection for bleeding PUD, with a 15% to 20% rebleeding rate [78]. Neither is recommended as monotherapy [48,49,79]. Failure of ablative

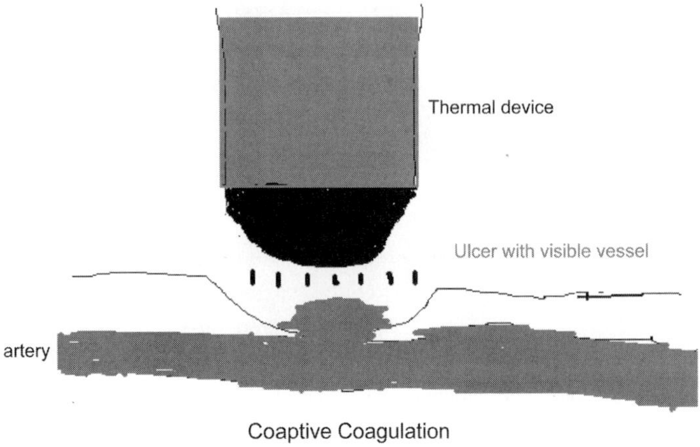


Fig. 4. Coaptive coagulation. Diagram shows a thermal probe (device) directly above a visible vessel within an ulcer. The thermal device would then be pressed firmly (coapted) on the visible vessel, under endoscopic guidance, while applying heat to close and seal the visible vessel to prevent rebleeding, just like a welder uses heat and applies force to fuse (weld) two pieces of metal together.

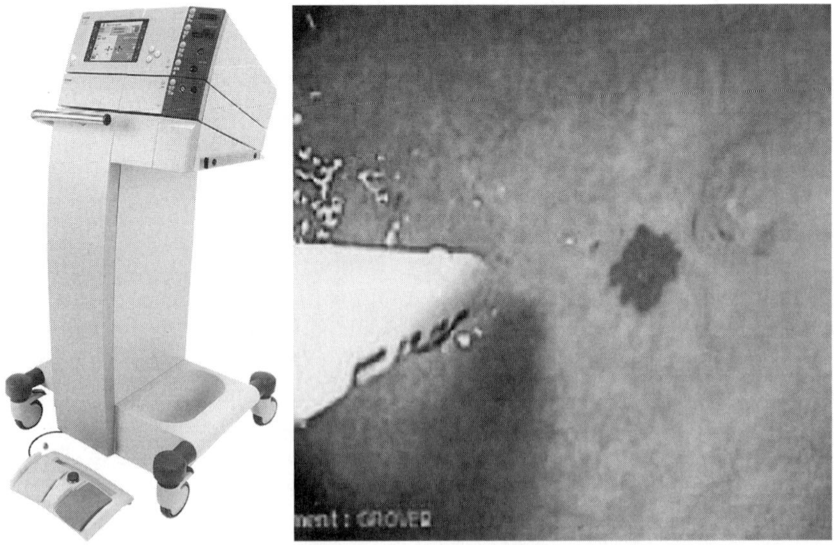

Fig. 5. Argon plasma coagulation (APC). Left photograph shows the apparatus, including the dials and monitor, together with the suction bottle mounted on a cart. The right endoscopic videophotograph shows an APC catheter in place within the channel of a therapeutic endoscope while applying ablative therapy to a large mucosal angiodysplasia. Note the catheter is not in direct contact with the lesion during APC application. (*Courtesy of* ERBE Elektromedizin GmbH, Tubingen, Germany; with permission.)

therapy is related to patient factors, such as significant comorbidities or coagulopathy, and ulcer factors, such as large, endoscopically inaccessible, or actively bleeding ulcers [11,57].

*Mechanical therapy*

In mechanical therapy, bleeding vessels are mechanically compressed to tourniquet the bleeding source. Mechanical therapy has a theoretic advantage in patients who have suboptimal hemostasis from cirrhosis, thrombocytopenia, or another coagulopathy. Metallic clips (endoclips) are the mechanical therapies of choice. They simulate surgical placement of hemostatic clips

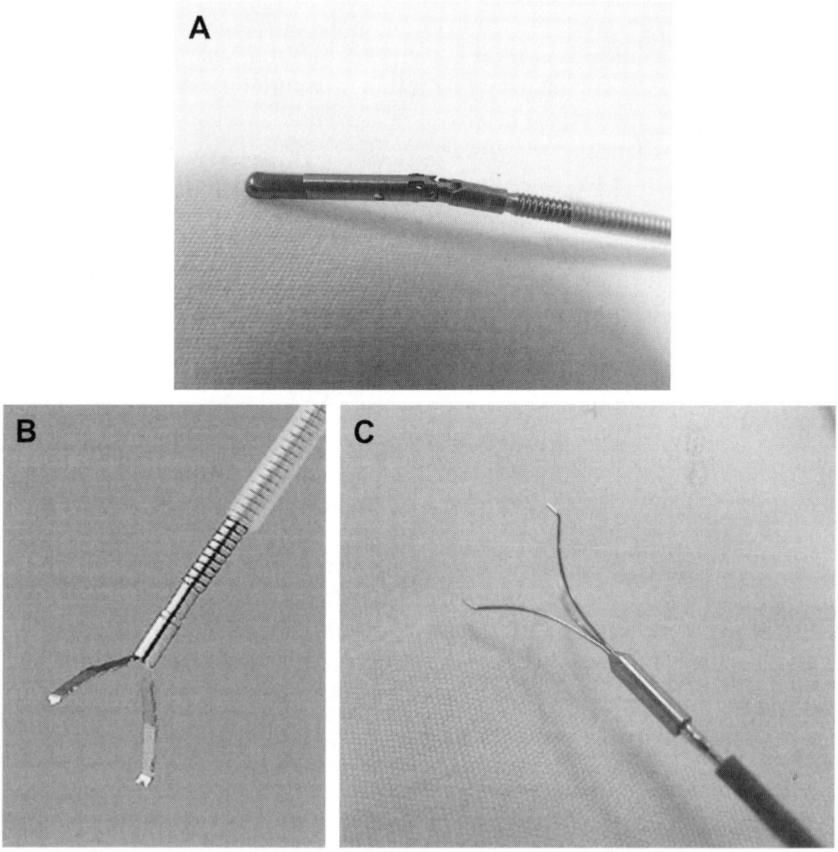


Fig. 6. Photographs illustrating the three different commercially available endoclips in the (*A*) closed state (*Courtesy of* Olympus America, Inc., Center Valley, PA; with permission) or (*B*) open state (*Courtesy of* Boston Scientific Co., Natick, MA; with permission). The manufactures are (*A*) Olympus Corporation, Center Valley, Pennsylvania; (*B*) Boston Scientific, Natick, Massachusetts; and (*C*) Wilson-Cook, Winston-Salem, North Carolina (*Courtesy of* Cook Endoscopy, Winston-Salem, NC; with permission). During endoscopy the completely opened endoclip is closed on a lesion and detached from the catheter.

(Fig. 6). Proper endoclip deployment requires a properly trained endoscopist and nurse-assistant. Deployment can be technically difficult in PUD because of a fibrotic ulcer base that is difficult to grasp, poor endoscopic visibility, awkward (acute) angle of deployment, and inadvertent clip dislodgment [74]. These technical problems can reduce efficacy [80,81]. Advanced patient age, proximal gastric lesions, and duodenal lesions are also associated with failed endoclip hemostasis [82].

Some studies report that endoclips are superior to ablative monotherapy, or even combined ablative and injection therapy, for ulcer hemostasis [83,84]. Endoclips provide useful markers to direct angiographic and surgical therapy [85]. Endoclips are being increasingly applied to various bleeding lesions, including iatrogenic bleeding after polypectomy, EMR, or sphincterotomy; and for bleeding from esophageal varices, or arterial lesions, such as the Dieulafoy lesion [86]. Some of these applications are insufficiently established. The efficacy of the three proprietary versions of endoclips is currently the subject of comparative clinical trials [87,88].

In endoscopic banding or ligation, a rubber band is deployed and contracts around a lesion that has been raised by endoscopic suction into a specially fitted, transparent endoscopic cap. It simulates surgical ligation for hemorrhage [89]. Banding is useful to treat larger (>2 mm) bleeding vessels. It is the endoscopic method of choice for bleeding esophageal varices [90]. The experience with banding for PUD, Mallory-Weiss tear, and Dieulafoy lesion is currently limited [91].

The detachable snare was developed for use before or after endoscopic polypectomy to prevent or to stop postpolypectomy bleeding, respectively. This device is being applied for hemostasis of other gastrointestinal lesions. These snares are tightly closed and left in situ around a lesion, without applying electrocautery, to tamponade internal vessels. Detachable snares are excellent for lesions that project into the lumen and are easily snared, such as pedunculated polyps, but are difficult to deploy on flat or excavated lesions, such as a typical ulcer. These devices have been successfully used to treat gastric varices, and have been used in scattered case reports for other causes of NVUGIB [92].

*Combination hemostasis*

Injection, ablative, and mechanical monotherapy have comparable efficacy for ulcer hemorrhage. Dual therapy is theoretically attractive to increase efficacy, but supporting evidence has only slowly accumulated. Although more effective than injection alone, dual therapy offers little advantage over ablative or mechanical monotherapy [7,49,84,93,94]. Combined epinephrine injection and thermocoagulation, using heater probe or bipolar electrocautery, reduces the rebleed rate to 5% to 15% from a 20% rate with injection monotherapy [49]. A meta-analysis has demonstrated the superiority of dual therapy over injection monotherapy in rebleeding, need for surgery, and mortality, but dual therapy had a moderate, but not statistically significant, trend toward increased gastrointestinal perforation, probably related to thermocoagulation [95]. Combining epinephrine injection with endoclips is effective for ulcer hemostasis [93,96]. Endoclips are usually not deployed after ablative therapy for ulcer hemorrhage, but can be considered as salvage therapy before surgery [57,58].

The newest trend is to combine two modes of endoscopic therapy in one device. The newest Gold probe model incorporates a needle for injection therapy together with traditional electrocautery (Fig. 7). A novel device, the Cograsper (Olympus), combines electrocautery with mechanical therapy.

## Non-ulcer upper gastrointestinal bleeding

### *Predominantly esophageal bleeding*

Potential sources of esophageal bleeding include hemorrhagic reflux esophagitis, reflux-induced ulcers, caustic ingestion, primary esophageal malignancies, malignancies extending from the mediastinum, NSAID-induced or other pill esophagitis, nasogastric tube trauma, and esophagitis from infections, such as Candida, herpes simplex, cytomegalovirus, or HIV [97,98]. In a large series of acute UGIB, 2% bled from esophageal ulcers; 60% of these were associated with a hiatal hernia and 50% were related to NSAIDs [99]. Endoscopic therapy for point sources of acute esophageal bleeding includes epinephrine injection or ablative therapy. With pill esophagitis, the offending drug should be discontinued. Specific antimicrobial therapy is recommended for infectious esophagitis.

#### *Reflux esophagitis*

Endoscopic findings with reflux esophagitis include mucosal erythema, hypervascularity, edema, exudation, erosions, hemorrhage, and ulceration [100]. The injury is characteristically most severe just proximal to the gastroesophageal

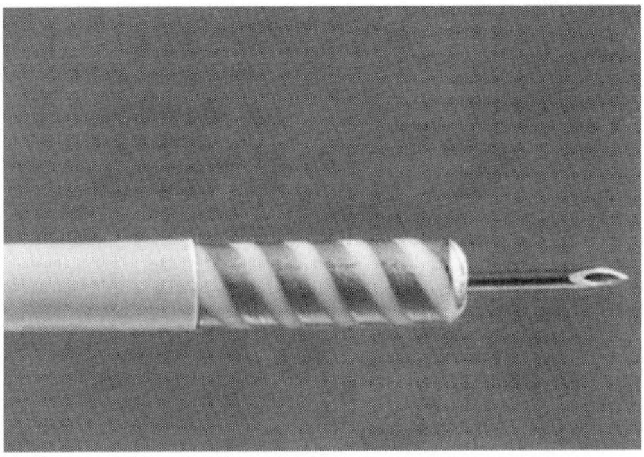

Fig. 7. Photograph shows a probe that provides for dual therapy. A central needle for injection therapy lies within a probe for electrical ablation therapy. (*Courtesy of* Boston Scientific Co. Natick, MA; with permission.)

junction. The severity of reflux esophagitis is classified, according to the Los Angeles grading system, as follows: A, one or more mucosal breaks less than 5 mm in length; B, at least one mucosal break greater than 5 mm but not continuous between the apices of adjacent mucosal folds; C, at least one mucosal break that is continuous between the tops of adjacent mucosal folds; and D, a mucosal break that involves at least three fourths of the luminal circumference [101].

Complications of reflux esophagitis include esophageal bleeding, Barrett esophagus, esophageal stricture, and esophageal ulcer. Barrett mucosa presents as islands or tongues of intensely erythematous mucosa extending from the gastroesophageal junction into the distal esophagus. It is associated with esophageal adenocarcinoma. An esophageal stricture from reflux esophagitis may be benign from acid-induced injury, or malignant from adenocarcinoma. Numerous biopsies should be obtained from a distal esophageal stricture to exclude severe dysplasia or adenocarcinoma.

Reflux esophagitis may cause bleeding from hemorrhagic esophagitis, benign esophageal ulcers, or an associated esophageal adenocarcinoma. Hemorrhagic esophagitis is difficult to treat with focal endoscopic therapy, such as epinephrine injection or thermocoagulation, because of the diffuse nature of the injury, but point sources of bleeding within hemorrhagic esophagitis may be considered for endoscopic therapy. Esophageal ulcers with high-risk SRH are amenable to injection or ablative therapy [102].

*Mallory-Weiss tear*

Tears at the gastroesophageal junction are a relatively common cause of NVUGIB. Patients typically present with hematemesis after repeated vomiting, retching, or coughing, often associated with an alcoholic binge, diabetic ketoacidosis, or emetogenic chemotherapy [103]. A Mallory-Weiss tear is rarely caused by EGD [23,104]. At EGD, a tear typically arises from the gastric side of the gastroesophageal junction; is linear and longitudinally arrayed; and manifests as a superficial ulcer, erosion, scab, or crevice depending on the stage of evolution and severity.

Bleeding from a Mallory-Weiss tear is typically mild to moderate, but can rarely be severe [105]. This mucosal laceration tends to heal rapidly because of its superficial nature and the abundant blood supply to esophageal mucosa. The bleeding spontaneously ceases in about 90% of cases [106]. Continued bleeding is often related to comorbidities, such as thrombocytopenia, other coagulopathies, or liver failure. The bleeding severity in cirrhotics correlates with the severity of liver dysfunction [105,107]. As for PUD, SRH include active hemorrhage, oozing, a visible vessel, or an adherent clot [108]. The indications for hemostasis are the same as for PUD [1,5,108,109]. Endoscopic hemostasis is unnecessary for relatively benign SRH, such as a pigmented flat spot [108]. The optimal endoscopic therapy for bleeding Mallory-Weiss tears (injection, ablative, or mechanical) is still being evaluated, and is likely to be influenced by technical factors and endoscopist preference [1,109]. Injection therapy, with epinephrine or a sclerosant, is effective [110,111], as is bipolar electrocautery [111]. Mechanical therapy is being increasingly used. Endoscopic band ligation is as effective as injection [97,98]. Endoclips have proved effective either as monotherapy or after injection therapy [99,108]. It is unclear whether combination therapy improves hemostasis. Rarely, recurrent bleeding requires selective angiographic vasopressin infusion and gelatin sponge embolization, or surgery [111].

*Esophageal varices*

Esophageal varices constitute about 10% to 15% of UGIB, depending on the catchment area [112]. They typically produce severe UGIB that is associated with a high mortality [113]. Octreotide has replaced vasopressin as the pharmacotherapy for acute variceal bleeding because of less frequent and less severe side effects [114]. Other therapies include endoscopic banding or sclerotherapy, balloon tamponade, transjugular intrahepatic portal shunts (TIPS), and portosystemic surgical shunts [115]. This subject is reviewed in detail in the article by Drs. Toubia and Sanyal elsewhere in this issue.

*Predominantly gastric lesions*

*Cameron lesion*

Cameron lesions are gastric erosions or ulcers located within a hiatal hernia. They are detected at EGD in about 5% of patients who have a hiatal hernia [116]. Lesions are frequently multiple and are frequently associated with peptic esophagitis [116]. Most are asymptomatic. Clinical manifestations include chronic blood loss and iron deficiency anemia. They rarely cause acute UGIB [117,118]. The endoscopic therapy is similar to that for ordinary PUD [23,118]. Other therapies include PPIs and iron repletion for patients who have iron deficiency anemia. Surgical repair of the hiatal hernia is considered for chronic refractory bleeding.

*Portal gastropathy*

At EGD, portal gastropathy appears as moderate to intense erythema in a mosaic or snakeskin pattern surrounded by a pale, white, fine, reticular network in the proximal stomach. The erythema is attributed to saccular dilatation of mucosal capillaries and veins. Portal gastropathy is strongly associated with portal hypertension. In a study of 222 cirrhotic patients, about 25% had portal gastropathy [119]. Lesion risk factors include severe liver disease, gastric varices, and prior sclerotherapy or banding of esophageal varices because of gastric venous congestion [120]. This lesion sometimes causes overt or occult gastrointestinal bleeding from rupture of the friable, small, ectatic superficial vessels. In a series of 315 patients, only 8 (2.5%) patients had acute bleeding, and 34 (10.8%) patients experienced chronic bleeding from portal gastropathy [121].

Portal gastropathy is not amenable to endoscopic therapy because of its diffuse nature. It is treated by reducing the portal hypertension pharmacologically with propranolol, radiologically with TIPS, or surgically with portosystemic shunts [122]. In one study, only 35% of patients treated with propranolol bled compared with 62% of patients treated with placebo [123]. In a study of 40 patients who mostly had mild portal gastropathy, the blood transfusion requirements decreased by 89% after TIPS [124]. Patients who bled from portal gastropathy associated with advanced liver failure should undergo liver transplantation [125].

*Benign and malignant gastric tumors*

Mesenchymal tumors, including gastrointestinal stromal tumors (GISTs) and leiomyomas, constitute about 1% of primary gastrointestinal tumors [126]. They most commonly occur in the stomach. GIST tumors nearly always express c-kit receptor, a membrane tyrosine kinase receptor, and are derived from the interstitial cells of Cajal, which function as the gastrointestinal pacemaker cells. Leiomyomas do not express this receptor and are derived from smooth muscle cells. Both tumors often present with overt UGIB. For example, in a series of 80 patients who had these tumors about 45% presented with acute UGIB [127]. At EGD, nonbleeding leiomyomas appear as a submucosal mass, covered by normal mucosa that has smooth margins and bulges into the lumen. Bleeding lesions, however, often have central mucosal ulceration from local mucosal ischemia. Lesions typically range from about 1 to 5 cm in diameter. Although usually benign, they are potentially malignant. Routine endoscopic biopsies are often nondiagnostic because of the deep lesion location within the bowel wall. The pathologic diagnosis requires deep endoscopic biopsies using the biopsy on biopsy (well) technique or endosonographic guidance. The endosonographic finding of a smooth mass localized to the muscularis propria is characteristic of leiomyoma. Microscopically, spindle or epithelioid cells occur in fascicles or whirls, without nuclear atypia and with rare mitoses. Possible malignancy is suggested by endosonographic findings of lesion size greater than 30 to 50 mm, tumor disruption of normal tissue planes, focal cystic lesions, and adjacent lymphadenopathy; and by histopathologic findings of abundant intracellular cytoplasm, presence of multinucleated giant cells, and an increased concentration of mitoses (>5 per high power field) [128]. Lesions usually require complete segmental resection [129].

Gastric lymphomas constitute about 5% of gastric tumors [130]. Gastric MALTomas (for mucosa-associated lymphoid tissue) are early B cell lymphomas. They commonly cause chronic occult gastrointestinal bleeding but rarely cause acute bleeding. Endoscopic findings include a polypoid mass; a gastric ulcer; or thickened cerebroid gastric folds. They may also present as relatively innocuous-appearing gastric nodularity. Gastric lymphomas, including MALTomas, can extend from the stomach across the pylorus into the duodenum, a growth pattern not exhibited by gastric adenocarcinomas.

Standard endoscopic biopsies are often nondiagnostic because of the deep submucosal location of MALTomas. The diagnostic yield of endoscopic biopsies is increased by use of jumbo biopsies or of biopsies on biopsies, using the well technique. Pathologically, MALToma is characterized by an infiltrate of lymphocytes and plasma cells that express the standard B cell antigens. Immunophenotyping can diagnose lymphoma and differentiate MALTomas from other lymphomas.

MALTomas are highly associated with chronic *H pylori* infection. Chronic *H pylori* infection stimulates proliferation of B lymphocytes that can result in genetic mutations, particularly chromosome 11:18 translocation, that leads to unregulated proliferation of transformed B cells. Early diagnosis is important because early lymphoma often responds to *H pylori* eradication. From 50% to 80% of MALTomas exhibit complete histologic regression after *H pylori* eradication [131,132].

Other primary or metastatic gastric malignancies can produce UGIB. Adenocarcinoma is the most common primary malignancy. It presents as a gastric mass, ulcerated mass, nonhealing ulcer, or stricture. Endoscopic differentiation of a malignant ulcer from a benign ulcer was considered under the section on PUD. In linitis plastica the stomach appears poorly motile and noncompliant because of diffuse infiltration of adenocarcinoma throughout the gastric wall. Gastric metastases most commonly arise from lung cancer, breast cancer, and cutaneous melanoma [133]. An eroded polypoid or submucosal mass is a common endoscopic appearance [133,134]. Endoscopic hemostasis of gastric malignancies is usually achieved by ablative therapy, epinephrine injection, or both [134]. These malignancies commonly rebleed, however, and generally have a poor long-term prognosis. UGIB after chemotherapy or radiotherapy for gastric malignancy is difficult to manage and often requires a multidisciplinary approach [135].

*Dieulafoy lesion*

A Dieulafoy lesion is a congenital, abnormally large, submucosal artery that has a potential to bleed through a small mucosal defect [136]. It accounts for about 2% of all NVUGIB [109,137]. Patients typically present with acute, severe UGIB, often associated with manifestations of hemodynamic compromise, such as hypotension or orthostasis. EGD reveals a pigmented protuberance, representing the vessel stump, with minimal surrounding erosion and no ulceration. In contrast, a pigmented protuberance within an ulcer is a visible vessel within a peptic ulcer. In 75% of cases the Dieulafoy lesion is located in the proximal stomach about 6 to 10 cm below the gastroesophageal junction along the lesser curvature, but it can occur throughout the gastrointestinal tract [136]. The lesion is typically only 2 to 5 mm in diameter. The lesion can be missed at EGD because it is so small and inconspicuous or because it is obscured by blood or clots. It may be associated with advanced liver disease [138]. Endoscopic biopsy of the lesion is contraindicated because of the risk of inducing bleeding.

Endoscopic therapy is particularly attractive for this point source of bleeding because of the propensity of this lesion to bleed frequently and massively, and its high mortality without endoscopic therapy. Hemostasis is accomplished with epinephrine injection; ablative therapy, including APC; or mechanical therapy, including band ligation or endoclips. In two large reviews, long-term hemostasis was achieved in about 90% of patients by various endoscopic therapies [139,140]. For example, endoscopic injection, with epinephrine or polidocanol, achieved hemostasis in 53 of 56 patients [54,55,141]. There is a recent trend toward mechanical therapy [109,138,142,143]. The lesion is particularly amenable to mechanical therapy because of its focal nature and protuberant shape. Band ligation and endoclips have comparable efficacy [143]. There is a concern about ulceration after mechanical therapy, especially after band ligation [109,144]. Up to 20% of patients require surgery because of recurrent hemorrhage [145]. A wide, wedge resection of the lesion and surrounding tissue is recommended [146]. The mortality of this lesion has declined from about 25% in the 1980s to about 10% now because of aggressive application of endoscopic therapy [147].

*Angiodysplasia*

Angiodysplasia accounts for about 2% to 5% of acute UGIB [148]. Upper gastrointestinal angiodysplasia occurs most commonly in the stomach, sometimes in the duodenum, and rarely in the esophagus [149]. Angiodysplasias are often multiple, and tend to be clustered when multiple [150]. Histologically, angiodysplasias consist of dilated, tortuous, and thin-walled vessels lined by endothelium with no or little smooth muscle and no inflammation, fibrosis, or atherosclerosis [151]. Angiodysplasia tends to occur in the elderly. Bleeding from angiodysplasia is believed to be associated with chronic renal failure [152], aortic stenosis [153], and CREST (calcinosis, Raynaud phenomenon, esophageal dysmotility, sclerodactyly, and telangiectasia) syndrome [154]. The nature and strength of the first two associations is somewhat controversial. The association with aortic stenosis likely arises from bleeding from previously clinically silent angiodysplasia caused by loss of large multimers of von Willebrand factor from high shear forces across a stenotic aortic valve [155].

At EGD, angiodysplasia appears as a dense, macular and reticular network of vessels (vascular tuft), which is typically 2 to 8 mm wide and is intensely red because of the high oxygen content of erythrocytes within vessels supplied by arteries without intervening capillaries [156]. Angiodysplasia may become inconspicuous at EGD in a patient who has hypotension or profound anemia, and may be obscured by meperidine administration [157]. Endoscopic biopsy is not recommended for the diagnosis because of the risk of inducing bleeding and the characteristic endoscopic appearance.

Angiodysplasias often are asymptomatic, incidental findings. For example, in a review of 41 patients who had upper gastrointestinal angiodysplasia, 21 (51%) were incidental endoscopic findings [158]. It is therefore important to assess at EGD whether an observed angiodysplasia is the source of UGIB. Up to 30% to 45% of patients who have angiodysplasia have other gastrointestinal lesions, which are more likely the cause of the bleeding [159]. Bleeding is attributed to angiodysplasia only when it is active bleeding, has an overlying clot, or all other causes are excluded. In a retrospective comparison of angiodysplasia with other causes of gastrointestinal bleeding, patients who had angiodysplasia had a milder hospital course with fewer transfusions of packed erythrocytes, shorter hospitalizations, and lower mortality [149].

An asymptomatic angiodysplasia, incidentally discovered at EGD, is generally not treated endoscopically because of a low likelihood of subsequent bleeding [148,160]. Endoscopic therapy may, however, be considered when an incidental angiodysplasia is exceptionally large or when prior bleeding from an angiodysplasia is suspected but undocumented. In other clinical situations, a graded approach to therapy is predicated on the likelihood of further bleeding from angiodysplasia [156]. Angiodysplasias that recently bled, as demonstrated by SRH, are treated at EGD. An angiodysplasia associated with otherwise unexplained iron deficiency anemia may be treated at EGD depending on the clinical scenario.

At EGD, actively bleeding angiodysplasias are sometimes first injected by epinephrine or alcohol, followed by thermocoagulation, electrocoagulation, or photocoagulation [161]. These endoscopic therapies are relatively safe and efficacious. For example, Gostout and colleagues [162] reported cessation of bleeding in 72 of 83 patients (87%) after laser photocoagulation during a mean follow-up of 12 months. Laser therapy, however, has a perforation rate of up to 4% attributable to deep mural injury [163]. Endoscopists therefore prefer thermocoagulation or electrocoagulation over photocoagulation.

APC is emerging as the endoscopic therapy of choice because of relatively low risks owing to the shallow depth of tissue injury and high efficacy because of the superficial, mucosal location of angiodysplasia. Among 100 patients undergoing APC for colonic angiodysplasia for either overt gastrointestinal bleeding or iron deficiency anemia and fecal occult blood, 90 patients (90%) did not require any blood transfusions during a mean follow-up of 20 months [164].

An actively bleeding angiodysplasia that is refractory to endoscopic therapy may be treated by angiographic embolization. This procedure has a high success rate [165,166]. Improved catheter design and superselective catheterization with more distal embolization have recently reduced the frequency of intestinal infarction from angiographic embolization. Surgery is reserved for severe bleeding from well-characterized and localized lesions refractory to endoscopic or angiographic therapy. EGD, colonoscopy, and capsule endoscopy should be performed preoperatively to exclude distant synchronous gastrointestinal angiodysplasia or other lesions [150].

*Hereditary hemorrhagic telangiectasia*

Hereditary hemorrhagic telangiectasia is a rare genetic vascular disorder caused by mutation of the *ENG* (endoligin) gene (type I) or the *ACVRL1* gene (type II) and characterized by multiple orocutaneous and mucosal telangiectasias, especially in the nose and gastrointestinal tract [167]. About 25% of affected patients experience clinically significant gastrointestinal bleeding, which typically begins during middle age [168]. Chronic gastrointestinal blood loss may cause iron deficiency anemia, whereas acute blood loss may cause hypovolemia and hypotension. The diagnosis is straightforward in patients who have the clinical triad of telangiectasia, recurrent epistaxis, and a compatible family history [169]. The site and source of UGIB is diagnosed by EGD. The endoscopic appearance of telangiectasia resembles that of nonsyndromic angiodysplasia or of cutaneous telangiectasia occurring in this syndrome. Lesions tend to be widespread throughout the gastrointestinal tract.

The endoscopic therapy resembles that for nonsyndromic angiodysplasia, but endoscopic therapy is complicated by lesion multiplicity, widespread dissemination, and progression over time. Isolated actively bleeding telangiectasias are usually successfully treated, but patients often rebleed from other, untreated gastrointestinal telangiectasias, and therefore require multiple endoscopic sessions [170]. A few small studies have suggested that estrogen-progesterone therapy may decrease the rate of chronic gastrointestinal bleeding from these telangiectasias [171], but this therapy is controversial [172]. Patients generally require iron supplementation because of recurrent gastrointestinal blood loss.

*Gastric antral vascular ectasia*

Gastric antral vascular ectasia (GAVE) usually occurs in females and in the elderly [173]. It commonly presents with iron deficiency anemia, sometimes presents as an incidental finding, and occasionally causes acute UGIB. The patient may have a long history of chronic gastrointestinal bleeding, with multiple prior blood transfusions, because of delayed diagnosis. GAVE is associated with chronic renal disease and, possibly, chronic liver disease, but is not associated with portal hypertension without liver disease [112]. EGD reveals parallel folds that radiate from the pylorus to the proximal antrum. The folds contain intensely erythematous linear streaks at their apices. GAVE is also called the watermelon stomach because these linear streaks resemble the stripes on a watermelon rind [174]. GAVE is differentiated from ordinary antral gastritis by its location on folds, blanching on pressure, and sharp lesion demarcation [173]. GAVE can be safely biopsied with only minimally increased and minor bleeding because of its low intravascular pressure. Biopsy may reveal characteristic findings of dilated, tortuous mucosal capillaries often occluded by bland fibrin thrombi and dilated submucosal veins without inflammatory infiltration [175].

Pharmacotherapy, including histamine-2 receptor antagonists and PPIs, are ineffective because this lesion is not acid related and patients often have hypochlorhydria from atrophic gastritis [176]. Endoscopic therapy is the primary therapy. From 87% to 100% of patients have stable hematocrits without blood transfusions for several years after endoscopic therapy [177]. Endoscopic thermal therapy used to be frequently performed, but it requires many sessions because of the large extent of the lesion. Although laser therapy is frequently successful and requires few endoscopic sessions, it is being used less frequently because of a modest risk for severe complications, high cost, and poor machine availability. APC therapy may become the therapy of choice because of the diffuse nature and superficial location of the lesion [178,179]. APC is well tolerated and safe because it produces only shallow tissue injury [180]. APC diminishes blood transfusion requirements, although several sessions are usually required [180,181]. Combining the results of four studies, 50 of 55 transfusion-dependent patients required no transfusions after APC therapy, during a mean follow-up of approximately 2 years [181–184]. It is important to differentiate GAVE from portal gastropathy because the former responds to endoscopic therapy but does not respond to portal pressure reduction [185], whereas the latter does not respond to endoscopic therapy but responds to portal pressure reduction [109]. Antrectomy is recommended if endoscopic hemostasis fails. It removes the lesion and nearly always cures the disease, but entails significant morbidity and 5% mortality [186].

*Gastritis*

Acute hemorrhagic gastritis can result from aspirin or NSAID use, radiation, toxic ingestion, and infection, such as cytomegalovirus or syphilis [187]. Stress-related mucosal disease (SRMD) refers to erosive gastritis in patients experiencing severe physiologic stress from critical diseases, especially overwhelming sepsis or respiratory failure requiring mechanical ventilation [188]. Patients often are in the ICU with multiple medical problems. The pathophysiology involves gastric mucosal ischemia and acid-mediated injury [188,189]. Patients who have SRMD usually experience mild bleeding [188,190]. EGD typically reveals multiple superficial ulcers with surrounding erythema. Treatment of the underlying disease that caused the SRMD is essential for lesion healing. PPIs have an established role in treating SRMD, but their role in preventing SRMD is not well validated [190,191]. Acid-suppressive agents do not diminish mortality or the already low rate of clinically significant UGIB in ICU patients, but might increase the risk for pneumonia [191]. Other medications, such as histamine-2 receptor antagonists, have a lower risk for causing pneumonia and are cheaper, but their use in SRMD has also not been validated [192]. The current consensus is not to routinely administer PPIs or other agents as prophylaxis against UGIB in ICU patients [188,190].

*Nasogastric tube erosions*

Nasogastric tube erosions occasionally cause gross UGIB, but this bleeding is characteristically mild and rarely requires blood transfusions. For example, in a review of 152 nasogastric tube insertions for gastrointestinal bleeding after myocardial infarction, only one patient had nasogastric tube–induced gastric erosions at EGD that required blood transfusions [29]. Nasogastric tube erosions appear at EGD as multiple, colinear, round, and relatively uniform erythematous erosions that are in register with the apertures of the nasogastric tube and that are at the same stage of evolution because of their simultaneous creation [193]. They typically occur in the stomach along the greater curve where the nasogastric tube tends to lodge. These erosions do not require endoscopic therapy. They are generally treated by nasogastric tube removal, if possible, and PPI therapy.

*Duodenal lesions*

*Anastomotic ulcers*

Marginal ulcers can develop distal to the gastrojejunal anastomosis after PUD surgery (Billroth II) and can cause UGIB. UGIB is being increasingly reported from marginal ulcers after gastric bypass surgery or vertical banded gastroplasty because of the increasing popularity of these bariatric surgeries [194]. Marginal ulcers occur in 4% to 7% of patients who have gastric bypass, and cause bleeding in 1% to 3% of patients after these surgeries [195,196]. The pathophysiology may be multifactorial, including bile reflux gastritis, inadequate prior surgery, local ischemia from vessel ligation, gastric stasis, and exposure to gastrotoxic medications, such as NSAIDs [197]. At EGD, the afferent and efferent loops of a Billroth II should be intubated and examined, and the anastomosis carefully inspected. Endoscopic intubation of a bypassed intestinal limb after bariatric surgery may be technically challenging and require an enteroscope or colonoscope for access [198]. Endoscopic manifestations of anastomotic injury include erosions, friability, ulcers, fibrosis, small polyps, and disrupted sutures [199]. The endoscopic therapy for bleeding from marginal ulcers is the same as for ordinary ulcers. Postprocedure management typically includes PPI therapy and investigation for *H pylori* infection [196].

*Aortoenteric fistula*

Aortoenteric fistula often presents with a mild "herald bleed" followed by massive bleeding [200]. It constitutes an indication for emergency EGD because of a high mortality with delayed diagnosis. It is rare. It is strongly associated with prior aortic surgery, aortic aneurysms, and severe atherosclerosis [201]. EGD should be performed up to the distal duodenum when this fistula is suspected because this fistula usually occurs at this location. At EGD a mesh from a prosthetic graft may be identified. If this lesion is identified at EGD, the EGD should be aborted without attempting endoscopic therapy because of the risk of massive bleeding when tampering with this lesion. The lesion is treated surgically. The mortality is high [202].

*Postprocedural bleeding*

Postprocedural bleeding is usually related to endoscopic biopsy or therapy [23]. Hemobilia, defined as blood coming from the bile ducts, usually occurs after a procedure, such as endoscopic sphincterotomy, liver biopsy, percutaneous transhepatic cholangiography, TIPS, or cholecystectomy, but may arise from hepatobiliary disease, such as malignancy, polyps, or cysts. Postsphincterotomy bleeding usually responds to balloon tamponade or epinephrine injection, but may require thermocoagulation or endoclip placement [203]. Blood in the gastrointestinal tract arising from the pancreas, or hemosuccus pancreaticus, usually results from chronic pancreatitis, pancreatic pseudocysts, pancreatic tumors, or blunt trauma to the pancreas, and from therapeutic endoscopy, including pancreatic stone removal, pseudocyst drainage, or pancreatic duct stenting.

*Small intestinal bleeding*

Small intestinal bleeding beyond the ligament of Treitz is most commonly caused by angiodysplasia, but may be caused by Crohn disease, Meckel diverticulum, jejunoileal ulcers, including ulcers related to NSAIDs or gastrinomas, ectopic varices, hemangiomas, masses, polyps, and submucosal lesions [204]. Hematemesis is unusual. The stool may appear bloody, melanotic, gray, or normal depending on the location and tempo of the bleeding [1,205].

Obscure gastrointestinal bleeding is defined as continuous or intermittent gastrointestinal bleeding that is not diagnosed by EGD and colonoscopy. It represents a diagnostic and therapeutic challenge [206]. Such bleeding is now evaluated by capsule endoscopy and single- or double-balloon enteroscopy [207,208]. Although it usually arises from small intestinal bleeding beyond the ligament of Treitz, occasionally repeat EGD or colonoscopy may reveal a previously missed lesion, such as a Dieulafoy lesion. The expanding therapeutic armamentarium available with double-balloon enteroscopy includes injection, ablative therapy (including APC), and variceal sclerotherapy [209]. Older technologies, including push enteroscopy, angiography, enteroclysis, and intraoperative endoscopy, are used to investigate obscure gastrointestinal bleeding when these new technologies are unavailable [206,210].

**Postendoscopy care**

EGD assists in patient triage. Those who have low-risk SRH may be downgraded to a lower level of hospital care or, rarely, even promptly discharged [2,11,109,211]. PPI therapy should be continued after EGD for

NVUGIB, but the optimal dose and route remains unclear [54,55,212]. Intravenous PPI therapy is expensive, but this cost is offset by its reducing the need for blood transfusions and the hospital length of stay [213]. All patients who have bleeding PUD and *H pylori* infection should receive triple therapy because infection eradication diminishes the rebleeding rate compared with PPI therapy alone [214]. The duration of PPI therapy after therapeutic EGD for PUD is unclear. The duration is much shorter if *H pylori* is eradicated and NSAIDs are avoided [214]. PPIs help prevent rebleeding from peptic ulcers in patients administered aspirin or NSAIDs, but these drugs should be avoided, if possible, in patients who have known PUD [215]. Mild to moderate anticoagulation only modestly increases the risk for severe rebleeding after endoscopic therapy for NVUGIB [216].

*Repeat esophagogastroduodenoscopy*

Repeat (second look) EGD after therapeutic endoscopy is controversial and not routinely recommended [109]. Repeat EGD has the greatest benefit for patients who have high-risk SRH, but this practice raises concerns about gastrointestinal perforation if ablative therapy is repeated [217]. A meta-analysis showed that systematic repeat EGD reduces the rebleeding rate but does not diminish the need for surgery or the mortality [218]. Most rebleeding occurs within 72 hours of the initial EGD [57]. Occasionally, the bleeding lesion is missed at the initial EGD and identified only at a repeat EGD [219,220].

*Refractory hemorrhage*

Overall, 5% to 15% of patients who have NVUGIB rebleed despite endoscopic therapy. Reversal of any severe coagulopathy, by platelet or fresh frozen plasma transfusions, is essential for endoscopic hemostasis. Patients who have refractory bleeding are candidates for angiography or surgery. The decision regarding a particular therapy requires a team approach with input by the gastroenterologist, surgeon, interventional radiologist, and intensivist. Even when endoscopic hemostasis fails, EGD is important before angiography or surgery to diagnose the site and cause of the bleeding. This information helps the angiographer plan which of the major mesenteric vessels, among the celiac axis, superior mesenteric artery, or inferior mesenteric artery, to first catheterize; which branches to selectively catheterize; and what hemostatic agents to use. This information helps the surgeon plan the surgical incision and approach, whether thoracic, upper abdominal, or lower abdominal; which organ to target for surgery; and what type of surgery to perform (eg, antiulcer surgery versus wedge resection for a Dieulafoy lesion).

The armamentarium of the interventional radiologist includes vasoconstrictor agents, such as vasopressin, or embolic agents, such as a gelatin sponge or microcoils, for selective occlusion of a bleeding artery. Rebleeding is common after radiologic intervention. Complications of radiologic intervention include gastrointestinal ischemia and infarction [221].

The specific operation for NVUGIB reflects the local expertise. Surgery for PUD optimally combines control of hemorrhage with acid-reduction procedures [222]. Peptic ulcer surgery is less commonly performed than previously because of endoscopic hemostasis, PPI therapy, and *H pylori* eradication, but it still constitutes a significant proportion of gastrointestinal surgery in urban and Veterans Administration hospitals. The mortality of this surgery is greater than 20% [223]. Patients often experience significant morbidity after gastrointestinal surgery [223].

## Future challenges and prospects

Aggressive endoscopic therapy for NVUGIB has resulted in a decreased need for surgery and blood transfusions, shorter hospital stays, and lower costs, but approximately 5% to 15% of patients rebleed [58,224]. Further research should clarify the clinical roles of the current endoscopic therapies and refine the therapeutic algorithm to further reduce the risk of rebleeding. Epinephrine remains the gold standard for injection therapy, until the technical and safety issues for endoscopic glues are clarified [69–71]. BICAP electrocautery and heater probe continue to be the principal ablative therapies, although APC is useful for diffuse lesions, such as GAVE, and is being increasingly applied for point sources of bleeding, such as the Dieulafoy lesion. Cryotherapy is still experimental for UGIB [225]. The clinical roles of the existing mechanical therapies need to be better defined and validated [48,58].

Regarding endoscopic therapy for SRH with PUD, the endoscopic approach to an adherent clot on an ulcer needs clarification [51–53]. The endoscopic therapy for many other upper gastrointestinal lesions, such as Mallory-Weiss tears and Dieulafoy lesions, needs to be standardized.

Exciting new mechanical therapies are being developed. NOTES (natural orifice transendoscopic surgery) is stimulating development of endoscopic suturing devices to close gastrointestinal perforations [226]. As such suturing devices become more sophisticated and versatile, they will be increasingly adapted to control gastrointestinal bleeding (eg, to endoscopically oversew bleeding ulcers). Experimental suturing devices may become a standard mechanical therapy for NVUGIB [226,227]. Novel devices that combine two therapies in one device, such as a probe that combines injection therapy with electrical ablation, or a device that combines electrocautery with mechanical therapy, need further study before achieving widespread clinical application. Undoubtedly, other devices offering multimodal therapy will be developed in the near future.

Doppler ultrasound evaluation of ulcer vessels may determine the need for and predict the effectiveness of endoscopic therapy [228]. Management of NVUGIB may be affected by the recent "pay for performance" trend which provides incentives for optimal triage and early discharge [229].

For low-risk patients, clinical assessment and endoscopic results should be better communicated and used for earlier discharge [15,17]. Clinical scoring systems will be further refined to improve patient prognostication and facilitate earlier patient discharge. PPIs have been validated for high-risk hemorrhage from PUD, but guidelines still need to be clarified concerning the PPI dosage, formulation, and duration of therapy [54,55].

## Summary

Acute UGIB is a relatively common, potentially life-threatening emergency that requires rapid patient assessment, proper triage, and rapid institution of resuscitative measures. EGD is the principal diagnostic, therapeutic, and prognostic modality for NVUGIB. Endoscopic therapy reduces the rate of rebleeding, blood transfusion requirements, and need for surgery. Administration of PPIs is important for NVUGIB.

## References

[1] Fallah MA, Prakash C, Edmundowicz S. Acute gastrointestinal bleeding. Med Clin North Am 2000;84(5):1183–208.
[2] Jiranek JC, Kozarek RA. A cost-effective approach to the patient with peptic ulcer bleeding. Surg Clin North Am 1996;76(1):83–103.
[3] Boonpongmanee S, Fleischer DE, Pezzulo JC, et al. The frequency of peptic ulcer disease as a cause of upper-GI bleeding is exaggerated. Gastrointest Endosc 2004;59(7):788–94.
[4] Palmer K. Acute upper gastrointestinal haemorrhage. Br Med Bull 2007;83:307–24.
[5] Kaplan RC, Heckbert SR, Koepsell TD, et al. Risk factors for gastrointestinal bleeding among older patients. Cardiovascular Health Study Investigators. J Am Geriatr Soc 2001;49(2):126–33.
[6] Peter DJ, Doughtery JM. Evaluation of the patient with gastrointestinal bleeding: an evidence based approach. Emerg Med Clin North Am 1999;17(1):239–61.
[7] Adler DG, Leighton JA, Davila RE, et al. ASGE guideline: the role of endoscopy in acute non-variceal upper-GI hemorrhage. Gastrointest Endosc 2004;60(4):497–504.
[8] Chak A, Cooper GS, Lloyd LE, et al. Effectiveness of endoscopy in patients admitted to the intensive care unit with upper GI hemorrhage. Gastrointest Endosc 2001;53(1):6–13.
[9] Hay JA, Lyubashevsky E, Elashoff J, et al. Upper gastrointestinal hemorrhage clinical guideline determining optimal hospital length of stay. Am J Med 1996;100(3):313–33.
[10] Rockall TA, Logan RF, Devlin HB, et al. Risk assessment after acute upper gastrointestinal hemorrhage. Gut 1996;38(3):316–21.
[11] Saeed ZA, Winchester CB, Michaletz PA, et al. A scoring system to predict rebleeding after endoscopic therapy of nonvariceal upper gastrointestinal hemorrhage, with a comparison of heat probe and ethanol injection. Am J Gastroenterol 1993;88(11):1842–9.
[12] Lewis JD, Shin EJ, Metz DC. Characterization of gastrointestinal bleeding in severely ill hospitalized patients. Crit Care Med 2000;28(1):261–2.
[13] Cooper GS, Chak A, Way L, et al. Early endoscopy in upper gastrointestinal hemorrhage: association with recurrent bleeding, surgery and length of hospital stay. Gastrointest Endosc 1999;49(1):145–52.
[14] Lau JY, Chung SC, Leung JW, et al. The evolution of stigmata of hemorrhage in bleeding peptic ulcers: a sequential endoscopic study. Endoscopy 1998;30(6):513–8.
[15] Bjorkman D, Zaman A, Fennerty B, et al. Urgent versus elective endoscopy for acute non-variceal upper GI bleeding: an effectiveness study. Gastrointest Endosc 2004;60(1): 1–8.

[16] Podilla PV, Ben-Manachem T, Batra SK, et al. Managing patients with acute nonvariceal upper gastrointestinal hemorrhage: development and effectiveness of a clinical care pathway. Am J Gastroenterol 2001;96(1):208–19.
[17] Romagnuolo J, Barkun AN, Enns R, et al. Simple clinical predictors may obviate urgent endoscopy in patients with nonvariceal upper gastrointestinal bleeding. Arch Intern Med 2007;167(3):265–70.
[18] Cipolletta L, Bianco MA, Rotondano G, et al. Outpatient management for low-risk nonvariceal GI bleeding: a randomized controlled trial. Gastrointest Endosc 2002;55(1):1–5.
[19] Gasporovic S, Rustemovic N, Opacic M, et al. Clinical safety of propofol deep sedation for 1,104 patients undergoing gastrointestinal endoscopic procedures: a three year prospective study. World J Gastroenterol 2006;12(2):327–30.
[20] Tohda G, Higashi S, Sakumoto H, et al. Efficacy and safety of nurse administered propofol during emergency upper endoscopy for emergency upper gastrointestinal bleeding: a prospective study. Endoscopy 2006;38(7):684–9.
[21] Rex DK, Heuss LT, Walker JA, et al. Trained registered nurses/endoscopy teams can administer propofol safely for endoscopy. Gastroenterology 2005;129(5):1384–91.
[22] VanNatta ME, Rex DK. Propofol alone titrated to deep sedation versus propofol in combination with opioids and/or benzodiazepines and titrated to moderate sedation for colonoscopy. Am J Gastroenterol 2006;101(10):2209–17.
[23] Cappell MS, Abdullah M. Management of gastrointestinal bleeding induced by gastrointestinal endoscopy. Gastroenterol Clin North Am 2000;29(1):125–67.
[24] Lin S, Konstance R, Jollis J, et al. The utility of upper endoscopy in patients with upper gastrointestinal bleeding and acute myocardial infarction. Dig Dis Sci 2006;51(12):2377–83.
[25] Cappell MS, Iacovone FM Jr. Safety and efficacy of esophagogastroduodenoscopy after myocardial infarction. Am J Med 1999;106(1):29–35.
[26] Cappell MS. Gastrointestinal bleeding associated with myocardial infarction. Gastroenterol Clin North Am 2000;29(2):423–44.
[27] Spiegel BM, Vakil NB, Ofman JJ. Endoscopy for acute nonvariceal upper–gastointestinal hemorrhage: is sooner better? A systematic review. Arch Intern Med 2001;161(11): 1393–404.
[28] Lim CH, Vani D, Shah SG, et al. The outcome of suspected upper gastrointestinal bleeding with 24-hour access to upper gastrointestinal endoscopy: a prospective cohort study. Endoscopy 2006;38(6):581–5.
[29] Cappell MS. Safety and efficacy of nasogastric intubation for gastrointestinal bleeding after myocardial infarction: an analysis of 125 patients at two tertiary cardiac referral hospitals. Dig Dis Sci 2005;50(11):2063–70.
[30] Lee JG. What is the value of early endoscopy in upper gastrointestinal bleeding? Nat Clin Pract Gastroenterol Hepatol 2006;3(10):534–5.
[31] Tai CM, Huang SP, Wang HP, et al. High risk ED patients with nonvariceal upper gastrointestinal hemorrhage undergoing emergency or urgent endoscopy: a retrospective analysis. Am J Emerg Med 2007;25(3):273–8.
[32] Da Silveira EB, Lam E, Martel M, et al, for the RUGBE investigators. The importance of process issues as predictors of time to endoscopy in patients with acute upper-GI bleeding using the RUGBE data. Gastrointest Endosc 2006;64(3):299–309.
[33] Parente F, Anderloni A, Bargiggia S, et al. Outcome of non-variceal acute upper gastrointestinal bleeding in relation to the time of endoscopy and experience of the endoscopist: a two year survey. World J Gastroenterol 2005;11(45):7122–30.
[34] Grossman MI. The Veterans Administration Cooperative Study on Gastric Ulcer: 10. Resume and comment. Gastroenterology 1971;61(4 Suppl 2):635–8.
[35] Graham DY, Schwartz JT, Cain GD, et al. Prospective evaluation of biopsy number in the diagnosis of esophageal and gastric carcinoma. Gastroenterology 1982;82(2):228–31.
[36] Bytzer P. Endoscopic follow-up of gastric ulcer to detect malignancy: is it worthwhile? Scand J Gastroenterol 1991;26(11):93–9.

[37] Borody TJ, George LL, Brandl S, et al. *Helicobacter pylori*-negative duodenal ulcer. Am J Gastroenterol 1991;86(9):1154–7.
[38] Kalaghchi B, Mekasha G, Jack MA, et al. Ideology of *Helicobacter pylori* prevalence in peptic ulcer disease in an inner-city minority population. J Clin Gastroenterol 2004; 38(3):248–51.
[39] Weels JF, van der Hulst RW, Gerrits Y, et al. The interrelationship between cytotoxin-associated gene A, vacuolating cytotoxin, and *Helicobacter pylori*-related diseases. J Infect Dis 1996;173(5):1171–5.
[40] Hopkins RJ, Girardi LS, Turney EA. Relationship between *Helicobacter pylori* eradication and reduced duodenal and gastric ulcer recurrence: a review. Gastroenterology 1996; 110(4):1244–52.
[41] Cappell MS, Schein JR. Diagnosis and treatment of nonsteroidal anti-inflammatory drug-associated upper gastrointestinal toxicity. Gastroenterol Clin North Am 2000;29(1): 97–124.
[42] Wilcox CM, Shalek KA, Cotsonis G. Striking prevalence of over-the-counter nonsteroidal anti-inflammatory drug use in patients with upper gastrointestinal hemorrhage. Arch Intern Med 1994;154(1):42–6.
[43] Lichtenstein DR, Syngal S, Wolfe MM. Nonsteroidal antiinflammatory drugs and the gastrointestinal tract: the double-edged sword. Arthritis Rheum 1995;38(1):5–18.
[44] Shiffman ML, Farrel MT, Yee YS. Risk of bleeding after endoscopic biopsy or polypectomy in patients taking aspirin or other NSAIDS. Gastrointest Endosc 1994;40(4): 458–62.
[45] Meko JB, Norton JA. Management of patients with Zollinger-Ellison syndrome. Annu Rev Med 1995;46:395–411.
[46] Berna MJ, Hoffmann KM, Serrano J, et al. Serum gastrin in Zollinger-Ellison syndrome: I. Prospective study of fasting serum gastrin in 309 patients from the National Institutes of Health and comparison with 2229 cases from the literature. Medicine 2006;85(6): 295–330.
[47] Berna MJ, Hoffmann KM, Long SH, et al. Serum gastrin in Zollinger-Ellison syndrome: II. Prospective study of gastrin provocative testing in 293 patients from the National Institutes of Health and comparison with 537 cases from the literature—evaluation of diagnostic criteria, proposal of new criteria, and correlations with clinical and tumoral features. Medicine 2006;85(6):331–64.
[48] Elta GH. Acute nonvariceal upper gastrointestinal hemorrhage. Curr Treat Options Gastroenterol 2002;5(2):147–52.
[49] Kovacs TO, Jensen DM. Endoscopic treatment of ulcer bleeding. Curr Treat Options Gastroenterol 2007;10(2):143–8.
[50] Amano Y, Moriyama N, Suetsugu H, et al. Which types of non-bleeding visible vessels in gastric peptic ulcers should be treated by endoscopic hemostasis? J Gastroenterol Hepatol 2004;19(1):13–7.
[51] Bleau BL, Gostout CJ, Sherman KE, et al. Recurrent bleeding from peptic ulcer associated with adherent clot: a randomized study comparing endoscopic treatment with medical therapy. Gastrointest Endosc 2002;56(1):1–6.
[52] Jensen DM, Kovacs TO, Jutabha R, et al. Randomized trial of medical or endoscopic therapy to prevent recurrent ulcer hemorrhage in patients with adherent clots. Gastroenterology 2002;123(2):407–13.
[53] Kahi CJ, Jensen DM, Sung JJ, et al. Endoscopic therapy versus medical therapy for bleeding peptic ulcer with adherent clot: a meta analysis. Gastroenterology 2005; 129(3):855–62.
[54] Andrews CN, Levy A, Fishman M, et al. Intravenous proton pump inhibitors in bleeding peptic ulcer disease with high-risk stigmata: a multicenter comparative study. Can J Gastroenterol 2005;19(11):667–71.

[55] Jensen DM, Pace SC, Soffer E, et al. Continuous infusion of pantoprazole versus ranitidine for prevention of ulcer rebleeding: a US multicenter randomized double-blind study. Am J Gastroenterol 2006;101(9):1991–9.
[56] Gupta PK, Fleischer DE. Nonvariceal upper gastrointestinal bleeding. Med Clin North Am 1993;77(5):973–92.
[57] Chung IK, Kim EJ, Lee MS, et al. Endoscopic factors predisposing to rebleeding following endoscopic hemostasis in bleeding peptic ulcers. Endoscopy 2001;33(11):969–75.
[58] Stiegman GV. Endoscopic approaches to upper gastrointestinal bleeding. Am Surg 2006; 72(2):111–5.
[59] Leung JW, Chung SC. Endoscopic injection of adrenaline in bleeding peptic ulcers. Gastrointest Endosc 1987;33(2):73–5.
[60] Oxner RB, Simmonds NJ, Gertner DJ, et al. Controlled trial of endoscopic injection therapy for bleeding from peptic ulcers with visible vessels. Lancet 1992;339(8799):966–8.
[61] Thomopoulos KC, Nikolopoulos VN, Katsakoulis EC, et al. The effect of endoscopic injection therapy on the clinical outcome of patients with benign peptic ulcer bleeding. Scand J Gastroenterol 1997;32(3):212–6.
[62] Chung SC, Leung JW, Leung FW. Effect of submucosal epinephrine injection on local gastric blood flow: a study using laser Doppler flowmetry and reflectance spectrophotometry. Dig Dis Sci 1990;35(8):1008–11.
[63] Lin HJ, Hsieh YH, Tseng GY, et al. A prospective randomized trial of large- versus small-volume endoscopic injection of epinephrine for peptic ulcer bleeding. Gastrointest Endosc 2002;55(6):615–9.
[64] Von Delius S, Thies P, Umgelter A, et al. Hemodynamics after endoscopic submucosal injection of epinephrine in patients with nonvariceal upper gastrointestinal bleeding: a matter of concern. Endoscopy 2006;38(12):1284–8.
[65] Sung JY, Chung SC, Low JM, et al. Systemic absorption of epinephrine after endoscopic submucosal injection in patients with bleeding peptic ulcers. Gastrointest Endosc 1993; 39(1):20–2.
[66] Villanueva C, Balanzo J, Espinos JC, et al. Prediction of therapeutic failure in patients with bleeding peptic ulcer treated with endoscopic injection. Dig Dis Sci 1993;38(11):2062–70.
[67] Church NI, Palmer KR. Injection therapy for endoscopic haemostasis. Baillieres Best Pract Res Clin Gastroenterol 2000;14(3):427–41.
[68] Kubba AK, Murphy W, Palmer KR. Endoscopic injection for bleeding peptic ulcer: a comparison of adrenaline alone with adrenaline plus human thrombin. Gastroenterology 1996; 111(3):623–8.
[69] Church NI, Dallal HJ, Masson J, et al. A randomized trial comparing heater probe plus thrombin with heater probe plus placebo for bleeding peptic ulcer. Gastroenterology 2003;125(2):396–403.
[70] Church NI, Palmer KR. Ulcers and nonvariceal bleeding. Endoscopy 2003;35(1):22–6.
[71] Lee KJ, Kim JH, Hahm KB, et al. Randomized trial of N-butyl-2 cyanoacrylate compared with injection of hypertonic saline-epinephrine in the endoscopic treatment of bleeding peptic ulcers. Endoscopy 2000;32(7):505–11.
[72] Repici A, Ferrari A, De Angelis C, et al. Adrenaline plus cyanoacrylate injection for treatment of bleeding peptic ulcers after failure of conventional endoscopic haemostasis. Dig Liver Dis 2002;34(5):349–55.
[73] Soon MS, Wu SS, Chen YY, et al. Monopolar coagulation versus conventional endoscopic treatment for high-risk peptic ulcer bleeding: a prospective randomized study. Gastrointest Endosc 2003;58(3):323–9.
[74] Laine L, Petersen WL. Bleeding peptic ulcer. N Engl J Med 1994;331(11):717–27.
[75] Cipolletti L, Bianco MA, Rotondano G, et al. Prospective comparison of argon plasma coagulator and heater probe in the endoscopic treatment of major peptic ulcer bleeding. Gastrointest Endosc 1998;48(2):191–5.

[76] Kanai M, Hamada A, Endo Y, et al. Efficacy of argon plasma coagulation in nonvariceal upper gastrointestinal bleeding. Endoscopy 2004;36(12):1085–8.

[77] Lin HJ, Wang K, Perng CL, et al. Heater probe thermocoagulation and multipolar electrocoagulation for arrest of peptic ulcer bleeding: a prospective, randomized comparative trial. J Clin Gastroenterol 1995;21(2):99–102.

[78] Lin HJ, Perng CL, Wang K, et al. Long-terms of heater probe thermocoagulation with massive peptic ulcer bleeding: a prospective study. Am J Gastroenterol 1995;90(1): 44–7.

[79] Llach J, Bordas JM, Salmeron JM, et al. A prospective randomized trial of heater probe thermocoagulation versus injection therapy in peptic ulcer hemorrhage. Gastrointest Endosc 1996;43(2):117–20.

[80] Lin HJ, Hsieh YH, Tseng GY, et al. A prospective randomized trial of endoscopic hemoclip versus heater probe thermocoagulation for peptic ulcer bleeding. Am J Gastroenterol 2002; 97(9):2250–4.

[81] Lin HJ, Perng CL, Sun IC, et al. Endoscopic haemoclip versus heater probe thermocoagulation plus hypertonic saline-epinephrine injection for peptic ulcer bleeding. Dig Liver Dis 2003;35(12):898 902.

[82] Peng YC, Chen SY, Tung CF, et al. Factors associated with failure of initial hemoclip hemostasis for upper gastrointestinal bleeding. J Clin Gastroenterol 2006;40(6):562–3.

[83] Cipolletta L, Bianco MA, Marmo R, et al. Endoclips versus heater probe in preventing early recurrent bleeding from peptic ulcer: a prospective and randomized trial. Gastrointest Endosc 2001;53(2):147–51.

[84] Saltman JR, Strate LL, Di Sena V, et al. Prospective trial of endoscopic clips versus combination therapy in upper GI bleeding (PROTECT-UGI bleeding). Am J Gastroenterol 2005;100(7):1503–8.

[85] Eriksson LG, Sundbom M, Gustavsson S, et al. Endoscopic marking with a metallic clip facilitates transcatheter arterial embolization in upper peptic ulcer bleeding. J Vasc Interv Radiol 2006;17(6):959–64.

[86] Raju GS, Gajula L. Endoclips for GI endoscopy. Gastrointest Endosc 2004;59(2): 267–79.

[87] Lin HJ, Lo WC, Cheng YC, et al. Endoscopic hemoclip versus triclip placement in patients with high-risk peptic ulcer bleeding. Am J Gastroenterol 2007;102(3):539–43.

[88] Jensen DM, Machicado GA, Hirabayashi K. Randomized controlled study of 3 different types of hemoclips for hemostasis of bleeding canine acute gastric ulcers. Gastrointest Endosc 2006;64(5):769–73.

[89] Hepworth CC, Kadirkamanathan SS, Gong F, et al. A randomized controlled comparison of injection, thermal and mechanical endoscopic methods of haemostasis on mesenteric methods. Gut 1998;42(4):462–9.

[90] Banares R, Albillos A, Rincon D, et al. Endoscopic treatment versus endoscopic plus pharmacologic treatment for acute variceal bleeding: a meta-analysis. Hepatology 2002;35(3): 609–15.

[91] Matsui S, Kamisako T, Kudo M, et al. Endoscopic band ligation for control of nonvariceal upper GI hemorrhage: comparison with bipolar electrocoagulation. Gastrointest Endosc 2002;55(2):214–8.

[92] Ljubicic N. Endoscopic detachable mini-loop ligation for treatment of gastroduodenal angiodysplasia: case study of 11 patients with long-term follow-up. Gastrointest Endosc 2004;59(3):420–3.

[93] Choa TS, Fock KM, Ng TM, et al. Epinephrine injection therapy versus a combination of epinephrine injection and endoscopic hemoclip in the treatment of bleeding ulcers. World J Gastroenterol 2005;11(7):1044–7.

[94] Barkun A, Bardou M, Marshall JK. Consensus recommendations for managing patients with nonvariceal upper GI bleeding. Ann Intern Med 2003;139(10):843–57.

[95] Marmo R, Rotondano G, Piscopo R, et al. Dual therapy versus monotherapy in the endoscopic treatment of high-risk bleeding ulcers: a meta-analysis of controlled trials. Am J Gastroenterol 2007;102(2):279–89.
[96] Lo CC, Hsu PI, Lo GH, et al. Comparison of hemostatic efficacy for epinephrine injection alone and injection combined with hemoclip therapy in treating high-risk bleeding ulcers. Gastrointest Endosc 2006;63(6):767–73.
[97] Murphy PP, Ballinger PJ, Massey BT, et al. Discrete ulcer in Barrett's esophagus: relationship to acute gastrointestinal bleeding. Endoscopy 1998;30(4):367–70.
[98] Kumar A. Massive bleeding due to Candidal esophagitis. South Med J 1994;87(6):669–71.
[99] Wolfsen HC, Wang KK. Etiology and course of acute bleeding esophageal ulcers. J Clin Gastroenterol 1992;14(4):342–6.
[100] Caletti GC, Ferrari A, Mattioli S, et al. Endoscopy versus endoscopic ultrasonography in staging reflux esophagitis. Endoscopy 1994;26(9):794–7.
[101] Kusano M, Ino K, Yamada T, et al. Interobserver and intraobserver variation in endoscopic assessment of GERD using the "Los Angeles" classification. Gastrointest Endosc 1994;49(6):700–4.
[102] Cappell MS. Clinical presentation, diagnosis, and management of gastroesophageal reflux disease. Med Clin North Am 2005;89(2):243–91.
[103] Kortas DY, Haas LS, Simpson WG, et al. Mallory-Weiss tear: predisposing factors and predictors of a complicated course. Am J Gastroenterol 2001;96(10):2863–5.
[104] Montalvo RD, Lee M. Retrospective analysis of iatrogenic Mallory-Weiss tears occurring during upper gastrointestinal endoscopy. Hepatogastroenterology 1996;43(7):174–7.
[105] Harris JM, DiPalma JA. Clinical significance of Mallory-Weiss tears. Am J Gastroenterol 1993;88(12):2056–8.
[106] Sugawa C, Benishek D, Walt AJ. Mallory-Weiss syndrome: a study of 224 patients. Am J Surg 1983;145(1):30–3.
[107] Schuman BM, Threadgill ST. The influence of liver disease and portal hypertension on bleeding in Mallory-Weiss syndrome. J Clin Gastroenterol 1994;18(1):10–2.
[108] Chung IK, Kim EJ, Hwang KY, et al. Evaluation of endoscopic hemostasis in upper gastrointestinal bleeding related to Mallory-Weiss syndrome. Endoscopy 2002;34(6): 474–9.
[109] DiMaio CJ, Stevens PD. Nonvariceal upper gastrointestinal bleeding. Gastrointest Endosc Clin N Am 2007;17(2):253–72.
[110] Llach J, Elizade JI, Guevara MC, et al. Endoscopic injection therapy in bleeding Mallory-Weiss syndrome: a randomized controlled trial. Gastrointest Endosc 2001;54(6):679–81.
[111] Morales P, Baum AE. Therapeutic alternatives for the Mallory-Weiss tear. Curr Treat Options Gastroenterol 2003;6(1):75–83.
[112] Jutabha R, Jensen DM. Management of upper gastrointestinal bleeding in the patient with chronic liver disease. Med Clin North Am 1996;80(5):1035–68.
[113] Habib A, Sanyal AJ. Acute variceal hemorrhage. Gastrointest Endosc Clin N Am 2007; 17(2):223–52.
[114] Thabut D, Bernard-Chabert B. Management of acute bleeding from portal hypertension. Best Pract Res Clin Gastroenterol 2007;21(1):19–27.
[115] Kupfer Y, Cappell MS, Tessler S. Acute gastrointestinal bleeding in the intensive care unit. The intensivist's perspective. Gastroenterol Clin North Am 2000;29(2):275–307.
[116] Weston AP. Hiatus hernia with Cameron ulcers and erosions. Gastrointest Endosc Clin N Am 1996;6(4):671–9.
[117] Panzuto F, Di Giulio E, Capurso G, et al. Large hiatus hernia in patients with iron deficiency anemia: a prospective study on prevalence and treatment. Aliment Pharmacol Ther 2004;19(6):663–70.
[118] Lin CC, Chen TH, Ho WC, et al. Endoscopic treatment of a Cameron lesion presenting as life-threatening gastrointestinal hemorrhage. J Clin Gastroenterol 2001;33(5):423–4.

[119] Merli M, Nicolini G, Angeloni S, et al. The natural history of portal hypertensive gastropathy in patients with liver cirrhosis and mild portal hypertension. Am J Gastroenterol 2004;99(10):1959–65.
[120] Sarin SK, Sreenivas DV, Lahoti D, et al. Factors influencing development of portal hypertensive gastropathy in patients with portal hypertension. Gastroenterology 1992;102(3): 994–9.
[121] Primignani M, Carpinelli L, Preatoni P, et al. Natural history of portal hypertensive gastropathy in patients with liver cirrhosis: the New Italian Endoscopic Club for the study and treatment of esophageal varices (NIEC). Gastroenterology 2000;119(1):181–7.
[122] Orloff MJ, Orloff MS, Orloff SL, et al. Treatment of bleeding from portal hypertensive gastropathy by portacaval shunt. Hepatology 1995;21(4):1011–7.
[123] Perez-Ayuso RM, Pique JM, Bosch J, et al. Propranolol in prevention of recurrent bleeding from severe portal hypertensive gastropathy in cirrhosis. Lancet 1991;337(8755): 1431–4.
[124] Trevino HH, Brady CE 3rd, Schenker S. Portal hypertensive gastropathy. Dig Dis 1996; 14(4):258–70.
[125] DeWeert TM, Gostout CJ, Wiesner RH. Congestive gastropathy and other upper endoscopic findings in 81 consecutive patients undergoing orthotopic liver transplantation. Am J Gastroenterol 1990;85(5):573–6.
[126] Miettinen M, Lasota J. Gastrointestinal stromal tumors: definition, clinical, histological, immunohistochemical, and molecular genetic features and differential diagnosis. Virchows Arch 2001;438(1):1–12.
[127] Chou FF, Eng HL, Sheen-Chen SM. Smooth muscle tumors of the gastrointestinal tract: analysis of prognostic factors. Surgery 1996;119(2):171–7.
[128] Demetri GD, Benjamin RS, Blanke C, et al. NCCN Task Force Report: management of patients with gastrointestinal stromal tumor (GIST)—update of the NCCN clinical practice guidelines. J Natl Compr Canc Netw 2007;5(Suppl 2):S1–29.
[129] Aparicio T, Boige V, Sabourin JC, et al. Prognostic factors after surgery of primary resectable gastrointestinal stromal tumors. Eur J Surg Oncol 2004;30(10):1098–103.
[130] Wotherspoon A. Gastric lymphoma of mucosa-associated lymphoid tissue and *Helicobacter pylori*. Annu Rev Med 1998;49:289–99.
[131] Chen LT, Lin JT, Tai JJ, et al. Long-term results of anti-*Helicobacter pylori* therapy in early-stage gastric high-grade transformed MALT lymphoma. J Natl Cancer Inst 2005; 97(18):1345–53.
[132] Wundisch T, Thiede C, Morgner A, et al. Long-term follow-up of gastric MALT lymphoma after *Helicobacter pylori* eradication. J Clin Oncol 2005;23(31):8018–24.
[133] Hsu CC, Chen JJ, Changchien CS. Endoscopic features of metastatic tumors in the upper gastrointestinal tract. Endoscopy 1996;28(2):249–53.
[134] Savides TJ, Jensen DM, Cohen J, et al. Severe gastrointestinal tumor bleeding: endoscopic findings, treatment and outcome. Endoscopy 1996;28(2):244–8.
[135] Imbesi JJ, Kurtz RC. A multidisciplinary approach to gastrointestinal bleeding in cancer patients. J Support Oncol 2005;3(2):101–10.
[136] Lee YT, Walmsley RS, Leong RW, et al. Dieulafoy's lesion. Gastrointest Endosc 2003; 58(2):236–43.
[137] Fockens P, Tytgat GN. Dieulafoy's disease. Gastrointest Endosc Clin N Am 1996;6(4): 739–52.
[138] Akhras J, Patel P, Tobi M. Dieulafoy's lesion-like bleeding: an underrecognized cause of upper gastrointestinal hemorrhage in patients with advanced liver disease. Dig Dis Sci 2007;52(3):722–6.
[139] Schmulewitz N, Baillie L. Dieulafoy lesions: a review of 6 years of experience at a tertiary referral center. Am J Gastroenterol 2001;96(6):1688–94.
[140] Norton ID, Petersen BT, Sorbi D, et al. Management and long term prognosis of Dieulafoy lesion. Gastrointest Endosc 1999;50(6):762–7.

[141] Kollef MH, O'Brien JD, Zuckerman GR, et al. BLEED: a classification to predict outcome in patients with acute upper and lower gastrointestinal hemorrhage. Crit Care Med 1997; 25(7):1101–2.
[142] Iacopini F, Petruzziello L, Marchese M, et al. Hemostasis of Dieulafoy's by argon plasma coagulation. Gastrointest Endosc 2007;66(1):20–6.
[143] Park CH, Joo YE, Kim HS, et al. A prospective randomized trial of endoscopic band ligation versus endoscopic hemoclip placement for bleeding gastric Dieulafoy's lesions. Endoscopy 2004;36(8):677–81.
[144] Yen HH, Chen YY. Endoscopic band ligation for Dieulafoy lesions: disadvantages and risks. Endoscopy 2006;38(6):651.
[145] Katsinelos P, Parotoglou G, Mimidis K, et al. Endoscopic treatment and follow-up of gastrointestinal Dieulafoy's lesions. World J Gastroenterol 2005;11(38):6022–6.
[146] Bech-Knudsen F, Toftgaard C. Exulceratio simplex Dieulafoy. Surg Gynecol Obstet 1993; 176(2):139–43.
[147] Romaozinho JM, Pontes JM, Lerias C, et al. Dieulafoy's lesion: management and long-term outcome. Endoscopy 2004;36(5):416–20.
[148] Foutch PG. Angiodysplasia of the gastrointestinal tract. Am J Gastroenterol 1993;88(6): 807–18.
[149] Cappell MS, Gupta A. Changing epidemiology of gastrointestinal angiodysplasia with increasing recognition of clinically milder cases: angiodysplasia tend to produce mild chronic gastrointestinal bleeding in a study of 47 consecutive patients admitted from 1980–1989. Am J Gastroenterol 1992;87(2):201–6.
[150] Cappell MS. Spatial clustering of simultaneous nonhereditary gastrointestinal angiodysplasia: small but significant correlation between nonhereditary colonic and upper gastrointestinal angiodysplasia. Dig Dis Sci 1992;37(7):1072–7.
[151] Boley SJ, Brandt LJ. Vascular ectasias of the colon-1986. Dig Dis Sci 1986;31(9 Suppl): 26S–42S.
[152] Chalasani N, Cotsonis G, Wilcox CM. Upper gastrointestinal bleeding in patients with chronic renal failure: role of vascular ectasia. Am J Gastroenterol 1996;91(11):2329–32.
[153] Cappell MS, Lebwohl O. Cessation of recurrent bleeding from gastrointestinal angiodysplasias after aortic valve replacement. Ann Intern Med 1986;105(1):54–7.
[154] Gates C, Morand EF, Davis M, et al. Sclerotherapy as treatment of recurrent bleeding from upper gastrointestinal telangiectasia in CREST syndrome. Br J Rheumatol 1993;32(8):760–1.
[155] Vincentelli A, Susen S, Le Tourneau T, et al. Acquired von Willebrand syndrome in aortic stenosis. N Engl J Med 2003;349(4):343–9.
[156] Cappell MS, et al. Gastrointestinal vascular malformations or neoplasms: arterial, venous, arteriovenous, and capillary. In: Yamada T, Alpers DH, Kaplowitz N, editors. Textbook of gastroenterology. 4th edition. Philadelphia: Lippincott Williams & Wilkins; 2003. p. 2722–41.
[157] Brandt LJ, Spinnell MK. Ability of naloxone to enhance the colonoscopic appearance of normal colon vasculature and colon vascular ectasias. Gastrointest Endosc 1999;49(1): 79–83.
[158] Marwick T, Kerlin P. Angiodysplasia of the upper gastrointestinal tract: clinical spectrum in 41 cases. J Clin Gastroenterol 1986;8(4):404–7.
[159] Richter JM, Christensen MR, Colditz GA, et al. Angiodysplasia: natural history and efficacy of therapeutic interventions. Dig Dis Sci 1989;34(10):1542–6.
[160] Tedesco FJ, Griffin JW Jr, Khan AQ. Vascular ectasia of the colon: clinical, colonoscopic, and radiographic features. J Clin Gastroenterol 1980;2(3):233–8.
[161] Askin MP, Lewis BS. Push enteroscopic cauterization: long-term follow-up of 83 patients with bleeding small intestinal angiodysplasia. Gastrointest Endosc 1996;43(6):580–3.
[162] Gostout CJ, Bowyer BA, Ahlquist DA, et al. Mucosal vascular malformations of the gastrointestinal tract: clinical observations and results of endoscopic neodymium: yttrium-aluminum-garnet laser therapy. Mayo Clin Proc 1988;63(10):993–1003.

[163] Buchi KN. Vascular malformations of the gastrointestinal tract. Surg Clin North Am 1992; 72(3):559–70.

[164] Olmos JA, Marcolongo M, Pogorelsky V, et al. Long-term outcome of argon plasma ablation therapy for bleeding in 100 consecutive patients with colonic angiodysplasia. Dis Colon Rectum 2006;49(10):1507–16.

[165] Gordon RL, Ahl KL, Kerlan RK, et al. Selective arterial embolization for the control of lower gastrointestinal bleeding. Am J Surg 1997;174(1):24–8.

[166] Guy GE, Shetty PC, Sharma RP, et al. Acute lower gastrointestinal hemorrhage: treatment by superselective embolization with polyvinyl alcohol particles. AJR Am J Roentgenol 1992;159(3):521–6.

[167] Abdalla SA, Geisthoff UW, Bonneau D, et al. Visceral manifestations in hereditary haemorrhagic telangiectasia type 2. J Med Genet 2003;40(7):494–502.

[168] Kjeldsen AD, Kjeldsen J. Gastrointestinal bleeding in patients with hereditary hemorrhagic telangiectasia. Am J Gastroenterol 2000;95(2):415–8.

[169] Haitjema T, Disch F, Overtoom TT, et al. Screening family members of patients with hereditary hemorrhagic telangiectasia. Am J Med 1995;99(5):519–24.

[170] Rutgeerts P, van Gompel F, Geboes K, et al. Long term results of treatment of vascular malformations of the gastrointestinal tract by neodymium Yag laser photocoagulation. Gut 1985;26(6):586–93.

[171] Hisada T, Kuwabara H, Tsunoda T, et al. Hereditary hemorrhagic telangiectasia showing severe anemia which was successfully treated with estrogen. Intern Med 1995;34(6):589–92.

[172] Longacre AV, Gross CP, Gallitelli M, et al. Diagnosis and management of gastrointestinal bleeding in patients with hereditary hemorrhagic telangiectasia. Am J Gastroenterol 2003; 98(1):59–65.

[173] Novitsky YW, Kercher KW, Czerniach DR, et al. Watermelon stomach: pathophysiology, diagnosis, and management. J Gastrointest Surg 2003;7(5):652–61.

[174] Ikeda M, Ishida H, Nakamura E, et al. An endoscopic follow-up study of the development of diffuse antral vascular ectasia. Endoscopy 1996;28(4):390–3.

[175] Gilliam JH 3rd, Geisinger KR, Wu WC, et al. Endoscopic biopsy is diagnostic in gastric antral vascular ectasia: the "watermelon stomach." Dig Dis Sci 1989;34(6):885–8.

[176] Jensen DM, Chaves DM, Grund KE. Endoscopic diagnosis and treatment of watermelon stomach. Endoscopy 2004;36(7):640–7.

[177] Gostout CJ, Viggiano TR, Ahlquist DA, et al. The clinical and endoscopic spectrum of the watermelon stomach. J Clin Gastroenterol 1992;15(3):256–63.

[178] Pavey DA, Craig PI. Endoscopic therapy for upper GI vascular ectasias. Gastrointest Endosc 2004;59(2):233–8.

[179] Ng I, Lai KC, Ng M. Clinical and histological features of gastric antral vascular ectasia: successful treatment with endoscopic laser therapy. J Gastroenterol Hepatol 1996;11(3): 270–4.

[180] Kwan V, Bourke MJ, Williams SJ, et al. Argon plasma coagulation in the management of symptomatic gastrointestinal vascular lesions: experience in 100 consecutive patients with long-term follow-up. Am J Gastroenterol 2006;101(1):58–63.

[181] Roman S, Saurin JC, Dumortier J, et al. Tolerance and efficacy of argon plasma coagulation for controlling bleeding in patients with typical and atypical manifestations of watermelon stomach. Endoscopy 2003;35(12):1024–8.

[182] Sebastian S, McLoughlin R, Qasim A, et al. Endoscopic argon plasma coagulation for the treatment of gastric antral vascular ectasia (watermelon stomach): long-term results. Dig Liver Dis 2004;36(3):212–7.

[183] Probst A, Scheubel R, Wienbeck M. Treatment of watermelon stomach (GAVE syndrome) by means of endoscopic argon plasma coagulation (APC): long-term outcome. Z Gastroenterol 2001;39(6):447–52.

[184] Yusoff I, Brennan F, Ormonde D, et al. Argon plasma coagulation for treatment of watermelon stomach. Endoscopy 2002;34(5):407–10.

[185] Kamath PS, Lacerdo M, Ahlquist DA, et al. Gastric mucosal responses to intrahepatic portosystemic shunting in patients with cirrhosis. Gastroenterology 2000;118(5):905–11.
[186] Bourke MJ, Hope RL, Boyd P, et al. Endoscopic laser therapy for watermelon stomach. J Gastroenterol Hepatol 1996;11(9):832–4.
[187] Chamberlain CE. Acute hemorrhagic gastritis. Gastroenterol Clin North Am 1993;22(4): 843–73.
[188] Harty RF, Ancha HB. Stress ulcer bleeding. Curr Treat Options Gastroenterol 2006;9(2): 157–66.
[189] Stollman N, Metz DC. Pathophysiology and prophylaxis of stress ulcer in intensive care unit patients. J Crit Care 2005;20(1):35–45.
[190] Janicki T, Stewart S. Stress ulcer prophylaxis for general medical patients: a review of the evidence. J Hosp Med 2007;2(2):86–92.
[191] Kantorova I, Svoboda P, Scheer P, et al. Stress ulcer prophylaxis in critically ill patients: a randomized controlled trial. Hepatogastroenterology 2004;51(57):757–61.
[192] Jung R, MacLaren R. Proton-pump inhibitors for stress ulcer prophylaxis in critically ill patients. Ann Pharmacother 2002;36(12):1929–37.
[193] Greene JF Jr, Sawicki JE, Doyle WF. Gastric ulceration: a complication of double-lumen nasogastric tubes. JAMA 1973;224(3):338–9.
[194] Yang CS, Lee WJ, Wang HH, et al. Spectrum of endoscopic findings in patients with upper gastrointestinal symptoms after laparoscopic bariatric surgery. Obes Surg 2006;16(9): 1232–7.
[195] Dallal RM, Bailey LA. Ulcer disease after gastric bypass surgery. Surg Obes Relat Dis 2006; 2(4):455–9.
[196] Gumbs AA, Duffy AJ, Bell RL. Incidence and management of marginal ulceration after laparoscopic Roux-Y gastric bypass. Surg Obes Relat Dis 2006;2(4):460–3.
[197] Shin JS, Chen KW, Lin XZ, et al. Active, bleeding marginal ulcer of Billroth II gastric resection: a clinical experience of 18 patients. Am J Gastroenterol 1994;89(10):1831–5.
[198] Cappell MS, Miller S. Gastric lesions in the excluded gastric segment undetected by endoscopy or radiography in patients status post vertical banded gastroplasty. Am J Gastroenterol 1992;87(5):639–44.
[199] Buchwald H, Avidor Y, Braunwald E, et al. Bariatric surgery: a systematic review and meta-analysis. JAMA 2004;292(14):1724–37.
[200] McGuirk TD, Coyle WJ. Upper gastrointestinal tract bleeding. Emerg Med Clin North Am 1996;14(3):523–45.
[201] Cappell MS, Friedel D. The role of esophagogastroduodenoscopy in the diagnosis and management of upper gastrointestinal disorders. Med Clin North Am 2002;86(6): 1165–216.
[202] Lemos DW, Raffetto JD, Moore TC, et al. Primary aortoduodenal fistula: a case report and review of the literature. J Vasc Surg 2003;37(3):686–9.
[203] Katsinelos P, Paroutoglou G, Beltsis A, et al. Endoscopic hemoclip placement for post-sphincterotomy bleeding refractory to injection therapy: report of two cases. Surg Laparosc Endosc Percutan Tech 2005;15(4):238–40.
[204] Lewis BS. Small intestinal bleeding. Gastroenterol Clin North Am 2000;29(1):67–95.
[205] Yavorski RT, Wong RK, Maydonovitch C, et al. Analysis of 3,294 cases of upper gastrointestinal bleeding in military medical facilities. Am J Gastroenterol 1995;90(4): 568–73.
[206] Concha R, Amaro R, Barkin JS. Obscure gastrointestinal bleeding: diagnostic and therapeutic approach. J Clin Gastroenterol 2007;41(3):242–51.
[207] Baichi MM, Arifuddin RM, Mantry PS. Capsule endoscopy for obscure GI bleeding: therapeutic yield of follow-up procedures. Dig Dis Sci 2007;52(5):1370–5.
[208] Hsu CM, Chiu CT, Su MY, et al. The outcome assessment of double balloon enteroscopy for diagnosing and managing patients with obscure gastrointestinal bleeding. Dig Dis Sci 2007;52(1):162–6.

[209] May A, Nachbar L, Pohl J, et al. Endoscopic interventions in the small bowel using double balloon enteroscopy: feasibility and limitations. Am J Gastroenterol 2007; 102(3):527–35.
[210] Heil U, Jung M. The patient with recidivant obscure gastrointestinal bleeding. Best Pract Res Clin Gastroenterol 2007;21(3):393–407.
[211] Tham TC, James C, Kelly M. Predicting outcome of acute non-variceal upper haemorrhage without endoscopy using the clinical Rockall Score. Postgrad Med J 2006;82(973): 757–9.
[212] Khuroo MS, Yattoo GN, Javid G, et al. A comparison of omeprazole and placebo for bleeding peptic ulcer disease. N Engl J Med 1997;336(15):1054–8.
[213] Leontiadis GI, Sharma VK, Howden CW. Systematic review and meta-analysis: proton-pump inhibitor treatment for ulcer bleeding reduces transfusion requirements and hospital stay—results from the Cochrane Collaboration. Aliment Pharmacol Ther 2005;22(3): 169–74.
[214] Gisbert JP, Khorrami S, Carballo F, et al. Meta-analysis: *Helicobacter pylori* eradication therapy vs. antisecretory non-eradication therapy for the prevention of recurrent bleeding from peptic ulcer. Aliment Pharmacol Ther 2004;19(6):617–29.
[215] Lanos A, Rodrigo L, Marquez JL, et al. Low frequency of upper gastrointestinal complications in a cohort of high-risk patients. Scand J Gastroenterol 2003;38(7):693–700.
[216] Wolf AT, Wasan SK, Saltzman JR. Impact of anticoagulation on rebleeding following endoscopic therapy for nonvariceal upper gastrointestinal hemorrhage. Am J Gastroenterol 2007;102(2):290–6.
[217] Lau JY, Sung JJ, Lam YH, et al. Endoscopic retreatment compared with surgery in patients with recurrent bleeding after initial endoscopic control of bleeding ulcers. N Engl J Med 1999;340(10):351–6.
[218] Marmo R, Rotondano G, Bianco MA, et al. Outcome for endoscopic treatment for peptic ulcer bleeding: is a second look endoscopy necessary? Gastrointest Endosc 2004;59(2): 329–30.
[219] Stollman NH, Putcha RV, Neustater BR, et al. The uncleared fundal pool in acute upper gastrointestinal bleeding: implications and outcomes. Gastrointest Endosc 1997;46(4): 324–7.
[220] Cheng CL, Lee CS, Liu NJ, et al. Overlooked lesions at emergency endoscopy for acute nonvariceal upper gastrointestinal bleeding. Endoscopy 2002;34(7):527–30.
[221] Lefkovitz Z, Cappell MS, Lookstein R, et al. Radiologic diagnosis and treatment of gastrointestinal hemorrhage and ischemia. Med Clin North Am 2002;86(6):1357–99.
[222] Smith BR, Stabile BE. Emerging trends in peptic ulcer disease and damage control surgery in the *H. pylori* era. Am Surg 2005;71(9):797–801.
[223] Sarosi GA Jr, Jaiswal KR, Nwariaku FE, et al. Surgical therapy of peptic ulcers in the twenty first century: more common than you think. Am J Surg 2005;190(5):775–9.
[224] Kwan V, Norton ID. Endoscopic management of non-variceal upper gastrointestinal haemorrhage. ANZ J Surg 2007;77(4):222–30.
[225] Kantsevov SV, Cruz-Correa MR, Vaughn CA, et al. Endoscopic cryotherapy for the treatment of bleeding mucosal vascular lesions of the GI tract: a pilot study. Gastrointest Endosc 2003;57(3):403–6.
[226] Hepworth CC, Swain CP. Mechanical endoscopic methods of haemostasis for bleeding peptic ulcers: a review. Bailleres Best Pract Res Clin Gastroenterol 2000;14(3):467–76.
[227] Chiu PW, Hu B, Lau JY, et al. Endoscopic plication of massively bleeding peptic ulcer by using the Eagle Claw VII device: a feasibility study in a porcine model. Gastrointest Endosc 2006;63(4):681–5.
[228] van Leerdam ME, Rauws EA, Geraedts MA, et al. The role of endoscopic Doppler US in patients with peptic ulcer bleeding. Gastrointest Endosc 2003;58(5):677–84.
[229] Epstein AM, Lee TH, Hamel MB. Paying physicians for high-quality care. N Engl J Med 2004;350(4):406–10.

ELSEVIER
SAUNDERS

Med Clin N Am 92 (2008) 551–574

THE MEDICAL CLINICS OF NORTH AMERICA

# Portal Hypertension and Variceal Hemorrhage

Nagib Toubia, MD, Arun J. Sanyal, MBBS, MD*

*Division of Gastroenterology, Hepatology and Nutrition, Virginia Commonwealth University School of Medicine, MCV, Box 980341, Richmond, VA 23298-0341, USA*

Portal hypertension, a major hallmark of cirrhosis, is defined as a portal pressure gradient exceeding 5 mm Hg [1]. In portal hypertension, portosystemic collaterals decompress the portal circulation and give rise to varices. Successful management of portal hypertension and its complications requires knowledge of the underlying pathophysiology, the pertinent anatomy, and the natural history of the collateral circulation, particularly the gastroesophageal varices.

## Hemodynamic principles and causes of portal hypertension

Portal hypertension is a pathologic increase in the portal venous pressure gradient between the portal vein and the inferior vena cava. It results from changes in portal resistance together with changes in portal inflow, as defined by Ohm's law:

$$P(\text{pressure}) = Q(\text{blood flow}) \times R(\text{resistance})$$

The mechanism of the increase in portal pressure depends on the site and the cause of portal hypertension (Box 1), cirrhosis being the most common cause in the Western world [2]. The initial event in the development of portal hypertension in cirrhosis is an increase in resistance to outflow from the portal venous bed. This results from a relatively fixed component from distortion of the intrahepatic vascular bed from the disruption of hepatic architecture and a dynamic component from impaired intrahepatic vasodilation. An estimated 30% of the increased portal resistance is due to the hemodynamic

This work was supported, in part, by a grant from the NIH (K24 DK 02755-08) to Dr. Sanyal.

* Corresponding author.
*E-mail address:* ajsanyal@vcu.edu (A.J. Sanyal).


doi:10.1016/j.mcna.2007.12.003 *medical.theclinics.com*

**Box 1. Causes of portal hypertension**

*Presinusoidal*
Prehepatic
- Portal vein thrombosis
- Superior mesenteric vein thrombosis
- Sinistral portal hypertension (splenic vein thrombosis)

Intrahepatic
- Idiopathic portal hypertension
- Primary biliary cirrhosis
- Primary sclerosing cholangitis

*Sinsuoidal*
Cirrhosis
Vitamin A toxicity
Infiltrative disorders (eg, lymphoproliferative and myeloproliferative diseases)

*Post-sinusoidal*
Veno-occlusive disease
Budd Chiari syndrome
Congestive heart failure

changes, characterized by hepatic vasoconstriction and impaired response to vasodilatory stimuli [3,4]. An intrahepatic decrease in the production of the vasodilator nitrous oxide (NO) [5], in combination with an increase in the production of the vasoconstrictor endothelin-1, is the major contributor to the dynamic increase in hepatic vascular resistance [6,7].

Cirrhosis is associated with a hyperdynamic circulatory state that is characterized by peripheral and splanchnic vasodilation, reduced mean arterial pressure, and increased cardiac output. NO-mediated splanchnic vasodilatation [8–16] produces an increase in inflow of systemic blood into the portal circulation, which causes an increase in portal pressure [17].

Portal pressure is most commonly determined by the hepatic vein pressure gradient (HVPG), which is the difference between the wedged hepatic venous pressure (reflecting the hepatic sinusoidal pressure) and free hepatic vein pressure [18,19]. In combination with venography, right-sided heart pressure measurements, and transjugular liver biopsy, measurement of the HVPG usually delineates the site of portal hypertension (ie, presinusoidal, sinusoidal, or postsinusoidal).

## Collateral circulation

Portal hypertension caused by cirrhosis persists and progresses due to (1) prominent obstructive resistance within the liver, (2) resistance within the collaterals, and (3) continued increase in portal vein inflow. This hypertension leads to the formation of collaterals that decompress the portal circulation by returning blood to the heart via the systemic venous circulation. The major sites of collaterals are:

Rectum, where the systemic inferior mesenteric vein connects with the portal pudendal vein and results in rectal varices

Umbilicus, where the vestigial umbilical vein communicates with the left portal vein and gives rise to prominent collaterals around the umbilicus (caput medusa)

Retroperitoneum, where collaterals, especially in women, communicate between ovarian vessels and iliac veins

Distal esophagus and proximal stomach, where gastroesophageal varices form major collaterals between the portal venous system and the systemic venous system

The following four zones of venous drainage are involved in the formation of gastroesophageal varices [20]:

The *gastric* zone is 2 to 3 cm below the gastroesophageal junction, where the veins meet at the upper end of the cardia of the stomach, drain into short gastric and left gastric veins, and then drain into the splenic and portal veins, respectively.

The *palisade* zone is 2 to 3 cm proximal to the gastric zone into the lower esophagus, where the veins communicate with extrinsic (periesophageal) veins in the distal esophagus. This zone forms the dominant watershed area between the portal and the systemic circulations.

More proximal to the palisade zone in the esophagus is the *perforating* zone, where a network of submucosal veins in the esophagus connects to the periesophageal veins, which drain into the azygous system and subsequently into the systemic circulation.

The *truncal* zone is approximately 10 cm in length and is located proximally to the perforating zone in the esophagus. It typically has four longitudinal veins in the lamina propria.

Most patients who have intrahepatic causes of portal hypertension have gastroesophageal varices because this provides the largest collateral flow via the short and left gastric veins.

Varices form only when the HVPG exceeds 10 mm Hg and bleed only when the HVPG exceeds 12 mm Hg [21,22]. Not all patients who have a HVPG greater than 12 mm Hg bleed. Other local factors that increase variceal wall tension are required [23]. The wall tension is defined by Frank's modification of Laplace's law [24]: T = (P varices – P esophageal lumen) × (radius of varix)/wall thickness. The varix ruptures when the tolerated wall tension is exceeded because the variceal wall thins and the varix increases in diameter and has an increased pressure. Larger varices at sites of limited soft tissue support, notably the gastroesophageal junction, are at greater risk for variceal rupture and bleeding in patients who have portal hypertension.

## Diagnosis of varices

Upper gastrointestinal endoscopy is the most common method to diagnose varices. Various criteria have been used to standardize the description of esophageal varices. The Japanese Research Society for Portal Hypertension described varices in terms of red color signs, color of the varix, form (size) of the varix, and location of the varix [25]. The Northern Italian Endoscopy Club simplified this scheme by classifying varices as F1, F2, or F3 (corresponding to small, medium, or large) with or without red signs. The clinically important decision is whether varices warrant therapeutic intervention. It is therefore useful to evaluate varices in terms of those that require treatment. It is recommended that varices be classified as small, which do not always warrant intervention, or large, which include those that were previously called large [26]. This provides a relatively simple and easily reproducible classification.

Gastric varices are classified by location, which correlates with their risk of hemorrhage. Varices in direct continuity with the esophagus along the lesser and greater curves of the stomach are called gastroesophageal varices (GOV) types 1 and 2, respectively. Isolated gastric varices in the fundus (IGV1) occur less frequently than GOVs (10% versus 90%) but are the most likely to bleed. They may be caused by splenic vein thrombosis or spontaneous splenorenal collaterals.

Endoscopic ultrasound (EUS) has been used to study esophageal varices and to identify a high risk of bleeding by assessment of the cross-sectional area of varices [24]; the size of and flow in the left gastric vein, azygous vein, and paraesophageal collaterals; the changes after endoscopic therapy; and the recurrence of esophageal varices after variceal ligation (collaterals >5 mm are at high risk for recurrent varices) [27]. It is unclear if EUS is superior to standard endoscopy.

Esophageal capsule endoscopy is a promising modality to assess varices. It may provide an accurate, less invasive alternative to EGD for the detection of esophageal varices or portal hypertensive gastropathy [28,29]. A large recent trial, reported only in abstract form, found excellent concordance with endoscopy. The role of capsule endoscopy in the management of varices is still evolving.

## Natural history of gastroesophageal varices

De novo varices develop in 5% to 15% of patients who have cirrhosis per annum and enlarge by 4% to 10% per annum. Most patients who have cirrhosis develop varices, but only one third of them experiences variceal bleeding. Only 40% to 50% of actively bleeding varices spontaneously stop bleeding.

Risk factors for variceal bleeding are listed in Table 1 [21]. When combined, these factors reasonably accurately predict the risk of bleeding (see Table 1) [30]. Varices with a high risk of bleeding include medium and large varices or small varices in patients who have advanced liver failure (Child-Pugh class C).

It is essential to identify and prophylactically treat high-risk patients because each episode of variceal hemorrhage carries a 15% to 20% mortality, and up to 70% of untreated patients die within 1 year of the initial bleeding episode [31]. All patients who have cirrhosis should undergo diagnostic endoscopy to document the presence of varices and to determine their risk for variceal hemorrhage. Recent data showed that a platelet count greater than 150,000 has a high negative predictive value (>90%) for the presence of high-risk esophageal varices [32] in patients who have hepatitis C and Ishak stage 3, 4, 5, or 6 fibrosis with compensated liver function. These data need to be corroborated in an independent population of subjects who have various causes of cirrhosis before applying them to alter screening strategies.

In patients who have cirrhosis without varices or with varices that do not require intervention, endoscopy must be periodically repeated. Patients who have cirrhosis without varices should be rescreened at 2- to 3-year intervals and at the time of hepatic decompensation; patients who have cirrhosis with small varices that do not warrant therapy should be rescreened at 1- to 2-year intervals [26]. Patients who have Child's class B or C with varices of any grade or Child's class A with medium-large varices should be considered for primary prophylaxis of variceal hemorrhage.

## Prophylactic treatment of esophageal varices

### *Pharmacologic therapy*

Nonselective beta-blockers (nadolol and propranolol) are the firstline treatment for primary prophylaxis. They block vasodilatory beta-adrenergic

Table 1
Risk factors for variceal hemorrhage

| | | | | |
|---|---|---|---|---|
| Portal pressure | HVPG > 12 mm Hg | | | |
| Varix size and location | Large esophageal varices | | Isolated cluster of varices in fundus of stomach | |
| Variceal appearance on endoscopy ("red signs") | Red wale marks (longitudinal red streaks on varices) | Cherry-red spots (red, discrete, flat spots on varices) | Hematocystic spots (discrete, red, raised spots) | Diffuse erythema |
| Degree of liver failure | Child-Pugh class C cirrhosis | | | |
| Presence of ascites | Tense ascites | | | |

*Abbreviation:* HVPG, hepatic vein pressure gradient.

receptors, permitting unopposed alpha-adrenergic vasoconstriction in the mesenteric arterioles, thereby reducing portal venous inflow and pressure. They also decrease cardiac output, which further decreases the portal inflow. Meta-analysis of clinical trials shows that the risk of bleeding is reduced by beta-blocker therapy versus placebo from 25% to 15% [33]. The effectiveness of beta-blockers is most accurately assessed by the HVPG. The best predictor of success is a sustained decrease in the HPVG to less than 12 mm Hg, whereas patients who have a sustained 20% decrease in HPVG to greater than 12 mm Hg have a risk of bleeding of less than 10% [34,35]. This approach is not widely applied to clinical practice. The efficacy of beta-blockers is clinically monitored by a decrease in the resting heart rate greater than 25% but not to a rate less than 55 beats/min. Only 20% to 30% of subjects achieve these endpoints, and 15% to 20% of subjects cannot tolerate and require discontinuation of this therapy.

Short-acting (nitroglycerin) or long-acting (isosorbide mononitrates) nitrates cause venodilatation, rather than arterial dilatation, and decrease portal pressure predominantly by decreasing portal venous blood flow. The effect on intrahepatic resistance is not impressive, and nitrates are no longer recommended for primary prophylaxis due to discrepant results of clinical trials.

Other agents that may decrease intrahepatic resistance include $\alpha_1$-adrenergic blockers and angiotensin II receptor antagonists. Prazosin, an $\alpha_1$-adrenergic blocker, caused worsening of the systemic hyperdynamic circulation and was associated with portal hypertension and consequent sodium retention and ascites [36]. Losartan, an angiotensin II receptor antagonist, caused a reduction in portal pressure without significant effects on the systemic circulation [37]. It did not significantly reduce portal pressure in randomized controlled trials, but it worsened the renal function [38,39]. Endothelin receptor blockers and liver-selective NO donors that target intrahepatic vascular resistance are promising investigational therapies [40].

*Endoscopic sclerotherapy*

Prophylactic endoscopic sclerotherapy (EST) was used in the 1980s. Although controlled trials initially reported that it significantly reduced the risk of a first variceal bleed and improved survival [41–43], subsequent trials did not show a survival benefit. EST may provoke bleeding that is difficult to control and may increase the mortality [44,45]. A meta-analysis showed a marked reduction in the risk for a first episode of bleeding, but the mortality was higher in certain studies [46]. Consequently, EST is not recommended for prophylaxis of esophageal varices.

*Endoscopic variceal ligation*

Endoscopic variceal ligation (EVL) is associated with fewer procedure-related complications than EST. EVL significantly reduces the risk of the first bleeding compared with no treatment [47–49] or compared with propranolol [50–52], with a relative risk reduction of almost 40% (Fig. 1). No survival benefit was seen compared with propranolol. One study did not reveal any benefit of EVL and propranolol versus EVL alone; however, given the low risk of bleeding after variceal eradication and the use of EVL when varices recurred, the investigators likely missed any chance of demonstrating a benefit of combined therapy because beta-blockers would be expected to prevent varices as their main effect.

In summary, nonselective beta-blockers or EVL are recommended first-line treatments for primary prophylaxis of variceal hemorrhage. EVL may be used in subjects who cannot tolerate beta-blockers. The authors use EVL in patients who are likely not to tolerate beta-blockers (eg, patients who have low blood pressure or asthma) and who have medium-large varices, whereas they preferentially use beta-blockers when the varices are small and technically difficult to band. This practice is based on evidence that up to 6% of subjects undergoing EVL may experience potentially life-threatening iatrogenic hemorrhage.

## Management of acute variceal bleed

The management of acute variceal bleeding includes hemodynamic resuscitation, general treatments, prevention of complications, and achievement of hemostasis. Intravenous access must be promptly secured (Box 2). Airway intubation is indicated in patients who are bleeding severely or who have mental status changes that preclude their ability to protect their airway. Intravascular volume loss is estimated and replaced with crystalloids

| AUTHOR | YEAR | BB | EBL |
|---|---|---|---|
| CHEN | 1998 | 2/26 | 1/26 |
| SARIN | 1999 | 12/44 | 4/45 |
| DE | 1999 | 1/15 | 2/15 |
| SONG | 2000 | 7/30 | 6/31 |
| DE LA MORA | 2000 | 2/12 | 1/12 |
| LUI | 2002 | 9/66 | 3/44 |
| GHEORGE | 2002 | 13/28 | 3/25 |
| LO | 2004 | 13/50 | 8/50 |
| DRASTICH | 2004 | 7/33 | 4/40 |
| SCHEPKE | 2004 | 22/77 | 19/75 |
| JUTABHA | 2005 | 6/31 | 0/31 |
| THULUVATH | 2005 | 1/15 | 2/16 |
| PSILOPOULOS | 2005 | 9/30 | 2/30 |
| LAY | 2006 | 12/50 | 11/50 |
| **Pooled (Fixed effect)** | | **116/509** | **66/490** |

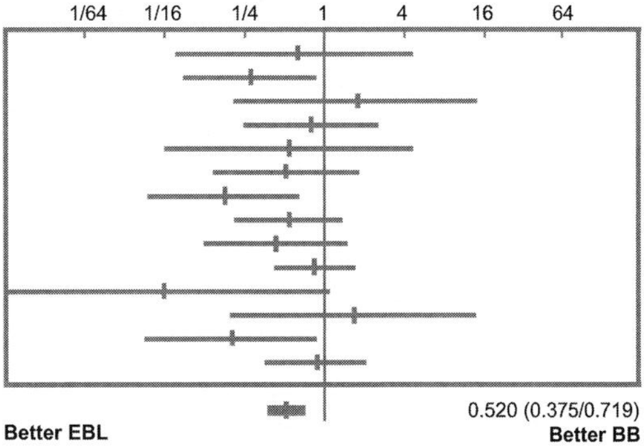


Fig. 1. A meta-analysis of trials of endoscopic variceal ligation versus beta-blockers for the primary prophylaxis of variceal hemorrhage. Each data point reflects the odds ratio for benefit of one treatment versus another for a given study. Horizontal bars represent the confidence limits for the data. Although most of the trials show a modest benefit for EVL, the confidence limits intersect the unit line indicating that these data did not reach significance for individual trials. (*From* Triantos CK, Burroughs AK. Prevention of the development of varices and first portal hypertensive bleeding episode. Best Pract Res Clin Gastroenterol 2007;21:31–42; with permission.)

**Box 2. General measures for the management of active variceal hemorrhage**

*Airway protection*
Endotracheal intubation if altered mental status or unconscious
Gastric aspiration

*Hemodynamic resuscitation*
Crystalloids and blood transfusion
Correction of coagulopathy and thrombocytopenia

*Antibiotic prophylaxis for spontaneous bacterial peritonitis*
Blood cultures and diagnostic paracentesis if ascites present
Third-generation cephalosporin intravenously and switch to oral quinolone when patient is stable and GI tract is functional

*Renal support*
Maintain urine output >50 mL/h
Avoid nephrotoxic drugs

*Metabolic support*
Inject thiamine when indicated
Monitoring blood glucose level
Monitor and treat for delerium tremens
Monitor and treat for acid base and electrolyte disturbances

*Neurologic support*
Monitor mental state
Avoid sedation

and packed red cells. The systolic blood pressure should be maintained at least at 90 to 100 mm Hg, and the heart rate should be maintained below 100 beats/min, with a hemoglobin level around 9 g/dL (hematocrit of 25–30), because overtransfusion can cause a rebound increase in portal pressure and precipitate early rebleeding [53,54]. Fresh frozen plasma and platelets (particularly for a platelet count <50,000/ml) are often used to correct a coagulopathy. They do not adequately correct the coagulopathy and can induce volume overload and rebound portal hypertension [55]. The use of recombinant factor VII has been shown to improve hemostasis rates, but it did not improve survival [56].

Bacteremia is often present on admission for acute variceal hemorrhage. Common bacterial infections include spontaneous bacterial peritonitis, urinary tract infection, and pneumonia. Infections are associated with an increased risk of rebleeding and higher mortality, likely secondary to a further increase in resistance to portal flow, further splanchnic arteriolar dilatation, and further coagulopathy [57,58]. A complete microbiological work-up, including blood cultures and diagnostic paracentesis when appropriate, should be performed. Empiric therapy with a third-generation cephalosporin (eg, ceftriaxone) should be uniformly instituted because several clinical trials have shown improvement in control of bleeding and in patient outcomes (Fig. 2) [59].

## Pharmacologic therapy

### *Vasopressin and its analogs*

Vasopressin is an endogenous nonopeptide that causes splanchnic vasoconstriction by acting on V1 receptors located in arterial smooth muscle, reduces portal venous inflow, and reduces portal pressure [60]. It has severe toxicity, including bowel necrosis from vasoconstriction. Terlipressin, a semisynthetic analog of vasopressin, has a lower rate of systemic side effects. It increases survival in patients who have variceal bleeding. It is not available in the United States [61].

### *Somatostatin and its analogs*

Somatostatin has a half-life in the circulation of 1 to 3 minutes. It decreases portal pressure and collateral blood flow by inhibiting the release of glucagon [62]. It also decreases portal hypertension by decreasing postprandial blood flow (blood perfusion of the gastrointestinal tract after a meal) [63]. Somatostatin is not available in the United States.

Octreotide, a somatostatin analog, has a half-life in the circulation of 80 to 120 minutes. Its effect on reducing portal pressure is not prolonged. Moreover, continuous infusion of octreotide does not decrease the baseline

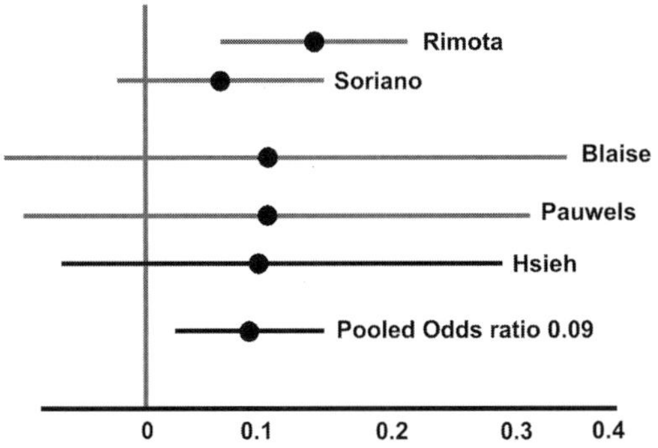


Fig. 2. A meta-analysis of studies of empiric antibiotic use in active variceal bleeding. Each data point reflects the odds ratio for the benefit of one treatment versus another for a given study. Horizontal bars represent the confidence limits for the data. There was a significant advantage for use of antibiotics (pooled odds ratio, 0.09). (*From* Bernard B, Grange JD, Khac EN, et al. Antibiotic prophylaxis for the prevention of bacterial infections in cirrhotic patients with gastrointestinal bleeding: a meta-analysis. Hepatology 1999;29(6):1655–61; with permission.)

portal pressure despite decreasing the postprandial increase in portal pressure [64]. Although some studies failed to prove the superiority of somatostatin or its analogs compared with placebo in the control of acute variceal bleeding [65], other studies showed efficacy [66]. Early administration of vapreotide may be associated with improved control of bleeding but without a significant reduction in mortality [67].

## Endoscopic therapy

### *Endoscopic sclerotherapy*

EST has largely been supplanted by EVL, except when poor visualization precludes effective band ligation of bleeding varices. Current evidence does not support emergency EST as first-line treatment of variceal bleeding [68]. The technique involves injection of a sclerosant into (intravariceal) or adjacent to (paravariceal) a varix. Complications of EST occurring during or after the procedure include chest discomfort, ulcers (and ulcer-related bleeding), strictures, and perforation. The risk of ulcers can be reduced by prescribing sucralfate after EST [69].

### *Endoscopic variceal ligation*

EVL is the preferred endoscopic modality for control of acute esophageal variceal bleeding and for prevention of rebleeding. Varices at the gastroesophageal junction are banded initially, and then more proximal varices are banded in a spiral manner at intervals of approximately every 2 cm. Varices in the middle or proximal esophagus do not need to be banded. EVL is associated with similar but fewer complications [70] than EST and requires fewer sessions to achieve variceal obliteration.

In summary, the first-line treatment for active esophageal variceal hemorrhage is a combination of pharmacologic treatment (ie, octerotide) and endoscopic treatment (EVL or EST) (Fig. 3) [71]. About 80% to 90% of patients achieve hemostasis with first-line therapy; the remaining patients fail to achieve hemostasis or experience early rebleeding [72].

Within the first 6 hours, failure to control bleeding is recognized by [73] (1) transfusion requirement of more than four units of packed red cells and (2) the inability to maintain the systolic blood pressure greater than 70 mm Hg or to raise it by 20 mm Hg or to reduce the resting pulse to less than 100/min or to decrease it by 20 beats/min.

After 6 hours, early rebleeding is defined by hematemesis together with (1) reduction in systolic blood pressure by 20 mm Hg from the level at 6 hours, (2) increase in pulse rate by 20/min from the rate at 6 hours on two consecutive readings 1 hour apart, or(3) the need to transfuse two or more units of packed red cells to increase the hematocrit to more than 27% or the hemoglobin to more than 9 g/dL.

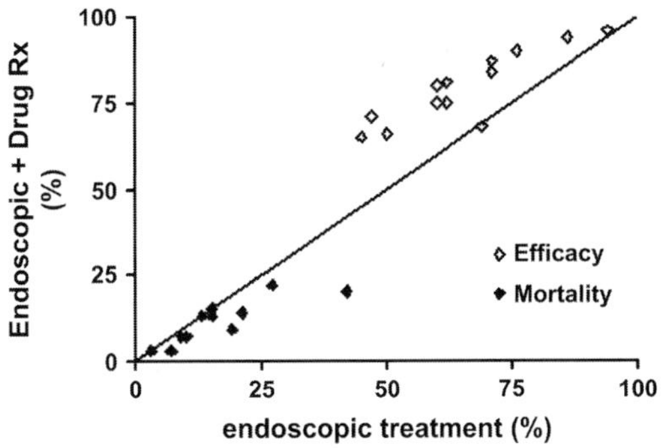


Fig. 3. A L'Abbe plot of trials of endoscopic and pharmacologic treatment of active esophageal variceal bleeding versus endoscopic treatment alone. There was a significantly better outcome of bleeding with combination therapy and a trend for better survival.

Bleeding that occurs more than 48 hours after the initial admission for variceal hemorrhage and is separated by at least a 24-hour bleed-free interval is considered as rebleeding. Specific factors have been associated with failure to control active bleeding and early rebleeding [74], including spurting varices, high Child-Pugh score, HPVG greater than 20 mm Hg [75], infection, and portal vein thrombosis (Box 3).

In patients who have uncontrolled active bleeding or early rebleeding, definitive salvage therapy must be performed before the onset of complications related to the bleeding. Balloon tamponade effectively produces hemostasis in 80% to 90% of cases [76]. Balloon tamponade requires airway protection, is associated with a high incidence of rebleeding when the balloon is deflated, and can cause pressure necrosis of the mucosa if the balloon remains inflated for more than 48 hours. It is therefore used to temporize until definitive treatment is instituted. EVL can be attempted once more for early rebleeding, but this decision must be individualized because of an absence of controlled trials in this setting. The salvage treatment in these patients is portal decompression, with transjugular intrahepatic portosystemic shunts (TIPS) being the procedure of choice.

## Transjugular intrahepatic portosystemic shunts

TIPS reduces elevated portal pressure by creating a communication between the hepatic vein and an intrahepatic branch of the portal vein. It produces hemostasis in more than 90% of cases [77,78]. Once complications from bleeding of aspiration pneumonia or multiorgan failure occur, the prognosis is dismal regardless of the achievement of hemostasis, as demonstrated by a 10% survival at 30 days in patients who have aspiration pneumonia [79]. In the absence of aspiration pneumonia, a 90% survival can be achieved. The best predictor of mortality after TIPS is the MELD (Model of End Stage Liver Disease) score.

**Box 3. Factors affecting risk of continued bleeding or recurrent bleeding**

*Factors associated with failure to control acute hemorrhage*
Spurting varices
High Child-Pugh score
High hepatic venous pressure gradient
Infection
Portal vein thrombosis

*Factors associated with early rebleeding*
Severe initial bleeding
Overly aggressive volume resuscitation
Infection
High hepatic venous pressure gradient
Complications of endoscopic therapy
Renal failure

*Factors associated with late rebleeding*
High Child-Pugh score
Large variceal size
Continued alcohol use
Hepatocellular carcinoma

Based on data from pooled sources.

Contraindications to TIPS include severe congestive heart failure, severe pulmonary hypertension, severe hepatic failure, portal vein thrombosis with cavernomatous transformation, and polycystic liver disease. In a decision in an individual patient, the risk of exsanguination must be weighed against the type of contraindication. Although hemostasis may be achieved with TIPS, patients who have multiorgan failure have a dismal prognosis in the authors' experience. After consultation with the next of kin, provision of only palliative care may often be appropriate in such patients.

Surgical decompression of the portal system via portosystemic shunts is another salvage modality. The use of surgical shunts has declined markedly due to the increasing availability of TIPS, the high morbidity of surgery, and the decline in the number of surgeons trained to perform these procedures.

## Secondary prophylaxis

Once acute variceal bleeding is controlled, prevention of recurrent bleeding should be emphasized. After an index bleed, 70% of patients experience recurrent variceal hemorrhage within 1 year [80], and these patients have a 70% 1-year mortality. The risk of rebleeding is greatest within the first 6 weeks, with more than 50% of rebleeding occurring within 3 to 4 days. Risk factors for rebleeding include severe initial bleeding as defined by a hemoglobin level less than 8 mg/dL, gastric variceal bleeding, active bleeding at endoscopy, and a high HPVG [81,82]. Age greater than 60 years, large esophageal varices, severe liver disease, continued alcoholism, renal failure, and the presence of a hepatoma also increase the risk of rebleeding [81,83]. It is important to prevent recurrent hemorrhage, preserve liver function, maintain a normal renal function, prevent ascites, and avoid alcohol consumption to prolong survival.

Orthotopic liver transplant is the only treatment that achieves most of these objectives and prolongs long-term survival. Some patients are unsuitable candidates for liver transplantation, and, even if orthotopic liver transplant is being considered, patients often have to wait several months before a donor liver becomes available. During this time, they are at risk for recurrent variceal hemorrhage and therefore require treatment to prevent this complication.

The first-line therapy for secondary prophylaxis of variceal hemorrhage is EVL and beta-blocker therapy (Fig. 4). A randomized controlled trial evaluated this combination therapy versus EVL alone [84]. After a median follow-up of 21 months, combination therapy was associated with a significantly lower rate of rebleeding (12% versus 29%) and of variceal recurrence (26% versus 50%). A meta-analysis of 13 studies of EVL versus EST demonstrated that EVL reduced the relative risk of rebleeding by 37% [70]. EVL does not provide a survival advantage over EST. On the other hand, nonselective beta-blockers alone reduce the risk of rebleeding from 63% to 42%, for a 33% relative risk reduction [33]. For mortality, the absolute risk reduction is 7%. Pharmacotherapy with beta-blockers and nitrates cannot be recommended due to discrepant results from clinical trials [84–86].

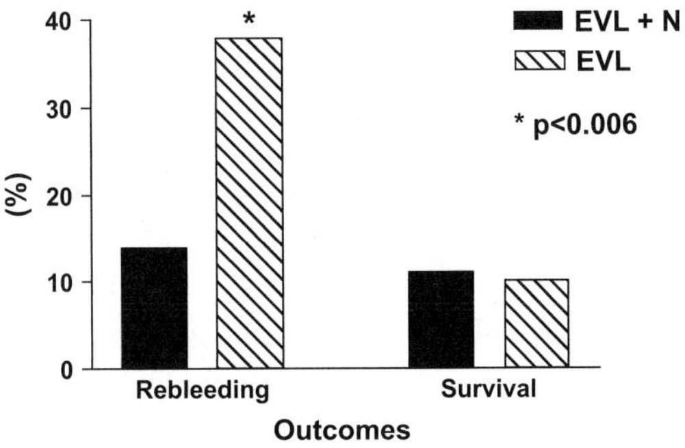


Fig. 4. The outcomes of a clinical trial of endoscopic variceal ligation and nadolol versus endoscopic variceal ligation alone. Combination therapy was associated with a significantly lower rebleeding rate, although survival was not significantly affected. (*Data from* de la Pena J, Brullet E, Sanchez-Hernandez E, et al. Variceal ligation plus nadolol compared with ligation for prophylaxis of variceal rebleeding: a multicenter trial. Hepatology 2005;41(3):572–8.)

A meta-analysis of 12 clinical trials of TIPS versus endoscopic treatment indicates that TIPS is superior to endoscopic treatment for the prevention of rebleeding (19% versus 47%) [87], but this advantage is offset by its failure to improve survival, its higher morbidity from the development of liver failure and encephalopathy (34% versus 19%), and its lack of a cost benefit [88]. Based on these considerations, TIPS is primarily used as a salvage treatment for patients who experience recurrent bleeding despite adequate endoscopic and pharmacologic treatment. In one recent study, subjects who had bleeding esophageal varices underwent early HVPG measurement after initial stabilization with band ligation. Patients who had a HVPG greater than 20 mm Hg were randomized to TIPS versus band ligation. In this high-risk subgroup, early, elective TIPS dramatically improved outcomes compared with EVL. These results await corroboration from other prospective trials.

In summary, the following regimen is recommended for secondary prophylaxis of esophageal variceal hemorrhage:

1. Eradication of esophageal varices by EVL (every 7–14 days until varices are eradicated) with concomitant use of nonselective beta-blockers (propranolol or nadolol)
2. Long-term endoscopic control and banding of recurrent varices every 3 to 6 months
3. If EVL is unavailable or contraindicated, nonselective beta-blockers can be used alone.
4. TIPS is considered if pharmacologic and endoscopic therapy faild (recurrence of variceal hemorrhage despite at least two sessions of endoscopic treatment performed not more than 2 weeks apart).

Always consider liver transplantation if the patient is Child-Pugh B or C.

## Gastric varices

Gastric varices most commonly are caused by portal hypertension, usually in patients who have cirrhosis. Patients who have splenic vein thrombosis or spontaneous splenorenal collaterals can develop isolated gastric varices, particularly IGV1. GOV1 disappears in approximately 58% and 70% after EST and EVL of esophageal varices, respectively [89,90]. The obliteration of varices at the gastroesophageal junction blocks the shunting veins in the palisade zone, leading to dilatation and the formation of new or secondary gastric varices [91]. These secondary varices occur at a rate of 9.7% to 15.3% [92–94] and have a higher frequency of bleeding compared with primary gastric varices. On the other hand, bleeding from primary gastric varices after endoscopic treatment of esophageal varices is uncommon.

The prevalence of gastric varices is 5% to 33% in patients who have portal hypertension, with an overall incidence of bleeding ranging from 3% to 30% [95,96]. Mortality associated with gastric variceal hemorrhage is 30% to 53%, with a 30% rebleeding rate.

Because GOV1 constitutes an extension of esophageal varices along the lesser curvature of the stomach, it is managed like esophageal varices. IGV1 secondary to splenic vein thrombosis is treated by splenectomy. There is no consensus on primary prophylaxis of bleeding GOV2 or IGV due to limited data.

EST controls active bleeding in 40% to 100% of cases of GOV1 [97–103]. The primary drawback is the high risk of recurrent bleeding. EST is frequently associated with ulceration, which bleeds in approximately 50% of cases [97,102,103]. Rebleeding rates have been reported to be 5.5% in GOV1, 19% in GOV2, and as high as 53% in IGV1 [102].

In prospective uncontrolled studies, EVL has been shown to achieve hemostasis rates of up to 89%, with a rebleeding rate of 18.5% [104]. These studies included all types of gastric varices. The major concern after gastric EVL is the potential of partial ligation of large gastric varices, which may produce bleeding [105,106]. EVL is generally not recommended for IGV1.

Compared with EST or EVL, endoscopic variceal occlusion with tissue adhesives, such as N-butyl-cyanoacrylate, isobutyl-2-cyanoacrylate, or thrombin, is more effective for acute fundal gastric variceal bleeding (Table 2). Successful obliteration leads to better control of the initial hemorrhage and lower rebleeding rates [107,108]. A prospective randomized trial of gastric variceal occlusion (GVO) with N-butyl-cyanoacrylate versus EVL in patients who had acute gastric variceal hemorrhage demonstrated that the control of active bleeding was similar in both groups but that rebleeding occurred significantly less frequently in the GVO group (23% versus 47%), with an average of only 1.5 therapy sessions (range 1–3) during a follow-up period of 1.6 to 1.8 years [109]. Therefore, GVO is preferred; however, no tissue adhesive is licensed for use in the United States. In an uncontrolled pilot study, 2-octyl cyanoacrylate, an agent approved for skin closure in the United States, has been described as effective for achieving initial hemostasis and preventing rebleeding from fundal varices [110].

TIPS is the major salvage or, perhaps, is even a primary therapeutic modality for gastric varices in the United States [111], with bleeding control rates greater than 90%. Balloon-occluded retrograde transvenous obliteration is a newly developed transvenous sclerotherapy technique performed for treating gastric fundal varices from spontaneous gastrorenal shunts

Table 2
Outcomes of trials of gastric variceal occlusion for gastric varices

| Author | Study comparison (n/n) | Control bleed (%) | Varices obliterated (%) | Rebleed (%) | AE (%) | Mortality (%) |
|---|---|---|---|---|---|---|
| Tan 2006 | GVO/EVL (48/49) | 93/93 | 62/67 | 22/44 | 22/22 | 15/15 |
| Lo 2001 | GVO/EVL (31/29) | 87/45 | 51/45 | 31/54 | 19/38 | 29/48 |
| Sarin 2002 | GVO/AA (8/9) | 89/62 | 100/44 | 22/25 | — | 11/25 |

*Abbreviations:* AA, Alcohol; AE, Adverse Events; EVL, esophageal variceal ligation; GVO, gastric variceal occlusion.

[112,113]. Shiba and colleagues [114] recently showed that balloon-occluded injection sclerotherapy is safe and effective even in patients who do not have gastrorenal shunts. Surgical shunts also control bleeding gastric varices and prevent recurrent bleeding.

## Ectopic varices

Ectopic varices are defined as portosystemic shunts, resulting from portal hypertension, that occur at any site in the gut or abdomen except in the gastroesophageal region. These sites include the duodenum, jejunum, ileum, colon, rectum, biliary tree, and ostomy sites [115,116]. It is important to differentiate anal varices from hemorrhoids: Anal varices collapse with digital pressure, whereas hemorrhoids do not [115].

Ectopic varices account for 1% to 5% of all variceal bleeding [117]. Patients who have ectopic variceal hemorrhage typically present with sudden, profuse melena or hematochezia. Because brisk upper gastrointestinal (UGI) bleeding can result in hematochezia, all subjects who have suspected variceal hemorrhage should initially undergo emergency upper endoscopy. If the upper endoscopy fails to reveal a source of UGI hemorrhage, colonoscopy is performed after a rapid colonic purge. If the colon looks normal and bleeding continues, angiography may be useful to identify varices or to localize a nonvariceal source of hemorrhage.

Several studies have reported successful therapy of duodenal varices with sclerosant injection [118] or with an occluding agent [119]. There are no data regarding band ligation of ectopic varices. The next treatment option is embolization. Unlike arterial embolization for gastrointestinal hemorrhage, the goal in this setting is to occlude the feeding vein (on the portal venous side) to the ectopic varices rather than to occlude the bleeding site. Balloon-occluded retrograde transvenous obliteration has been successfully used in several reported cases. If the patient continues to bleed despite embolization, options include TIPS or surgery. At our center, TIPS is the preferred approach for the treatment of bleeding ectopic varices.

## Gastric antral vascular ectasia

Gastric antral vascular ectasia (GAVE), or watermelon stomach, describes a vascular lesion of the gastric antrum that consists of ectatic and sacculated antral mucosal vessels radiating toward from the pylorus (Fig. 5). Its cause is unknown, but it has been proposed that gastric peristalsis causes prolapse of the loose antral mucosa into the duodenum with consequent elongation and ectasia of the mucosal vessels [120,121]. Microscopic features include dilated capillaries with focal thrombosis, dilated and tortuous submucosal venous channels, and fibromuscular hyperplasia of the muscularis mucosa. Most cases are idiopathic, but it has been associated

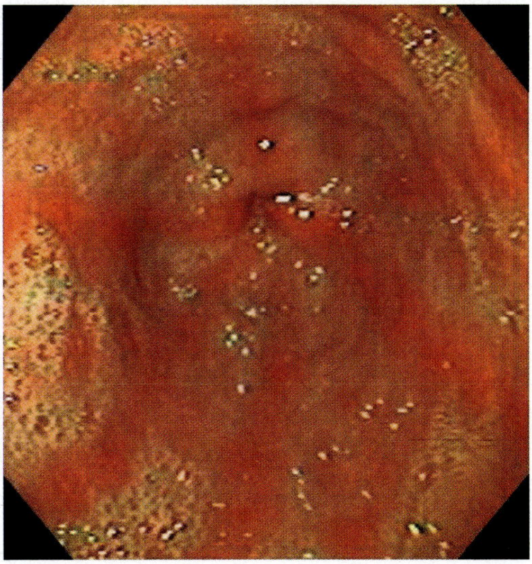

Fig. 5. The endoscopic appearance of gastric antral vascular ectasia with red streaks radiating in to the antrum from the pylorus and a section of the antrum demonstrating the submucosal thickening, hemorrhage, and thrombosis in GAVE. (*Courtesy of* A. Scott Mills, MD, Richmond, VA.)

with cirrhosis, achlorhydria, atrophic gastritis, and the CREST syndrome and has occurred after bone marrow transplantation [122]. The association with cirrhosis and portal hypertension is considered unreliable because GAVE with coexisting portal hypertension does not generally respond to reduction of the portal pressure [123].

GAVE may cause acute hemorrhage or chronic occult bleeding. It frequently occurs in middle-aged or older women. Treatment consists mainly of endoscopic coagulation with heater probe, Gold probe, argon plasma coagulator, or laser therapy. Chronic cases sometimes require periodic transfusions and iron therapy. Portal decompression with TIPS does not reduce the bleeding. Antrectomy prevents recurrent bleeding but is usually reserved for patients who fail endoscopic therapies.

## Portal hypertensive gastropathy

Portal hypertensive gastropathy (PHG) is characterized endoscopically by three patterns: (1) fine red speckling of gastric mucosa; (2) superficial reddening, especially on the tips of the gastric rugae; and, most commonly, (3) the presence of a mosaic pattern with red spots (snake-skin appearance) in the gastric fundus or body. Histologically, the stomach in PHG contains dilated, tortuous, irregular veins in the mucosa and submucosa, sometimes with intimal thickening, usually in the absence of significant inflammation

[124]. PHG is correlated with the severity of liver disease [125]. It is diagnosed by endoscopy. It is an uncommon cause of significant UGI bleeding in patients who have portal hypertension. In one study [126], acute bleeding from PHG was observed in only 2.5% of patients.

Treatment is directed at decreasing portal pressure. Propranolol has been shown to significantly reduce the rate of recurrent bleeding compared with placebo (35% versus 62% at 1 year) [127]. Vasopressin, terlipressin, somatostatin, and octerotide have not been studied for this indication. TIPS is the next therapy. It is associated with significant improvement in the endoscopic findings and a decrease in the transfusion requirements. If bleeding continues, surgical portal decompression is performed. Liver transplantation is indicated for decompensated liver disease. Endoscopic thermal coagulation is not effective for controlling or preventing this diffuse form of bleeding.

## Downhill varices

Esophageal veins form a plexus on the outer surface of the esophagus. The lower part drains into the short and left gastric veins of the portal system, whereas the upper part drains into the azygous, thyroid, and internal mammary veins and then into the superior vena cava. "Downhill" esophageal varices (DEV) form in the upper third of the esophagus as collateral branches directing blood flow "downward" to bypass superior vena cava (SVC) obstruction via the azygous vein or to drain the systemic superior venous system via the portal vein when the SVC and the azygous vein are obstructed.

DEV are mostly due to SVC syndrome secondary to mass effects (external compression of the SVC) from lung cancer, intrathoracic goiter, mediastinal lymphoma, thyroid carcinoma, thymoma, or mediastinal lymphadenopathy secondary to head and neck cancers. DEV usually disappear after treatment of the underlying condition. Several cases have been associated with gastrointestinal hemorrhage, which can be life threatening [128]. Due to its rarity, neither controlled trials nor a general consensus exists on the best therapeutic approach. Isolated case reports have suggested success with EST, EBL, or balloon tamponade.

## References


[1] Bosch J. The sixth Carlos E. Rubio Memorial Lecture. Prevention and treatment of variceal hemorrhage. P R Health Sci J 2000;19:57–67.

[2] Garcia-Tsao G. Portal hypertension. Curr Opin Gastroenterol 2006;22:254–62.

[3] Gupta PS, Toruner M, Chung M, et al. Endothelial dysfunction and decreased production of nitric oxide in the intrahepatic microcirculation of cirrhotic rats. Hepatology 1998;41:926–31.

[4] Shah V, Garcia-Cardena G, Sessa W, et al. The hepatic circulation in health and in disease: report of a single-topic symposium. Hepatology 1998;27:279–88.

[5] Sarin S, Groszmann RT, Mosca P. Propranolol ameliorates the development of portal-systemic shunting in a chronic murine schistosomiasis model of portal hypertension. J Clin Invest 1991;87:1032–6.
[6] Pinzani M, Milani S, De Franco R, et al. Endothelin 1 is overexpressed in human cirrhotic liver and exerts multiple effects on activated hepatic stellate cells. Gastroenterology 1996; 110:534–48.
[7] Rockey DC, Weisiger RA. Endothelin induced contractility of stellate cells from normal and cirrhotic rat liver: implications for regulation of portal pressure and resistance. Hepatology 1996;59:233–40.
[8] Atucha NM, Shah V, Garcia-Cardena G, et al. Role of endothelium in the abnormal response of mesenteric vessels in rats with portal hypertension and liver cirrhosis. Gastroenterology 1996;111:1627–32.
[9] Cahill PA, Foster C, Redmond EM, et al. Enhanced nitric oxide synthase activity in portal hypertensive rabbits. Hepatology 1995;22:598–606.
[10] Cahill PA, Redmond EM, Hodges R, et al. Increased endothelial nitric oxide synthase activity in the hyperemic vessels of portal hypertensive rats. J Hepatol 1996;25:370–8.
[11] Garcia-Pagan JC, Fernandez M, Bernadich C, et al. Effects of continued NO inhibition on portal hypertensive syndrome after portal vein stenosis in rat. Am J Phys 1994;267: G984–90.
[12] Niederberger M, Gines P, Martin PY, et al. Comparison of vascular nitric oxide production and systemic hemodynamics in cirrhosis versus prehepatic portal hypertension in rats. Hepatology 1996;24:947–51.
[13] Sieber CC, Groszmann RJ. In vitro hyporeactivity to methoxamine in portal hypertensive rats: reversal by nitric oxide blockade. Am J Phys 1992;262:G996–1001.
[14] Sieber CC, Groszmann RJ. Nitric oxide mediates hyporeactivity to vasopressors in mesenteric vessels of portal hypertensive rats. Gastroenterology 1992;103:235–9.
[15] Sieber CC, Lopez-Talavera JC, Groszmann RJ. Role of nitric oxide in the in vitro splanchnic vascular hyporeactivity in ascitic cirrhotic rats. Gastroenterology 1993;104:1750–4.
[16] Sogni P, Sabry S, Moreau R, et al. Hyporeactivity of mesenteric resistance arteries in portal hypertensive rats. J Hepatol 1996;24:487–90.
[17] Vorobioff J, Bredfeldt JE, Groszmann RJ. Increased blood flow through the portal system in cirrhotic rats. Gastroenterology 1984;87:1120–6.
[18] Garcia-Pagan JC, Groszmann RJ, Bosch J. Measurement of portal pressure. Clin Gastroenterol Hepatol 2005;981.
[19] Groszmann RJ, Glickman M, Blei AT. Wedged and free hepatic venous pressure measured with a balloon catheter. Gastroenterology 1979;76:253–8.
[20] Vianna A, Hayes PC, Moscoso G, et al. Normal venous circulation of the gastroesophageal junction: a route to understanding varices. Gastroenterology 1987;93:876–89.
[21] Garcia-Tsao G, Groszmann RJ, Fisher RL, et al. Portal pressure, presence of gastroesophageal varices and variceal bleeding. Hepatology 1985;5:419–24.
[22] Groszmann RJ, Garcia-Tsao G, Bosch J, et al. Beta-blockers to prevent gastroesophageal varices in patients with cirrhosis. N Engl J Med 2005;353:2254–61.
[23] Escorsell A, Gines A, Llach J, et al. Increasing intra-abdominal pressure increases pressure, volume, and wall tension in esophageal varices. Hepatology 2002;36:936–40.
[24] Rigau J, Bosch J, Bordas JM, et al. Endoscopic measurement of variceal pressure in cirrhosis: correlation with portal pressure and variceal hemorrhage. Gastroenterology 1989;96:873–80.
[25] Beppu K, Inokuchi K, Koyanagi N, et al. Prediction of variceal hemorrhage by esophageal endoscopy. Gastrointest Endosc 1981;27:213–8.
[26] Garcia-Tsao G, Sanyal AJ, Grace ND, et al, and the Practice Guidelines Committee of the Americal Association for the Study of Liver Diseases, the Practice Parameters Committee of the American College of Gastroenterology. Prevention and management of gastroesophageal varices and variceal hemorrhage in cirrhosis. Hepatology 2007;46:922–38.

[27] Konishi Y, Nakamura T, Kida H, et al. Catheter US probe EUS evaluation of gastric cardia and perigastric vascular structures to predict esophageal variceal recurrence. Gastrointest Endosc 2002;55:197–203.

[28] Eisen GM, Eliakim R, Zaman A. The accuracy of PillCam ESO capsule endoscopy versus conventional upper endoscopy for the diagnosis of esophageal varices: a prospective three-center pilot study. Endoscopy 2006;38:31–5.

[29] Lapalus MG, Dumortier J, Fumex F, et al. Esophageal capsule endoscopy versus esophagogastroduodenoscopy for evaluating portal hypertension: a prospective comparative study of performance and tolerance. Endoscopy 2006;38:36–41.

[30] Prediction of the first variceal hemorrhage in patients with cirrhosis of the liver and esophageal varices: a prospective multicenter study. The North Italian Endoscopic Club for the Study and Treatment of Esophageal Varices. N Engl J Med 1988;319:983–9.

[31] Smith JL, Graham DY. Variceal hemorrhage: a critical evaluation of survival analysis. Gastroenterology 1982;82:968–73.

[32] Sanyal AJ, Fontana R, Di Bisceglie AM. The prevalence and risk factors associated with esophageal varices in subjects with hepatitis C and advanced fibrosis. Gastrointest Endosc 2006;64:855–64.

[33] D'Amico G, Pagliaro L, Bosch J. Pharmacological treatment of portal hypertension: an evidence-based approach. Semin Liver Dis 1999;19:475–505.

[34] Feu F, Garcia-Pagan JC, Bosch J, et al. Relation between portal pressure response to pharmacotherapy and risk of recurrent variceal haemorrhage in patients with cirrhosis. Lancet 1995;346:1056–9.

[35] Groszmann RJ, Bosch J, Grace ND, et al. Hemodynamic events in a prospective randomized trial of propranolol versus placebo in the prevention of a first variceal hemorrhage. Gastroenterology 1990;99:1401–7.

[36] Albillos A, Lledo JL, Rossi I, et al. Continuous prazosin administration in cirrhotic patients: effects on portal hemodynamics and on liver and renal function. Gastroenterology 1995;109:1257–65.

[37] Schneider AW, Kalk JF, Klein CP. Effect of losartan, an angiotensin II receptor antagonist, on portal pressure in cirrhosis. Hepatology 1999;29:334–9.

[38] Gonzalez-Abraldes J, Albillos A, Banares R, et al. Randomized comparison of long-term losartan versus propranolol in lowering portal pressure in cirrhosis. Gastroenterology 2001; 121:382–8.

[39] Schepke M, Werner E, Biecker E, et al. Hemodynamic effects of the angiotensin II receptor antagonist irbesartan in patients with cirrhosis and portal hypertension. Gastroenterology 2001;121:389–95.

[40] Fiorucci S, Antonelli E, Morelli O, et al. NCX-1000, a NO-releasing derivative of ursodeoxycholic acid, selectively delivers NO to the liver and protects against development of portal hypertension. Proc Natl Acad Sci U S A 2001;98:8897–902.

[41] Paquet KJ. Prophylactic endoscopic sclerosing treatment of the esophageal wall in varices: a prospective controlled randomized trial. Endoscopy 1982;14:4–5.

[42] Piai G, Cipolletta L, Claar M, et al. Prophylactic sclerotherapy of high-risk esophageal varices: results of a multicentric prospective controlled trial. Hepatology 1988;8:1495–500.

[43] Witzel L, Wolbergs E, Merki H. Prophylactic endoscopic sclerotherapy of oesophageal varices: a prospective controlled study. Lancet 1985;1:773–5.

[44] Prophylactic sclerotherapy for esophageal varices in men with alcoholic liver disease: a randomized, single-blind, multicenter clinical trial. The Veterans Affairs Cooperative Variceal Sclerotherapy Group. N Engl J Med 1991;324:1779–84.

[45] Santangelo WC, Dueno MI, Estes BL, et al. Prophylactic sclerotherapy of large esophageal varices. N Engl J Med 1988;13:814–8.

[46] Fardy JM, Laupacis A. A meta-analysis of prophylactic endoscopic sclerotherapy for esophageal varices. Am J Gastroenterol 1994;89:1938–48.

[47] Lay CS, Tsai YT, Teg CY, et al. Endoscopic variceal ligation in prophylaxis of first variceal bleeding in cirrhotic patients with high-risk esophageal varices. Hepatology 1997;25: 1346–50.
[48] Lo GH, Lai KH, Cheng JS, et al. Prophylactic banding ligation of high-risk esophageal varices in patients with cirrhosis: a prospective, randomized trial. J Hepatol 1999;31:451–6.
[49] Sarin SK, Guptan RK, Jain AK, et al. A randomized controlled trial of endoscopic variceal band ligation for primary prophylaxis of variceal bleeding. Eur J Gastroenterol Hepatol 1996;8:337–42.
[50] De BK, Ghoshal UC, Das T, et al. Endoscopic variceal ligation for primary prophylaxis of oesophageal variceal bleed: preliminary report of a randomized controlled trial. J Gastroenterol Hepatol 1999;14:220–4.
[51] Imperiale TF, Chalasani N. A meta-analysis of endoscopic variceal ligation for primary prophylaxis of esophageal variceal bleeding. Hepatology 2001;33:802–7.
[52] Sarin SK, Lamba GS, Kumar M, et al. Comparison of endoscopic ligation and propranolol for the primary prevention of variceal bleeding. N Engl J Med 1999;340:988–93.
[53] Kravetz D, Bosch J, Arderiu M, et al. Hemodynamic effects of blood volume restitution following a hemorrhage in rats with portal hypertension due to cirrhosis of the liver: influence of the extent of portal-systemic shunting. Hepatology 1989;9:808–14.
[54] Kravetz D, Sikuler E, Groszmann RJ. Splanchnic and systemic hemodynamics in portal hypertensive rats during hemorrhage and blood volume restitution. Gastroenterology 1986; 90:1232–40.
[55] Youssef WI, Salazar F, Dasarathy S, et al. Role of fresh frozen plasma infusion in correction of coagulopathy of chronic liver disease: a dual phase study. Am J Gastroenterol 2003; 98:1391–4.
[56] Bosch J, Thabut D, Bendtsen F, et al. Recombinant factor VIIa for upper gastrointestinal bleeding in patients with cirrhosis: a randomized, double-blind trial. Gastroenterology 2004;127:1123–30.
[57] Bernard B, Cardanel JF, Valla. Prognostic significance of bacterial infection in bleeding cirrhotic patients: a prospective study. Gastroenterology 1995;108:1828–34.
[58] Goulis J, Armonis A, Patch D, et al. Bacterial infection is independently associated with failure to control bleeding in cirrhotic patients with gastrointestinal hemorrhage. Hepatology 1998;27:1207–12.
[59] Bernard B, Grange JD, Khac EN, et al. Antibiotic prophylaxis for the prevention of bacterial infections in cirrhotic patients with ascites: a meta-analysis. Digestion 1998; 59(Suppl 2):54–7.
[60] Reichen J. Liver function and pharmacological considerations in pathogenesis and treatment of portal hypertension. Hepatology 1990;11:1066–78.
[61] Escorsell A, Ruiz del Arbol L, Planas R, et al. Multicenter randomized controlled trial of terlipressin versus sclerotherapy in the treatment of acute variceal bleeding: the TEST study. Hepatology 2000;32:471–6.
[62] Bosch J, Kravetz D, Rodes J. Effects of somatostatin on hepatic and systemic hemodynamics in patients with cirrhosis of the liver: comparison with vasopressin. Gastroenterology 1981;80:518–25.
[63] Villanueva C, Ortiz J, Minana J, et al. Somatostatin treatment and risk stratification by continuous portal pressure monitoring during acute variceal bleeding. Gastroenterology 2001;121:110–7.
[64] Buonamico P, Sabba C, Garcia-Tsao G, et al. Octreotide blunts postprandial splanchnic hyperemia in cirrhotic patients: a double-blind randomized echo-Doppler study. Hepatology 1995;21:134–9.
[65] Abraldes JG, Bosch J. Somatostatin and analogues in portal hypertension. Hepatology 2002;35:1305–12.
[66] Jenkins SA, Baxter JN, Corbett W, et al. Efficacy of somatostatin and vasopressin in the control of acute variceal hemorrhage. Hepatology 1985;5:344–5.

[67] Cales P, Masliah C, Bernard B, et al. Early administration of vapreotide for variceal bleeding in patients with cirrhosis. N Engl J Med 2001;344:23–8.
[68] D'Amico G, Pietrosi G, Tarantino I, et al. Emergency sclerotherapy versus vasoactive drugs for variceal bleeding in cirrhosis: a Cochrane meta-analysis. Gastroenterology 2003;124:1277–91.
[69] Kahn D, Jones B, Bornman PC. Incidence and management of complications of injection sclerotherapy: a ten-year prospective evaluation. Surgery 1989;105:160–5.
[70] Laine L, Cook D. Endoscopic ligation compared with sclerotherapy for treatment of esophageal variceal bleeding: a meta-analysis. Ann Intern Med 1995;123:280–7.
[71] Banares R, Albillos A, Rincon D, et al. Endoscopic treatment versus endoscopic plus pharmacologic treatment for acute variceal bleeding: a meta-analysis. Hepatology 2002;35: 609–15.
[72] D'Amico G, Pagliaro L, Bosch J. The treatment of portal hypertension: a meta-analytic review. Hepatology 1995;22:332–54.
[73] de Franchis R. Updating consensus in portal hypertension: report of the Baveno III Consensus Workshop on definitions, methodology and therapeutic strategies in portal hypertension. J Hepatol 2000;33:846–52.
[74] D'Amico G, De Franchis R. Upper digestive bleeding in cirrhosis: post-therapeutic outcome and prognostic indicators. Hepatology 2003;38:599–612.
[75] Moitinho E, Escorsell A, Bandi JC, et al. Prognostic value of early measurements of portal pressure in acute variceal bleeding. Gastroenterology 1999;117:626–31.
[76] Cook D, Laine L. Indications, technique, and complications of balloon tamponade for variceal gastrointestinal bleeding. J Intensive Care Med 1992;7:212–8.
[77] Azoulay D, Castaing D, Majno P, et al. Salvage transjugular intrahepatic portosystemic shunt for uncontrolled variceal bleeding in patients with decompensated cirrhosis. J Hepatol 2001;35:590–7.
[78] Sanyal AJ, Freedman AM, Luketic VA, et al. Transjugular intrahepatic portosystemic shunts for patients with active variceal hemorrhage unresponsive to sclerotherapy. Gastroenterology 1996;111:138–46.
[79] Malinchoc M, Kamath PS, Gordon FD, et al. A model to predict poor survival in patients undergoing transjugular intrahepatic portosystemic shunts. Hepatology 2000;31:864–71.
[80] Graham DY, Smith JL. The course of patients after variceal hemorrhage. Gastroenterology 1981;80:800–9.
[81] de Franchis R, Primignani M. Why do varices bleed? Gastroenterol Clin North Am 1992; 21:85–101.
[82] McCormick PA, Jenkins SA, McIntyre N, et al. Why portal hypertensive varices bleed and bleed: a hypothesis. Gut 1995;36:100–3.
[83] de Dombal FT, Clarke JR, Clamp SE, et al. Prognostic factors in upper G.I. bleeding. Endoscopy 1986;18(Suppl 2):6–10.
[84] Lo GH, Lai KH, Cheng JS, et al. Endoscopic variceal ligation plus nadolol and sucralfate compared with ligation alone for the prevention of variceal rebleeding: a prospective, randomized trial. Hepatology 2000;32:461–5.
[85] Patch D, Sabin CA, Goulis J. A randomized, controlled trial of medical therapy versus endoscopic ligation for the prevention of variceal re-bleeding in patients with cirrhosis. Gastroenterology 2002;123:1013–9.
[86] Villanueva C, Minana J, Ortiz J, et al. Endoscopic ligation compared with combined treatment with nadolol and isosorbide mononitrate to prevent recurrent variceal bleeding. N Engl J Med 2001;345:647–55.
[87] Luca A, D'Amico G, La Galla R, et al. TIPS for prevention of recurrent bleeding in patients with cirrhosis: meta-analysis of randomized clinical trials. Radiology 1999;212:411–21.
[88] Meddi P, Merli M, Lionetti R, et al. Cost analysis for the prevention of variceal rebleeding: a comparison between transjugular intrahepatic portosystemic shunt and endoscopic sclerotherapy in a selected group of Italian cirrhotic patients. Hepatology 1999;29:1074–7.

[89] Kage M, Korula J, Harada A, et al. Effects of sodium tetradecyl sulfate endoscopic variceal sclerotherapy on the esophagus: a prospective clinical and histopathologic study. J Clin Gastroenterol 1987;9:635–43.
[90] Sarin SK, Sachdev G, Nanda R. Follow-up of patients after variceal eradication: a comparison of patients with cirrhosis, noncirrhotic portal fibrosis, and extrahepatic obstruction. Ann Surg 1986;204:78–82.
[91] Korula J, Ralls P. The effects of chronic endoscopic variceal sclerotherapy on portal pressure in cirrhotics. Gastroenterology 1991;101:800–5.
[92] Hashizume M, Kitano S, Yamago H. Endoscopic classification of gastric varices. Gastrointest Endosc 1990;36:276–80.
[93] Hosking SW, Johnson AG. Gastric varices: a proposed classification leading to management. Br J Surg 1988;75:195–6.
[94] Korula J, Chin K, Ko Y, et al. Demonstration of two distinct subsets of gastric varices: observations during a seven-year study of endoscopic sclerotherapy. Dig Dis Sci 1991;36: 303–9.
[95] Ryan BM, Stockbrugger RW, Ryan JM. A pathophysiologic, gastroenterologic, and radiologic approach to the management of gastric varices. Gastroenterology 2004;126: 1175–89.
[96] Sarin SK, Lahoti D, Saxena SP, et al. Prevalence, classification and natural history of gastric varices: a long-term follow-up study in 568 portal hypertension patients. Hepatology 1992;16:1343–9.
[97] Chang KY, Wu CS, Chen PC. Prospective, randomized trial of hypertonic glucose water and sodium tetradecyl sulfate for gastric variceal bleeding in patients with advanced liver cirrhosis. Endoscopy 1996;28:481–6.
[98] Ciuh KW, Changchien CS, Chuah SK. Endoscopic imjection sclerotherapy with 1.5% sotradecol for bleeding gastric varices. J Clin Gastroenterol 1997;24:161–4.
[99] Gimson AE, Westaby D, Williams R. Endoscopic sclerotherapy in the management of gastric variceal haemorrhage. J Hepatol 1991;13:274–8.
[100] Ogawa K, Ishikawa S, Naritaka Y, et al. Clinical evaluation of endoscopic injection sclerotherapy using n-butyl-2-cyanoacrylate for gastric variceal bleeding. J Gastroenterol Hepatol 1999;14:245–50.
[101] Oho K, Iwao T, Sumino M, et al. Ethanolamine oleate versus butyl cyanoacrylate for bleeding gastric varices: a nonrandomized study. Endoscopy 1995;27:349–54.
[102] Sarin SK. Long-term follow-up of gastric variceal sclerotherapy: an eleven-year experience. Gastrointest Endosc 1997;46:8–14.
[103] Trudeau W, Prindiville T. Endoscopic injection sclerosis in bleeding gastric varices. Gastrointest Endosc 1986;32:264–8.
[104] Shiha G, El-Sayed SS. Gastric variceal ligation: a new technique. Gastrointest Endosc 1999; 49:437–41.
[105] Takeuchi M, Nakai Y, Syu A. Endoscopic ligation of gastric varices. Lancet 1996;348:1038.
[106] Vitte RL, Eugene C, Fingerhut A. Fatal outcome following endoscopic fundal variceal ligation. Gastrointest Endosc 1996;43:82.
[107] Lo GH, Lai KH, Cheng JS, et al. A prospective, randomized trial of butyl cyanoacrylate injection versus band ligation in the management of bleeding gastric varices. Hepatology 2001;33:1060–4.
[108] Sarin SK, Jain AK, Jain M, et al. A randomized controlled trial of cyanoacrylate versus alcohol injection in patients with isolated fundic varices. Am J Gastroenterol 2002;97: 1010–5.
[109] Tan PC, Hou MC, Lin HC, et al. A randomized trial of endoscopic treatment of acute gastric variceal hemorrhage: N-butyl-2-cyanoacrylate injection versus band ligation. Hepatology 2006;43:690–7.
[110] Rengstorff DS, Binmoeller KF. A pilot study of 2-octyl cyanoacrylate injection for treatment of gastric fundal varices in humans. Gastrointest Endosc 2004;59:553–8.

[111] Boyer TD. Transjugular intrahepatic portosystemic shunt: current status. Gastroenterology 2003;124:1700–10.
[112] Chikamori F, Kuniyoshi N, Shibuya S. Eight years of experience with transjugular retrograde obliteration for gastric varices with gastrorenal shunts. Surgery 2001;129:414–20.
[113] Kanagawa H, Mima S, Kouyama H, et al. Treatment of gastric fundal varices by balloon-occluded retrograde transvenous obliteration. J Gastroenterol Hepatol 1996;11:51–8.
[114] Shiba M, Higuchi K, Nakamura K, et al. Efficacy and safety of balloon-occluded endoscopic injection sclerotherapy as a prophylactic treatment for high-risk gastric fundal varices: a prospective, randomized, comparative clinical trial. Gastrointest Endosc 2002; 56:522–8.
[115] Hosking SW, Smart HL, Johnson AG, et al. Anorectal varices, haemorrhoids, and portal hypertension. Lancet 1989;1:349–52.
[116] Weisner RH, LaRusso NF, Dozois RR. Peristomal varices after proctocolectomy in patients with primary sclerosing cholangitis. Gastroenterology 1986;90:316–22.
[117] Kinkhabwala M. Bleeding ileal varicosity demonstrated by transhepatic portography. Am J Roentgenol 1977;129:514–6.
[118] Barbish AW, Ehrinpreis MN. Successful endoscopic injection sclerotherapy of a bleeding duodenal varix. Am J Gastroenterol 1993;88:90–2.
[119] Bhasin DK, Sharma BC, Sriram PV, et al. Endoscopic management of bleeding ectopic varices with histoacryl. HPB Surg 1999;11:171–3.
[120] Jabbari M, Cherry R, Lough JO. Gastric antral vascular ectasia: the watermelon stomach. Gastroenterology 1984;87:1167–70.
[121] Toyota M, Hinoda Y, Nakagawa N. Gastric antral vascular ectasia causing severe anemia. J Gastroenterol 1996;31:710–3.
[122] Fisher NC. Gastric antral vascular ectasia and its relation with portal hypertension. Gut 2000;46:441–2.
[123] Spahr L, Villeneuve JP, Dufresne MP, et al. Gastric antral vascular ectasia in cirrhotic patients: absence of relation with portal hypertension. Gut 1999;44:739–42.
[124] Iwao T, Toyonaga A, Sumino M, et al. Portal hypertensive gastropathy in patients with cirrhosis. Gastroenterology 1992;102:2060–5.
[125] Primignani M, Carpinelli L, Preatoni P, et al. Natural history of portal hypertensive gastropathy in patients with liver cirrhosis. The New Italian Endoscopic Club for the study and treatment of esophageal varices (NIEC). Gastroenterology 2000;119:181–7.
[126] Perez-Ayuso RM, Pique JM, Bosch J, et al. Propranolol in prevention of recurrent bleeding from severe portal hypertensive gastropathy in cirrhosis. Lancet 1991;337:1431–4.
[127] Trevino HH, Brady CE 3rd, Schenker S. Portal hypertensive gastropathy. Dig Dis 1996; 14:258–70.
[128] Fleig W. Upper gastrointestinal hemorrhage from "downhill" esophageal varices. Dig Dis Sci 1982;27:23–7.

ELSEVIER
SAUNDERS

Med Clin N Am 92 (2008) 575–597

THE MEDICAL
CLINICS
OF NORTH AMERICA

# Mechanical Obstruction of the Small Bowel and Colon

Mitchell S. Cappell, MD, PhD*, Mihaela Batke, MD

*Division of Gastroenterology, Department of Medicine, William Beaumont Hospital, MOB 233, 3601 West Thirteen Mile Road, Royal Oak, MI 48073, USA*

A clinical review of mechanical intestinal obstruction is important and timely. First, it is a relatively common cause of hospitalization. It composes 15% of all emergency admissions for abdominal pain, constituting more than 300,000 hospitalizations per year in the United States [1,2]. It is an important cause of mortality, responsible for about 30,000 deaths per annum. It directly costs more than 3 billion dollars in medical care per annum in the United States [1]. Second, surgical therapy is occasionally inappropriately delayed because of misdiagnosis of total mechanical obstruction as partial mechanical obstruction or pseudo-obstruction, resulting in increased morbidity and mortality. Third, new diagnostic modalities, such as CT enteroclysis, and new minimally invasive therapies, such as endoscopic stents, have been recently introduced. Clinicians have to be familiar with the new therapeutic modalities for mechanical obstruction and the clinical manifestations and radiologic techniques for the diagnosis. This article reviews the pathophysiology, etiology, diagnosis, and therapy of small and large bowel mechanical obstruction, with attention to the role of the internist, intensivist, gastroenterologist, radiologist, and surgeon in the clinical management, including a focus on the newest therapies.

## Terminology

The definition and nosology of intestinal obstruction has been confusing, because of incomplete understanding of the pathophysiology and application of different meanings to the same term. For example, gallstone ileus is a misnomer, because it actually represents mechanical obstruction by an impacted gallstone, rather than a functional obstruction or ileus. The

* Corresponding author.
*E-mail address:* mscappell@yahoo.com (M.S. Cappell).


doi:10.1016/j.mcna.2008.01.003 **medical.theclinics.com**

following is a clear, generally accepted classification of intestinal obstruction based on physiologic and pathophysiologic principles. Intestinal transit is acutely impaired by mechanical obstruction or by functional obstruction (pseudo-obstruction) from attenuated or uncoordinated intestinal muscle contractions. Mechanical obstruction can arise from intrinsic lesions, such as colon cancer, that block the lumen; obturator lesions, such as gallstones, that become impacted in the lumen; or extrinsic lesions, such as hernias or adhesions, that indirectly block flow by compressing the lumen. Adynamic ileus constitutes an acute functional obstruction attributable to intestinal hypomotility. Acute colonic pseudo-obstruction (ACPO) is a form of ileus characterized by massive colonic dilatation [3].

Mechanical obstruction is classified as small bowel obstruction (SBO) versus large bowel obstruction (LBO), according to the level of the obstruction. SBO is generally caused by benign lesions, whereas LBO is often caused by cancer [4]. Mechanical obstruction is categorized as partial when gas or liquid stool can pass through the point of narrowing and as total when no substance can pass. Partial obstruction is further characterized as high grade or low grade according to the severity of the narrowing. Complete bowel obstruction requires surgery, whereas partial bowel obstruction is often managed conservatively.

## Pathophysiology

In simple obstruction the bowel is occluded at one point. Fluid and chyme accumulates proximal to intestinal obstruction because of impaired intestinal water and electrolyte absorption and enhanced intestinal secretion, which leads to volume depletion. Luminal stasis results in bacterial overgrowth and a marked increase in the concentration of anaerobic bacteria that in turn leads to bacterial fermentation and increased production of gas [5]. Bowel dilatation from accumulated liquid and gas induces local inflammation and neuroendocrine reflexes that initially increase enteric propulsive activity to attempt to overcome the obstruction [6]. Bowel motility then decreases as bowel muscle gradually fatigues. Bowel dilatation gradually compromises vascular perfusion because of increasing intraluminal pressure and intramural tension. Orthograde arterial flow is severely compromised when the intraluminal pressure reaches the diastolic pressure, and ceases when the intraluminal pressure reaches the systolic pressure. Venous obstruction causes increased intraluminal fluid transudation and intramural edema. Bowel mucosa is highly sensitive to ischemia because of its perfusion by end arteries and its high metabolic activity.

In closed-loop obstruction, a bowel segment is occluded at two points. Common forms of closed loops include an incarcerated hernia, in which a loop of bowel is compressed at both ends within a hernial sac, and volvulus, in which a loop of bowel is mechanically compressed at both ends of a twist [7]. If the ileocecal valve is competent, an LBO forms a closed loop—from one pathologic mechanical obstruction and one physiologic occlusion at the ileocecal valve. If the ileocecal valve is incompetent, LBO produces simple obstruction as the colon is decompressed by way of the small bowel. A closed loop of bowel rapidly dilates because of a lack of both a proximal and a distal outlet for accumulated gas and liquid. The mucosa consequently rapidly develops ischemia. Extrinsic compression that strangulates mesenteric vessels (eg, at a point of volvulus or at the neck of a hernial sack) exacerbates the ischemia and rapidly produces bowel necrosis and perforation [4].

In LBO, the mural tension increases in proportion with the colonic radius, according to Laplace's Law. The tension is therefore greatest in the cecum, where the colonic radius is greatest. The cecum is therefore most often the site of colonic ischemia or perforation when it is involved in a mechanical obstruction with a competent ileocecal valve.

## General principles

Differentiation between total mechanical obstruction versus partial obstruction or pseudo-obstruction is critical because the first is generally treated surgically, whereas the latter two entities are generally treated medically [8]. Differentiating between these entities, however, is often difficult, especially early in the course of an illness. Clinical differences between these entities are summarized in Table 1. The differential diagnosis of these entities is considered in detail in the article on colonic pseudo-obstruction and adynamic ileus by Batke and Cappell elsewhere in this issue. After differentiating total mechanical obstruction from these other entities, the diagnostic evaluation centers on determining the level of the obstruction, particularly distinguishing small intestinal versus colonic obstruction; determining the cause of the obstruction, particularly distinguishing malignant from nonmalignant obstruction; and determining the presence of complications, such as closed-loop obstruction, bowel necrosis, or perforation. The clinical presentation and course of mechanical obstruction are determined by all these factors along with the duration of the obstruction and the presence of comorbidities [9].

Because of the complexity of these clinical decisions, suspected mechanical obstruction is best handled by a team of specialists, with specialized expertise and experience, including an intensivist to treat metabolic and hemodynamic abnormalities, a surgeon to monitor the abdominal findings and treat the surgical complications, a gastroenterologist to assist in the diagnosis and to administer the medical and colonoscopic therapy for colonic pseudo-obstruction or volvulus, and a gastrointestinal radiologist for specialized imaging. Moreover, because of these complexities, patients are serially and closely monitored clinically and radiologically. Patients who have an uncertain diagnosis of total versus partial mechanical obstruction may prove to have partial obstruction by gradually improving clinically with

Table 1
Differentiation between mechanical and functional intestinal obstruction

| | Mechanical obstruction | Ileus | Acute colonic pseudo-obstruction | Chronic intestinal pseudo-obstruction |
|---|---|---|---|---|
| Impaired intestinal transit | Yes (secondary) | Yes (primary) | Yes (primary) | Yes (primary) |
| Obliterated lumen | Yes | No | No | No |
| Acute | Yes | Yes | Yes | No |
| Dilatation | Yes, proximal to the obstruction | ± | Yes, massive | Yes |
| Predominant involvement | Any bowel segment | Small bowel | Colon | Small bowel, colon |
| Air/fluid levels | Yes | No | ± | No |
| Digestive progression | Typically rapid | Gradual | Gradual | Chronic, intermittent |

conservative therapy. Contrariwise, patients initially misdiagnosed with partial obstruction or pseudo-obstruction may manifest obvious clinical or radiographic signs of mechanical obstruction as the disease progresses. The abdominal examination is followed serially to diagnose progressive mechanical obstruction and to identify supervening complications of intestinal necrosis or perforation.

## Small bowel obstruction

### *Etiology*

SBO accounts for about 300,000 or more hospitalizations annually in the United States [1]. Postoperative peritoneal adhesions account for 75% of SBO in adults [9,10]. The incidence of SBO from adhesions has increased during the last 30 years because of the increasing number of laparotomies [10]. Overall about 5% of abdominopelvic surgeries are complicated by SBO from postoperative adhesions, but the rate ranges widely, from 0.05% for cesarean section, to 1% for appendectomy [11], and to 10% for colorectal surgery [12–16]. The risk of SBO from adhesions peaks in the first few years after an index surgery, but SBO can still occur 30 years after an index surgery [12–15,17].

The relative frequency of SBO from hernias has decreased from 30% to 15% during the last 30 years because of increasing elective prophylactic herniorrhaphy [18–21]. External hernias much more commonly cause SBO than internal hernias [22,23]. Femoral, inguinal, midventral, periumbilical, and incisional hernias are all classified as external. Congenital internal hernias include obturator hernias that occur through the pelvic obturator canal, and paraduodenal, transmesenteric, and transomental hernias [24]. Acquired internal hernias develop from mesenteric defects or other foramina created during prior surgery. Neoplasms account for 5% to 10% of SBO, but make up half of the cases without prior laparotomy and without clinical evidence of an incarcerated hernia [25]. Neoplastic SBO most commonly arises from extrinsic bowel compression by advanced gastrointestinal or gynecologic cancers, particularly colon or ovarian cancer [26,27], and most uncommonly arises from primary small bowel cancer [22]. Infrequent causes of SBO include strictures caused by Crohn disease, drugs, such as nonsteroidal anti-inflammatory medications (NSAIDs) or enteric-coated potassium chloride tablets, radiation enteritis, and ischemia; obturator obstruction from gallstone ileus, phytobezoars, and foreign bodies; intussusception; and infections, such as peritoneal tuberculosis, actinomycosis, and enteric parasites. In children, intussusception, intestinal atresia, and meconium ileus are common causes of SBO [22].

*Clinical presentation*

The clinical presentation varies depending on the severity, duration, and type of obstruction. The clinical presentation, described herein, emphasizes the more severe form, which manifests the most characteristic findings. Less severe forms present with less characteristic findings. The classical clinical tetrad is colicky abdominal pain, nausea and emesis, abdominal distention, and progressive obstipation. The pain is relatively sudden in onset, sharp, and periumbilical. The pain may progressively diminish because of bowel fatigue. Emesis may temporarily ameliorate the pain by deflating distended bowel. The pain becomes more intense and unremitting if intestinal ischemia or perforation occurs. Closed-loop obstruction often presents with pain out of proportion to the abdominal signs because of concurrent mesenteric ischemia. Proximal intestinal obstruction typically produces epigastric pain that occurs every 3 to 4 minutes, with frequent bilious emesis. Distal intestinal obstruction typically produces periumbilical pain that occurs every 15 to 20 minutes, with infrequent feculent emesis.

The medical history should include prior episodes of SBO, abdominal surgery, abdominal cancer, or abdominopelvic radiation; symptoms of external hernias; and history of inflammatory bowel disease or pelvic inflammatory disease. The last menstrual period should be noted in women. Failure to pass flatus may signal transition from partial to complete SBO [4]. The development of rigors, high fever, or systemic toxicity suggests that the obstruction may be complicated by intestinal necrosis or perforation. Intussusception typically presents in infants with episodic abdominal pain, currant jelly stools, and bilious vomiting [28].

Physical examination typically reveals an acutely ill, restless, and febrile patient. Signs of intravascular volume depletion include tachycardia, orthostatic hypotension, dry mucous membranes, and poor skin turgor. Jaundice suggests possible gallstone ileus or malignant obstruction. Malignant obstruction is also suggested by hepatomegaly, splenomegaly, a palpable abdominal mass, or periumbilical (Sister Mary Joseph node), inguinal, and right supraclavicular (Virchow node) lymphadenopathy. The abdomen is variably distended, ranging from moderate with proximal obstruction to severe with distal obstruction. Inspection occasionally reveals visible peristalsis. Air-filled bowel loops produce abdominal tympany. Palpation reveals mild generalized abdominal tenderness. Peritoneal signs, such as rebound tenderness and guarding, are typically absent, unless bowel necrosis or perforation supervenes. Bowel sounds are initially high-pitched (tinkling) and hyperactive, with audible rushes or borborygmi corresponding to paroxysms of abdominal pain, but become progressively hypoactive and softer, and then disappear because of bowel fatigue. Abdominal scars and external incarcerated femoral, inguinal, umbilical, or incisional hernias should be identified. Rectal examination is mandatory to exclude obstruction from fecal impaction or a rectal mass. Digital examination of the stoma should be performed in patients who have a colostomy or ileostomy. Urgent surgical consultation is indicated for suspected intestinal obstruction.

### *Diagnosis*

Laboratory tests are generally nonspecific. Patients may have electrolyte imbalances and azotemia because of third-spacing of fluids. A serum bicarbonate level, arterial blood pH, and lactic acid level assist in the diagnosis of intestinal ischemia. Marked leukocytosis, neutrophilia, and hyperamylasemia also suggest possible intestinal ischemia, but no laboratory test reliably detects intestinal ischemia. A coagulation profile, including prothrombin time (with international normalized ratio), partial thromboplastin time, and platelet count, should be determined because of the potential need for surgery. Women of childbearing age should be screened for pregnancy with a β-HCG (human chorionic gonadotrophin) test. Patients who have ascites should undergo diagnostic paracentesis with fluid analysis for erythrocyte count, leukocyte count, and leukocyte differential; for Gram stain and bacterial cultures; and for glucose, total protein, and albumin levels. A simultaneous serum albumin is needed to determine the serum-to-ascites albumin gradient.

Radiologic studies are essential for the diagnosis because the clinical presentation is nonspecific. A plain abdominal roentgenogram in the supine and upright position is diagnostic in 50% to 70% of cases [29]. The radiologic diagnosis requires a dilated, gas-filled, proximal bowel and a collapsed, gasless, distal bowel. A transition zone between dilated and nondilated bowel is a highly specific, but insensitive, sign of SBO. Small bowel loops greater than 3 cm in diameter are considered dilated. Abdominal roentgenograms can be normal in patients who have complete, closed-loop, or strangulated obstructions [30]. A closed-loop obstruction may produce a gasless abdomen because the obstructed loops are fluid-filled [29,30]. The diagnostic accuracy improves with the radiologist's experience [31]. In one study, plain abdominal roentgenograms were correctly diagnosed by 60% of radiology residents compared with 90% of attending radiologists [32]. Ascites produces a hazy, ground-glass appearance in the central abdomen. SBO is differentiated from ACPO by an absence of rectal air. Pneumoperitoneum indicates bowel perforation.

Differentiation between large bowel and small bowel obstruction on the basis of plain abdominal roentgenograms may be problematic. Air-filled loops of small bowel are distinguished from those of large bowel by their more central abdominal location, by their narrower caliber even when dilated, and by the presence of valvulae conniventes that extend across the entire luminal diameter as opposed to the colonic haustral folds that extend only partially across the luminal diameter. When SBO is clinically suspected and the abdominal roentgenogram is inconclusive, a small bowel follow-through (SBFT), enteroclysis, abdominal CT, ultrasound, or fast MRI should be performed.

Abdominal ultrasound is as sensitive and is more specific than a plain abdominal roentgenogram, but is infrequently used for suspected SBO because other tests are more accurate [33,34]. It is used in critically ill patients because it can be performed at the bedside without administration of intravenous contrast. Abdominal ultrasound is useful to differentiate mechanical obstruction from postoperative ileus [35]. It is particularly helpful when the plain abdominal roentgenogram is unrevealing, the obstruction is proximal, or an incarcerated femoral hernia is clinically suspected. A high resistive index and a decrease in the end-diastolic velocity of the superior mesenteric artery by pulse Doppler ultrasonography suggest strangulation [36].

SBFT is widely used in patients treated conservatively. It changes the diagnosis in about half of cases [37]. In a recent meta-analysis, passage of a water-soluble contrast agent into the colon on SBFT predicted resolution of the obstruction with a sensitivity of 97% and specificity of 96%; the SBFT did not reduce the need for surgery, but did reduce the length of hospitalization in nonsurgical patients by a mean of 1.8 days [38]. The major disadvantages of SBFT are the long duration of the test and the inadequate resolution of mucosal details because of dilution of ingested contrast in the fluid-filled, dilated bowel. In enteroclysis, contrast is injected directly into the jejunum by way of a nasoenteral tube to achieve a higher intraluminal concentration of contrast and better resolution of mucosal details. Although it is more accurate than SBFT, with a 100% sensitivity and 88% specificity in diagnosing SBO, it has disadvantages of requiring a radiologist who has special expertise in this technique, and requiring nasoenteral intubation [39].

Abdominal ultrasound, SBFT, and enteroclysis are being superceded by CT for more rapid and more accurate diagnosis. Nonvisualization of oral contrast in the colon on CT 12 hours after administration is a reliable indicator of complete obstruction, whereas visualization of oral contrast in the colon indicates incomplete SBO. In a meta-analysis conventional CT had a sensitivity of 92% (range 81%–100%) and specificity of 93% (range 68%–100%) in detecting complete obstruction [40]. Intravenous contrast helps in diagnosing strangulation, in identifying the specific cause of an

SBO, and in characterizing other pathology, such as superior mesenteric artery or superior mesenteric vein thrombosis, which can produce an ileus that mimics mechanical obstruction [29].

Closed-loop SBO should be diagnosed promptly to facilitate early surgery to prevent bowel strangulation. CT is only about 60% sensitive in identifying this complication. CT signs of a closed loop include: (1) radial distribution of the incarcerated bowel (like the rim of a bicycle wheel), with mesenteric vessels converging toward a central point of torsion (like the spokes of a bicycle wheel); (2) a coffee bean C or V loop; (3) two adjacent collapsed, round, oval, or triangular loops in an arrowhead configuration; (4) the beak sign; and (5) the whirl sign [41].

The CT signs of strangulation, like those of intestinal ischemia, include: a thickened bowel wall because of bowel wall edema, inflammation, or intramural hemorrhage; mural thumbprinting from intramural hemorrhage or edema; pneumatosis intestinalis from intramural gas produced by bacteria; absence of enhancement with intravenous contrast because of vascular hypoperfusion; hazy or streaky mesentery or "dirty" fat from inflammatory infiltration; portal venous gas; target sign; and ascites [29]. A serrated beak sign is occasionally present. In a meta-analysis, CT had a sensitivity of 83% (range 63%–100%) and specificity of 92% (range 61%–100%) in detecting intestinal ischemia [40]. Characteristic CT findings of gallstone ileus include pneumobilia, because of a choledochointestinal fistula created during gallstone passage, together with radiographic signs of intestinal obstruction [42]. The obstructing gallstone is sometimes visualized.

CT enteroclysis or multidetector helical CT enteroclysis is more accurate than conventional CT in defining the cause of SBO (89% versus 50%) and the site of SBO (100% versus 94%), but are currently available only at tertiary centers [43,44]. These tests are particularly valuable in patients managed conservatively. The nasoenteral tube can be left in the small bowel for intestinal decompression after CT enteroclysis.

Conventional or fast MRI with T2-weighted images is more accurate than contrast-enhanced helical CT in localizing the point of obstruction (96% versus 93%) and in determining the cause (88% versus 57%) [45,46]. Magnetic resonance enteroclysis is a promising, emerging technique that needs further evaluation before becoming a standard test [47]. Double-balloon enteroscopy has been studied in incomplete SBO in selected patients, with encouraging results [48], but is currently experimental and reserved for tertiary care centers. It is generally contraindicated when the SBO is complete. Videocapsule endoscopy is not used to evaluate suspected SBO because of the risk of videocapsule impaction at the site of obstruction that would require surgery.

### *Treatment*

Supportive treatment is initiated early, with aggressive intravenous rehydration, antiemetics, and bowel rest. Patients who have borderline blood pressure should have a central venous catheter to guide fluid replacement, whereas patients who have congestive heart failure or renal failure may require a Swan-Ganz catheter to guide fluid replacement. Nasogastric decompression may be diagnostically useful to sample gastric contents, and may be therapeutically useful to clear gastric contents to prevent aspiration pneumonia and to decompress the proximal bowel. A feculent gastric aspirate is characteristic of distal SBO. Long enteral tubes are infrequently used because of difficulty in placement, patient discomfort, and their tendency to become kinked [49]. A Foley catheter is inserted to continuously monitor urine output; urine output less than 0.5 mL/kg/h suggests dehydration and inadequate fluid resuscitation.

About 90% of partial SBOs resolve spontaneously with conservative therapy [50]. Patients who have acute obstruction from inflammatory Crohn disease often clinically resolve with conservative management [51]. SBO from impacted food, bezoars, foreign bodies, or gallstones may be treated endoscopically when the obstructing object is accessible by push enteroscopy [52]. Mechanical obstruction less than 30 days after surgery is usually caused by adhesions and is usually managed nonoperatively because early postoperative adhesions tend to be thin and to spontaneously dissolve [53].

Complete obstruction, peritonitis, pneumatosis intestinalis, or strangulation mandate emergency surgery. A chronic fibrotic stricture from Crohn disease often requires limited segmental resection or stricturoplasty. If an SBO does not resolve after 24 to 48 hours of conservative management, it is likely total rather than partial and laparotomy is indicated. Delaying surgery more than 24 hours after the onset of symptoms in patients who have strangulation increases the mortality by threefold [10,54]. Do not let the sun set on an SBO. Preoperative antibiotic therapy should provide broad coverage for anaerobic and Gram-negative bacteria. A diagnostic and therapeutic algorithm for SBO is presented in Fig. 1.

Intraoperative evaluation of bowel viability, although difficult, is essential. Retention of poorly viable bowel can lead to a postoperative anastomotic leak, intra-abdominal abscess, or chronic stricture, whereas removing truly viable bowel can increase operative mortality and increase postoperative morbidity from the short bowel syndrome. Bowel viability is conventionally determined at surgery by inspection of bowel color, observation of intestinal contractions, and palpation of local mesenteric pulses. A fluorescein dye study helps assess bowel viability: bowel with patchy or no dye uptake is likely nonviable and should be resected [55]. Doppler flowmetry helps assess vascular flow after relief of mechanical compression of blood vessels (eg, after reducing a strangulated hernia or detorting a volvulus). At surgery all definitely necrotic and likely necrotic bowel is resected. If questionably viable bowel is retained, a second-look laparotomy may be performed 24 hours after the initial laparotomy to reassess bowel viability [51].

Most patients undergo conventional open laparotomy, including patients who have distal obstruction, advanced or complete obstruction, matted

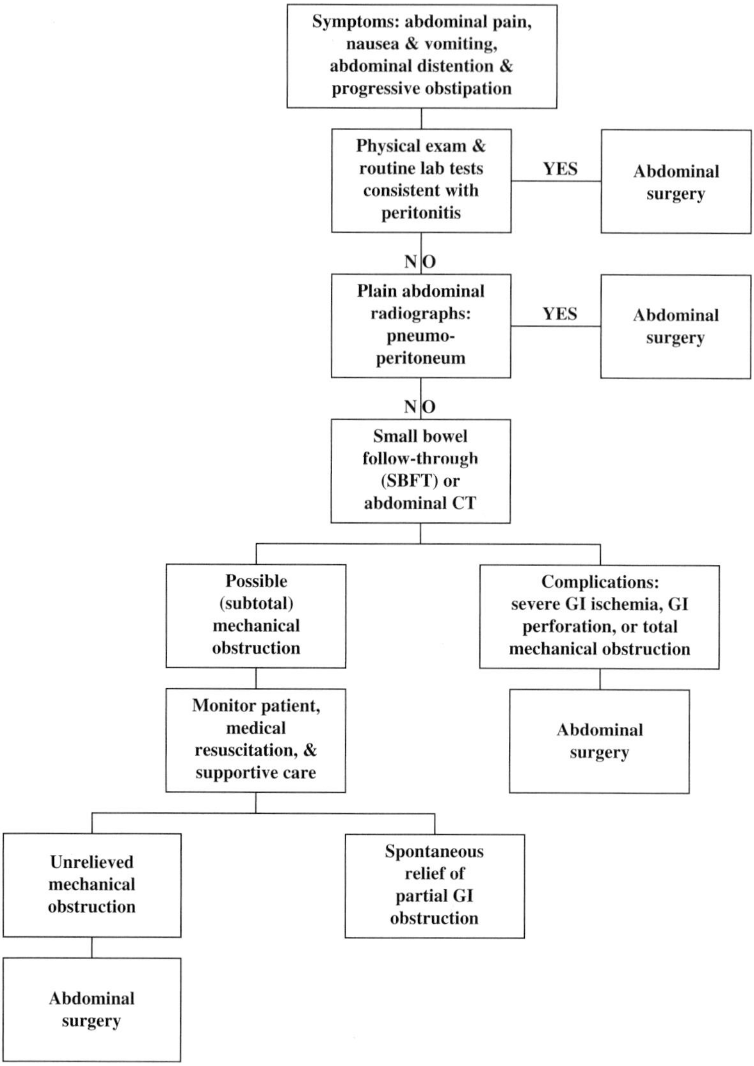


Fig. 1. Management algorithm for a patient with possible or suspected small bowel obstruction. The diagnostic evaluation, as shown on the left, is urgently interrupted at any time if the complications of severe gastrointestinal ischemia/necrosis or gastrointestinal perforation supervene. If an (incomplete) mechanical obstruction is not relieved by medical management, with supportive care and medical resuscitation, within about 24 hours of clinical presentation, the patient is strongly considered for emergency surgery to relieve the mechanical obstruction. (CT, computerized tomography; GI, gastrointestinal.)

adhesions, carcinomatosis, and persistent significant abdominal distention despite nasogastric decompression. Less invasive surgery is occasionally feasible, such as an inguinal incision for inguinal hernias. Patients who have external hernias that can be reduced preoperatively can then undergo elective herniorrhaphy. Laparoscopic abdominal exploration is feasible in selected patients, such as patients who have proximal obstruction, partial obstruction, anticipated single-band adhesion, and mild abdominal distention. Laparoscopy results in a shorter hospitalization [56]. Intra-abdominal malignancy, Crohn disease, complicated SBO, and more than one prior episode of SBO from adhesions are relative contraindications to laparoscopy.

SBO therapy in patients who have prior cancer is challenging. Prior abdominal malignancy should not deter aggressive surgery for SBO. In a retrospective review, one third of patients who had prior intra-abdominal malignancy had a benign and potentially curable cause for SBO [57]. Even in patients who have obstruction from recurrent malignancy, surgical intervention improves the in-hospital mortality and the quality of life after discharge [27,58]. Symptoms of SBO in patients who have terminal cancer are palliated with octreotide, hyoscine, or corticosteroids [59,60]. In a comparative study, both octreotide (a somatostatin analog) and palliative surgery controlled the symptoms of SBO in patients who had terminal cancer, but survival was significantly longer after surgery [61]. Octreotide was more effective than hyoscine in reducing nausea and vomiting in a study of 18 patients [62]. Intravenous corticosteroids can resolve SBO in patients who have terminal cancer, but do not improve survival [63].

### *Complications/prognosis*

Strangulation occurs in 30% of SBOs and bowel necrosis in 15% of cases [10,20]. Strangulation usually arises in closed-loop obstruction, usually from hernias [29]. Strangulation is definitively diagnosed at surgery. Postoperative morbidity and mortality from SBO is 23% and 5%, respectively [10]. Risk factors for mortality include old age, comorbidity, nonviable strangulated bowel, and delayed surgery [10]. For example, mortality increases from 4% in uncomplicated SBO to 16% in strangulated bowel.

### *Recurrence/prophylaxis*

SBO recurs after an index surgery for adhesions in about 15% of cases within 5 years [21,64,65], but the risk for recurrence extends up to 30 years after an index surgery [65]. The number of prior episodes of SBO is the strongest predictor of recurrence [66]. After a second episode the risk of recurrence increases to 85%. Recurrence occurs sooner and more frequently when an SBO is managed nonoperatively [66]. Young patients are at greater risk for recurrent SBO [64], as are patients who have matted (dense and multiple) bowel adhesions as compared with patients who have a single adhesive band [19].

Given the frequency, morbidity, and costs of SBO, strategies to prevent bowel adhesions are important [13]. Prudent surgical technique includes gentle handling of abdominal tissue, avoidance of irritating materials, careful hemostasis, avoidance of bowel ischemia or tissue desiccation, and early surgery before sepsis occurs. Although numerous agents decrease adhesion formation in animals, evidence of efficacy in humans is mostly inconclusive, and many agents have unacceptable side effects, such as an increased risk for peritonitis with high molecular weight dextran solutions [67]. Barrier methods, including sodium hyaluronate–based or cellulose-based bioresorbable membranes, significantly decrease the frequency of adhesions [68–70] and may reduce the rate of SBO [69]. Laparoscopic surgery seems to decrease the rate of adhesions and the risk of SBO [71]. For example, only 6 (2%) of 306 patients undergoing laparoscopic colorectal surgery had obstruction from adhesions during a mean follow-up of 38 months [72].

### *Summary*

The most common causes of SBO are adhesions and incarcerated hernias, with a relative increase in the incidence of adhesions during the last few decades. Complications include bowel ischemia and perforation, the incidence of which is higher in closed-loop obstruction. SBO is diagnosed by clinical examination and radiographic studies. Patients appear acutely ill, complaining of colicky abdominal pain, emesis, abdominal distention, and progressive obstipation. The plain abdominal roentgenogram usually provides useful, but limited, information. Although SBFT is still widely used, its diagnostic role is being superceded by abdominal CT. The initial treatment is supportive, with intravenous fluid resuscitation, correction of electrolyte disorders, bowel rest, and nasogastric decompression. If an SBO is complete or if intestinal ischemia or peritonitis is evident, the patient should be administered antibiotics and undergo emergency surgery. If an SBO is partial, conservative management is maintained for 24 to 48 hours. If the patient does not improve with conservative management or develops signs of peritonitis, laparotomy is indicated. The mortality from SBO has recently decreased to 5%. The recurrence rate of SBO from adhesions is high, ranging from 15% to 50% at 10 years.

## Large bowel obstruction

### *Etiology*

About 60% of LBOs are attributable to neoplasms, mostly colon cancer. About 10% of colon cancers present with LBO [73]. The descending colon and rectosigmoid are the most common sites of malignant obstruction because of the narrow colonic lumen in these segments [73]. Colonic volvulus causes another 10% to 15% of LBO [74]. It arises from axial torsion of the colon around its mesentery. Volvulus occurs in the sigmoid colon in 76% of cases and in the cecum in 22% of cases [75]. Cecal bascule is an uncommon variant of cecal volvulus in which the cecum folds in an anterior and medial direction, without a twist [76]. Strictures from chronic diverticular disease cause about 10% of LBO. Acute diverticulitis can also cause colonic obstruction from external compression by a pericolonic abscess and colonic spasm. Uncommon causes of LBO include Crohn disease, intussusception, extrinsic tumors, and fecal impaction. Rare causes include infections, such as actinomycosis, *Taenia saginata*, botulism, or *Salmonella* enterocolitis; vasculitides, such as Churg-Strauss disease; eosinophilic gastroenteritis; colonic hemangioma; endometriosis; and migrated duodenal stent.

Patients who have cecal volvulus are younger than patients who have sigmoid volvulus, suggesting that cecal volvulus may be attributable to a congenitally abnormally lax attachment of the right colon to the abdominal wall, whereas sigmoid volvulus is attributable to an acquired mesenteric laxity. Risk factors for acquiring sigmoid volvulus include a high-fiber diet, which is more common in developing countries, African American heritage, institutionalization, previous abdominal surgery, laxative abuse, pregnancy, Chagas disease, Parkinsonism, and Hirschsprung disease [77].

### *Clinical presentation*

Colonic obstruction presents with abdominal pain, abdominal distention, and progressive obstipation [77]. Emesis is less prominent and occurs later with LBO than with SBO. The clinical presentation varies with the cause. Volvulus presents acutely, with sudden onset of marked abdominal distention, whereas obstructing carcinomas present subacutely, with gradual development of symptoms.

Physical examination reveals an acutely ill patient. Pyrexia suggests possible complications of sepsis, ischemia, or perforation. Signs of dehydration include tachycardia, orthostatic hypotension, and dry mucous membranes. The abdomen is distended with abdominal tympany. Bowel sounds are usually present and hyperactive initially, but become progressively hypoactive. The bowel may be diffusely tender, but localized direct tenderness, guarding, or rebound tenderness suggest peritonitis. A mass is occasionally palpable on abdominal or rectal examination. Ascites and hepatomegaly in a patient who had prior malignancy suggests metastases. As for SBO, the laboratory tests are nonspecific. The blood tests are obtained as for SBO, and blood test abnormalities have the same clinical significance as for SBO.

### *Complications*

Complications include bowel ischemia and peritonitis. Colonic perforation can occur from massive colonic distention in the presence of a competent ileocecal valve or from tumor penetration through the serosa with subsequent necrosis.

### *Diagnosis*

The diagnosis is frequently evident on the plain abdominal roentgenogram. In a review of 140 cases of suspected LBO, the plain abdominal roentgenogram had 84% sensitivity and 72% specificity in diagnosing LBO [78]. About one third of patients diagnosed with LBO on clinical examination and plain abdominal roentgenograms have ACPO, however, whereas about one fifth of patients diagnosed with ACPO have LBO [74]. Patients usually require additional radiologic imaging. A water-soluble contrast enema has 96% sensitivity and 98% specificity in diagnosing LBO [78]. Multidetector abdominopelvic CT has a sensitivity and specificity of about 90% in the diagnosis [79]. Turning the patient during the CT to the decubitus or prone position improves diagnostic accuracy by shifting of colonic air. Administration of intravenous contrast provides additional information regarding associated intra-abdominal pathology [79,80]. Other imaging tests include ultrasonography or MRI. Flexible sigmoidoscopy can be a useful diagnostic (and therapeutic) tool.

In sigmoid volvulus the most sensitive and specific radiologic signs are: finding the apex of the loop under the left hemidiaphragm, inferior convergence on the left abdomen, and the left flank overlap sign [81]. In half the cases of cecal volvulus, the cecum is located in the left upper quadrant [74]. Other radiologic signs include the bent inner tube sign or the whirl pattern for sigmoid volvulus, and the coffee bean sign for cecal volvulus.

## *Treatment*

### *Supportive measures*

LBO is an abdominal emergency with high morbidity and significant mortality. The initial treatment is supportive, with aggressive administration of intravenous fluid and correction of electrolyte derangements. A central venous line is necessary if fluid overload is a concern. An indwelling Foley catheter can monitor urinary output. A nasogastric tube may help suppress nausea and emesis by gastric decompression, but has limited efficacy in deflating a dilated colon. A rectal tube can decompress the very distal colon, but has minimal efficacy in deflating the proximal colon.

Laparotomy is required for suspected perforation or ischemia, and for a lack of clinical improvement or increasing cecal diameter with conservative therapy [77]. Perioperative management includes administration of antibiotics with coverage for Gram-negative and anaerobic bacteria, prophylaxis for deep vein thrombosis, and stomal marking. The surgical technique depends on the cause and site of the LBO, the viability of the colon, comorbidities, and the technical skill of the surgeon (Table 2).

### *Malignant obstruction*

Right-sided colon cancer generally requires emergency right hemicolectomy. A primary anastomosis can be performed in relatively stable patients with a less than 10% risk for anastomotic leakage [82]. Highly unstable patients—those who have colonic perforation, severely distended bowel, or generalized peritonitis—undergo emergent ileostomy with an elective

Table 2
Treatment of the common causes of large bowel obstruction

| Causes of LBO | Preferred treatment |
|---|---|
| CRC | |
| Right-sided obstruction | • Right colectomy with primary anastomosis<br>• Right colectomy with Hartmann procedure if perforation or gangrene present |
| Left-sided obstruction | • Intraoperative lavage followed by resection with primary anastomosis<br>• Intraoperative lavage followed by resection with Hartmann procedure if perforation or gangrene present<br>• Subtotal colectomy with primary anastomosis or without primary anastomosis if synchronous cancer or cecal perforation is present<br>• Proximal stoma if patient is unstable or surgical team is inexperienced, with subsequent staged resection |
| Disseminated primary CRC | • Resection, or limited palliation |
| Recurrent CRC | • Bypass or proximal stoma<br>• Colonoscopic stenting or laser therapy |
| Colonic volvulus | |
| Sigmoid | • Preoperative decompressive sigmoidoscopy, and resection and primary anastomosis<br>• Preoperative decompression, resection and Hartmann procedure if perforation or gangrene present |
| Cecal | • Resection with primary anastomosis<br>• Resection with end-ileostomy and exteriorization of the proximal colon if perforation or gangrene is present |
| Diverticular disease | |
| Abscess | • Percutaneous drainage, antibiotics, resection with primary anastomosis<br>• Percutaneous drainage, antibiotics, resection with Hartmann procedure if perforation or gangrene present |
| Fibrous stricture | • Intraoperative lavage, resection and primary anastomosis |
| Crohn fibrous stricture | • Stricturoplasty or segmental resection |
| Radiation-induced stricture | • Preoperative colonoscopy<br>• Colostomy or segmental colectomy and primary anastomosis if the entire injured segment can be excised |
| Fecal impaction | • Manual disimpaction via rectal exam and enemas<br>• Prevent recurrence by adequate dietary oral intake, ambulation, gentle laxatives and stool softeners |
| Single colonic adhesions without colonic ischemia | • Adhesiolysis |
| Pseudo-obstruction | • Colonoscopic decompression<br>• Blow-hole colostomy if nonoperative management fails<br>• Resection with end-ileostomy and exteriorization of the proximal colon if perforation or gangrene is present |

*Abbreviation:* CRC, colorectal cancer.

reanastomosis performed several months later. The operative technique for LBO from left-sided colon cancer is controversial. Many surgeons advocate a single-stage resection and primary anastomosis, with or without intraoperative lavage [83]. This surgery entails a risk for anastomotic leakage of at least 5% [84]. Subtotal colectomy with primary anastomosis is often performed when a synchronous right-sided cancer is present or when the colon is ischemic. The Hartmann procedure remains a popular alternative for patients in poor medical condition or those who have colonic perforation or necrosis. The stoma is never reversed in 40% of patients undergoing this procedure for malignant left-sided obstruction [85].

When surgery is performed on an unprepared colon, a primary end-to-end anastomosis is generally avoided because of an increased risk for anastomotic leakage and infection. Mortality of emergency surgery for acute malignant colonic obstruction is as high as 20%, but the mortality decreases to 1% to 6% when the surgery is elective. Likewise, the mortality is only about 10% when the bowel is viable, but increases to about 30% with bowel infarction [86].

Colonoscopic deployment of self-expandable metallic stents is used to palliate obstruction from advanced colon cancer or for emergency decompression that can convert the required surgery from an emergency two-step procedure, involving a temporary colostomy on an unprepped colon, into a one-step elective procedure, with a primary anastomosis on a prepped colon [87]. Stent placement also permits preoperative colonoscopy in patients who have resectable cancer. In a prospective Italian study, preoperative colonoscopy made possible by stent deployment detected a synchronous cancer in 10% of patients, a finding that changed the planned surgery [88]. Stenting is technically successful in 76% to 96% of patients, usually resulting in rapid resolution of symptoms [73,89–95]. Stents can function for 6 months or longer in the colon in 75% of cases. Major complications include colonic perforation or enteric fistulae in about 5% to 10% of cases [73,90], and recurrent obstruction from stent migration or from cancer growth into the stent in about 17% of cases [91–95]. A coaxial stent can be deployed by repeat colonoscopy if the stent occludes and the obstruction recurs [96].

When used as a bridge to elective surgery, the mean interval between stent placement and surgery was 7 days, with a range of 2 to 20 days [90,97]. Although perioperative morbidity and mortality is improved by bridging with colonic stents, long-term survival is similar for patients who have stents followed by subsequent resection versus patients who undergo emergency bowel resection [89]. Median survival after palliative stent placement varies from 6 weeks to 12 months [92,93,97]. Colonoscopic decompression can also be achieved by way of a through-the-scope balloon dilator [98], a long tube passed over a colonoscopically placed guidewire [99], or colonoscopic laser ablation of the tumor [100–103]. These techniques are used to palliate symptoms in patients who have widespread metastases or who are poor surgical candidates because of underlying comorbidities. Laser therapy entails a 3.5% risk of colonic perforation [100,102].

*Volvulus therapy*

Flexible sigmoidoscopy successfully detorts and decompresses sigmoid volvulus in about 75% of cases [104]. Contraindications to sigmoidoscopy include clinical findings of sepsis, such as high fever, marked leukocytosis, bacteremia, or rebound tenderness. Likewise, the sigmoidoscopy should be aborted if gangrenous bowel is encountered. At sigmoidoscopy the torsion appears as a spiral narrowing with proximal dilatation. After successful sigmoidoscopic decompression, definitive elective surgical therapy is strongly considered because of the approximately 60% risk of volvulus recurrence with sigmoidoscopic decompression alone [77]. If sigmoidoscopy is unsuccessful, the patient requires urgent surgery. At surgery, if the sigmoid is viable, surgical detorsion is combined with colopexy to prevent recurrent volvulus. If the sigmoid is questionably viable or shows patchy ischemia, the sigmoid is resected. Sigmoid resection with a Hartmann procedure is recommended in the presence of colonic necrosis or perforation. Subtotal colectomy with ileorectal anastomosis may be required in the presence of a megacolon. Recurrent sigmoid volvulus can be prevented in debilitated patients, who are poor surgical candidates, by left-sided percutaneous sigmoidoscopic colostomy. Complications of this procedure include intra-abdominal sepsis, fecal leakage, and fecal peritonitis [105].

Nonoperative decompression is rarely successful for cecal volvulus. The surgical approach depends on colonic viability. Patients who have a viable colon usually undergo segmental resection with primary anastomosis, but can undergo detorsion with cecopexy or cecostomy [106]. These two latter alternatives have a lower operative mortality but a higher postoperative morbidity than resection with primary anastomosis. Patients who have compromised colonic viability undergo end-ileostomy and a proximal colostomy [107].

*Therapy for other causes*

In LBO from acute diverticulitis, the initial treatment is medical, directed at controlling the diverticulitis by intravenous antibiotics, bowel rest, and percutaneous drainage of any loculated collection. Surgical resection with primary anastomosis is performed after control of the acute diverticulitis. LBO from a benign stricture after multiple bouts of diverticulitis is generally treated by segmental colonic resection [77].

A chronic benign fibrotic stricture from Crohn colitis is treated by stricturoplasty or limited segmental resection. Preoperative colonoscopy, if feasible, is important to exclude a malignant stricture. Radiation proctitis can produce a stricture from chronic ischemia. Preoperative colonoscopy should be performed to determine the extent and severity of the radiation injury. A radiation-induced stricture usually requires a colostomy, but can be treated by segmental colectomy and primary anastomosis provided that the entire injured segment can be excised [77].

Complications of fecal impaction include distal LBO or stercoral ulcers. Fecal impaction is generally treated medically by digital disimpaction and enema instillation. Recurrence should be prevented by a regimen of an appropriate diet, including adequate oral fluid intake, ambulation, and medications to promote regular, soft stools. Colonic obstruction from simple adhesions is usually treated by adhesiolysis.

The overall in-hospital mortality of LBO is about 10%, but the rate varies according to the cause and the promptness of the surgery. Poor postoperative prognostic indicators include an American Society of Anesthesiologists score of III or IV, preoperative renal failure, peritonitis, and proximal colonic ischemia [83].

*Summary*

The most common cause of LBO is colorectal carcinoma, followed by colonic volvulus and diverticular disease. The clinical presentation is variable, but patients commonly present with abdominal distention, abdominal pain, progressive obstipation, and nausea and emesis. Pyrexia and marked leukocytosis suggest possible bowel ischemia or perforation. LBO is usually diagnosed by clinical presentation, plain abdominal roentgenogram, and specialized radiographic tests. LBO is an abdominal emergency associated with high morbidity and significant mortality. Initial therapy includes aggressive fluid replacement, correction of electrolyte abnormalities, and broad-spectrum antibiotics. Right-sided colon cancer is usually treated by a single-stage resection with primary anastomosis. The management of left-sided colon cancer is controversial, with commonly used alternatives of single-stage resection versus initial decompression with staged resection. Hartmann procedure is preferred in the presence of bowel ischemia or perforation. A primary anastomosis is avoided on an unprepped colon. Poor surgical candidates may undergo colonoscopic palliation by laser ablation, stenting, or balloon dilatation of the stricture. Sigmoid volvulus is initially treated with sigmoidoscopic decompression, followed by consideration of definitive elective surgery. Cecal volvulus is usually treated by segmental resection if nonviable colon is present, or by detorsion with cecopexy or cecostomy when the colon is viable.

## References

[1] Ray NF, Denton WG, Thamer M, et al. Abdominal adhesiolysis: inpatient care and expenditures in the United States in 1994. J Am Coll Surg 1998;186(1):1–9.

[2] Irvin TT. Abdominal pain: a surgical audit of 1190 emergency admissions. Br J Surg 1989; 76(11):1121–5.

[3] Soreide O, Bjerkeset T, Fossdal JE. Pseudo-obstruction of the colon (Ogilvie's syndrome), a genuine clinical condition? Review of the literature (1948–1975) and report of five cases. Dis Colon Rectum 1977;20(6):487–91.

[4] Helton WS, Fisichella PM. Intestinal obstruction. In: Wilmore DW, editor. ACS surgery: principles & practice 2007. New York: WebMD Corp.; 2007. Section 5, Chapter 4.
[5] Sykes PA, Boulter KH, Schofield PF. The microflora of obstructed bowel. Br J Surg 1976; 63(9):721–5.
[6] Fraser I. Motility changes associated with large bowel obstruction and its surgical relief. Ann R Coll Surg Engl 1984;66(5):321–6.
[7] Ihedioha U, Alani A, Modak P, et al. Hernias are the most common causes of strangulation in patients presenting with small bowel obstruction. Hernia 2006;10(4):338–40.
[8] Saunders MD, Cappell MS. Endoscopic management of acute colonic pseudo-obstruction. Endoscopy 2005;37(8):760–3.
[9] Kahi CJ, Rex DK. Bowel obstruction and pseudo-obstruction. Gastroenterol Clin North Am 2003;32(4):1229–47.
[10] Fevang BT, Fevang J, Stangeland L, et al. Complications and death after surgical treatment of small bowel obstruction: a 35-year institutional experience. Ann Surg 2000;231(4): 529–37.
[11] Ahlberg G, Bergdahl S, Rutqvist J, et al. Mechanical small-bowel obstruction after conventional appendectomy in children. Eur J Pediatr Surg 1997;7(1):13–5.
[12] Parker MC, Ellis H, Moran BJ, et al. Postoperative adhesions: ten-year follow-up of 12,584 patients undergoing lower abdominal surgery. Dis Colon Rectum 2001;44(6): 822–9.
[13] MacLean AR, Cohen Z, MacRae HM, et al. Risk of small bowel obstruction after ileal pouch-anal anastomosis. Ann Surg 2002;235(2):200–6.
[14] Beck DE, Opelka FG, Bailey HR, et al. Incidence of small-bowel obstruction and adhesiolysis after open colorectal and general surgery. Dis Colon Rectum 1999;42(2):241–8.
[15] Parker MC, Wilson MS, Menzies D, et al. The SCAR-3 study: 5-year adhesion-related readmission risk following lower abdominal surgical procedures. Colorectal Dis 2005; 7(6):551–8.
[16] Nieuwenhuijzen M, Reijnen MM, Kuijpers JH, et al. Small bowel obstruction after total or subtotal colectomy: a 10 year retrospective review. Br J Surg 1998;85(9):1242–5.
[17] Ellis H, Moran BJ, Thompson JN, et al. Adhesion-related hospital readmissions after abdominal and pelvic surgery: a retrospective cohort study. Lancet 1999;353:1476–80.
[18] Miller G, Boman J, Shrier I, et al. Natural history of patients with adhesive small bowel obstruction. Br J Surg 2000;87(9):1240–7.
[19] Miller G, Boman J, Shrier I, et al. Etiology of small bowel obstruction. Am J Surg 2000; 180(1):33–6.
[20] Lo OS, Law WL, Choi HK, et al. Early outcomes of surgery for small bowel obstruction: analysis of risk factors. Langenbecks Arch Surg 2007;392(2):173–8.
[21] Foster NM, McGory ML, Zingmond DS, et al. Small bowel obstruction: a population-based appraisal. J Am Coll Surg 2006;203(2):170–6.
[22] Turnage RH, Heldmann M, Cole P. Intestinal obstruction and ileus. In: Feldman M, Friedman LS, Brandt LJ, et al, editors. Sleisenger and Fordtran's gastrointestinal and liver disease: pathophysiology, diagnosis, and management. 8th edition. Philadelphia: Elsevier Saunders; 2006. p. 2653–78.
[23] Ghiassi S, Nguyen SQ, Divino CM, et al. Internal hernias: clinical findings, management and outcomes in 49 nonbariatric cases. J Gastrointest Surg 2007;11(3):291–5.
[24] Newsom BD, Kukora JS. Congenital and acquired internal hernias: unusual causes of small bowel obstruction. Am J Surg 1986;152(3):279–85.
[25] McCloy C, Brown T, Bolton JS, et al. The etiology of intestinal obstruction in patients without prior laparotomy or hernia. Am Surg 1998;64(1):19–22.
[26] Ripamonti C, De Conno F, Ventafridda V, et al. Management of bowel obstruction in advanced and terminal cancer patients. Ann Oncol 1993;4(1):15–21.
[27] Miller G, Boman J, Shrier I, et al. Small-bowel obstruction secondary to malignant disease: an 11-year audit. Can J Surg 2000;43(5):353–8.

[28] Stringer MD, Pablot SM, Brereton RJ. Paediatric intussusception. Br J Surg 1992;79(9): 867–76.
[29] Frager D. Intestinal obstruction role of CT. Gastroenterol Clin North Am 2002;31(3): 777–99.
[30] Gough IR. Strangulating adhesive small bowel obstruction with normal radiographs. Br J Surg 1978;65(6):431–4.
[31] Thompson WM, Kilani RK, Smith BB, et al. Accuracy of abdominal radiography in small-bowel obstruction: does reviewer experience matter? AJR Am J Roentgenol 2007;188(3): W233–8.
[32] Lee PW. The plain X-ray in the acute abdomen: a surgeon's evaluation. Br J Surg 1976; 63(10):763–6.
[33] Ko YT, Lim JH, Lee DH, et al. Small bowel obstruction: sonographic evaluation. Radiology 1993;188(3):649–53.
[34] Suri S, Gupta S, Sudhakar PJ, et al. Comparative evaluation of plain films, ultrasound and CT in the diagnosis of intestinal obstruction. Acta Radiol 1999;40(4):422–8.
[35] Meiser G, Meissner K. Ileus and intestinal obstruction: ultrasonographic findings as a guideline to therapy. Hepatogastroenterology 1987;34(5):194–9.
[36] Okada T, Yoshida H, Iwai J, et al. Pulsed Doppler sonography for the diagnosis of strangulation in small bowel obstruction. J Pediatr Surg 2001;36(3):430–5.
[37] Brochwicz-Lewinski MJ, Paterson-Brown S, Murchison JT. Small bowel obstruction: the water-soluble follow-through revisited. Clin Radiol 2003;58(5):393–7.
[38] Abbas SM, Bisset IP, Parry BR. Meta-analysis of oral water-soluble contrast agent in the management of adhesive small bowel obstruction. Br J Surg 2007;94(4):404–11.
[39] Maglinte DD, Kelvin FM, Sandrasegaran K, et al. Radiology of small bowel obstruction: contemporary approach and controversies. Abdom Imaging 2005;30(2): 160–78.
[40] Mallo RD, Salem R, Lalani T, et al. Computed tomography diagnosis of ischemia and complete obstruction in small bowel obstruction: a systematic review. J Gastrointest Surg 2005;9(5):690–4.
[41] Balthazar EJ, Birnbaum BA, Megibow AJ, et al. Closed-loop and strangulating intestinal obstruction. Radiology 1992;185(3):769–75.
[42] Cappell MS, Davis M. Characterization of Bouveret's syndrome: a comprehensive review of 128 cases. Am J Gastroenterol 2006;101(9):2139–46.
[43] Maglinte DD, Bender GN, Heitkamp DE, et al. Multidetector-row helical CT enteroclysis. Radiol Clin North Am 2003;41(2):249–62.
[44] Rajesh A, Maglinte DD. Multislice CT enteroclysis: technique and clinical applications. Clin Radiol 2006;61(1):31–9.
[45] Matsuoka H, Takahara T, Masaki T, et al. Preoperative evaluation by magnetic resonance imaging in patients with bowel obstruction. Am J Surg 2002;183(6):614–7.
[46] Beall DP, Fortman BJ, Lawler BC, et al. Imaging bowel obstruction: a comparison between fast magnetic resonance imaging and helical computed tomography. Clin Radiol 2002; 57(8):719–24.
[47] Maglinte DD, Heitkamp DE, Howard TJ, et al. Current concepts in imaging of small bowel obstruction. Radiol Clin North Am 2003;41(2):263–83.
[48] Sun B, Shen R, Cheng S, et al. The role of double-balloon enteroscopy in diagnosis and management of incomplete small-bowel obstruction. Endoscopy 2007;39(6):511–5.
[49] Fleshner PR, Siegman MG, Slater GI, et al. A prospective, randomized trial of short versus long tubes in adhesive small-bowel obstruction. Am J Surg 1995;170(4):366–70.
[50] Brolin RE, Krasna MJ, Marst BA. Use of tubes and radiographs in the management of small bowel obstruction. Ann Surg 1987;206(2):126–33.
[51] Evers BM. Small intestine. In: Townsend CM, Beauchamp RD, Evers BM, et al, editors. Sabiston textbook of surgery: the biologic basis of modern surgical practice. 17th edition. Philadelphia: Elsevier Saunders; 2004. p. 1323–80.

[52] Lubbers H, Mahike R, Lankisch PG. Gallstone ileus: endoscopic removal of a gallstone obstructing the upper jejunum. J Intern Med 1999;246(6):593–7.
[53] Pickleman J, Lee RM. The management of patients with suspected early postoperative small bowel obstruction. Ann Surg 1989;210(2):216–9.
[54] Shelton AA, Chang G, Welton ML. Small intestine. In: Doherty GM, Way LW, editors. Current surgical diagnosis and treatment. 12th edition. New York: Lange Medical Books; 2006. p. 654–84.
[55] Redaelli CA, Schilling MK, Carrel TP. Intraoperative assessment of intestinal viability by laser Doppler flowmetry for surgery of ruptured abdominal aortic aneurysms. World J Surg 1998;22(3):283–9.
[56] Leon EL, Metzger A, Tsiotos GG, et al. Laparoscopic management of small bowel obstruction: indications and outcome. J Gastrointest Surg 1998;2(2):132–40.
[57] Ellis CN, Boggs HW Jr, Slagle GW, et al. Small bowel obstruction after colon resection for benign and malignant diseases. Dis Colon Rectum 1991;34(5):367–71.
[58] Woolfson RG, Jennings K, Whalen GF. Management of bowel obstruction in patients with abdominal cancer. Arch Surg 1997;132(10):1093–7.
[59] Mangili G, Franchi M, Mariani A, et al. Octreotide in the management of bowel obstruction in terminal ovarian cancer. Gynecol Oncol 1996;61(3):345–8.
[60] Matulonis UA, Seiden MV, Roche M, et al. Long-acting octreotide for the treatment and symptomatic relief of bowel obstruction in advanced ovarian cancer. J Pain Symptom Manage 2005;30(6):563–9.
[61] Mangili G, Aletti G, Frigerio L, et al. Palliative care for intestinal obstruction in recurrent ovarian cancer: a multivariate analysis. Int J Gynecol Cancer 2005;15(5):830–5.
[62] Mercadante S, Ripamonti C, Casuccio A, et al. Comparison of octreotide and hyoscine butylbromide in controlling gastrointestinal symptoms due to malignant inoperable bowel obstruction. Support Care Cancer 2000;8(3):188–91.
[63] Feuer DJ, Broadley KE. Corticosteroids for the resolution of malignant bowel obstruction in advanced gynaecological and gastrointestinal cancer. Cochrane Database Syst Rev 2000;(2) CD001219.
[64] Duron JJ, Silva NJ, du Montcel ST, et al. Adhesive postoperative small bowel obstruction: incidence and risk factors of recurrence after surgical treatment: a multicenter prospective study. Ann Surg 2006;244(5):750–7.
[65] Fevang BT, Fevang J, Lie SA, et al. Long-term prognosis after operation for adhesive small bowel obstruction. Ann Surg 2004;240(2):193–201.
[66] Barkan H, Webster S, Ozeran S. Factors predicting the recurrence of adhesive small-bowel obstruction. Am J Surg 1995;170(4):361–5.
[67] Fabri PJ, Ellison EC, Anderson ED, et al. High molecular weight dextran: effect on adhesion formation and peritonitis in rats. Surgery 1983;94(2):336–41.
[68] Adams JTY. Adynamic ileus of the colon: an indication for cecostomy. Arch Surg 1974; 109(4):503–7.
[69] Fazio VW, Cohen Z, Fleshman JW, et al. Reduction in adhesive small-bowel obstruction by Seprafilm adhesion barrier after intestinal resection. Dis Col Rectum 2006;49(1):1–11.
[70] Beck DE, Cohen Z, Fleshman JW, et al. A prospective, randomized, multicenter controlled study of the safety of Seprafilm adhesion barrier in abdominopelvic surgery of the intestine. Dis Col Rectum 2003;46(10):1310–9.
[71] Gutt CN, Oniu T, Schemmer P, et al. Fewer adhesions induced by laparoscopic surgery? Surg Endosc 2004;18(6):898 906.
[72] Rosin D, Zmora O, Hoffman A, et al. Low incidence of adhesion-related bowel obstruction after laparoscopic colorectal surgery. J Laparoendosc Adv Surg Tech A 2007;17(5): 604–7.
[73] Athreya S, Moss J, Urquhart G, et al. Colorectal stenting for colonic obstruction: the indications, complications, effectiveness and outcome- 5-year review. Eur J Radiol 2006; 60(1):91–4.

[74] Taourel P, Kessler N, Lesnik A, et al. Helical CT of large bowel obstruction. Abdom Imaging 2003;28(2):267–75.
[75] Ballantyne GH. Review of sigmoid volvulus: clinical patterns and pathogenesis. Dis Col Rectum 1982;25(8):823–30.
[76] Pousada L. Cecal bascule: an overlooked diagnosis in the elderly. J Am Geriatr Soc 1992; 40(1):65–7.
[77] Lopez-Kostner F, Hool GR, Lavery IC. Management and causes of acute large-bowel obstruction. Surg Clin North Am 1997;77(6):1265–90.
[78] Chapman AH, McNamara M, Porter G. The acute contrast enema in suspected large bowel obstruction: value and technique. Clin Radiol 1992;46(4):273–8.
[79] Beattie GC, Peters RT, Guy S, et al. Computed tomography in the assessment of suspected large bowel obstruction. ANZ J Surg 2007;77(3):160–5.
[80] Sinha R, Verma R. Multidetector row computed tomography in bowel obstruction. Part 2. Large bowel obstruction. Clin Radiol 2005;60(10):1068–75.
[81] Burrell HC, Baker DM, Wardrop P, et al. Significant plain film findings in sigmoid volvulus. Clin Radiol 1994;49(5):317–9.
[82] Phillips RKS, Hittinger R, Fry JS, et al. Malignant large bowel obstruction. Br J Surg 1985; 72(4):296–302.
[83] Biondo S, Pares D, Frago R, et al. Large bowel obstruction: predictive factors for postoperative mortality. Dis Col Rectum 2004;47(11):1889–97.
[84] Thomson WH, Carter SS. On-table lavage to achieve safe restorative rectal and emergency left colonic resection without covering colostomy. Br J Surg 1986;73(1):61–3.
[85] Deans GT, Krukowski ZH, Irwin ST. Malignant obstruction of the left colon. Br J Surg 1994;81(9):1270–6.
[86] Lynch CR, Jones RG, Hilden K, et al. Percutaneous endoscopic cecostomy in adults: a case series. Gastrointest Endosc 2006;64(2):279–82.
[87] Targownik LE, Spiegel BM, Sack J, et al. Colonic stent vs. emergency surgery for management of acute left-sided malignant colonic obstruction: a decision analysis. Gastrointest Endosc 2004;60(6):865–74.
[88] Vitale MA, Villotti G, D'Alba L, et al. Preoperative colonoscopy after self-expandable metallic stent placement in patients with acute neoplastic colon obstruction. Gastrointest Endosc 2006;63(6):814–9.
[89] Tilney HS, Lovegrove RE, Purkayastha S, et al. Comparison of colonic stenting and open surgery for malignant large bowel obstruction. Surg Endosc 2007;21(2):225–33.
[90] Soto S, Lopez-Roses L, Gonzalez-Ramirez A, et al. Endoscopic treatment of acute colorectal obstruction with self-expandable metallic stents: experience in a community hospital. Surg Endosc 2006;20(7):1072–6.
[91] Canon CL, Baron TH, Morgan DE, et al. Treatment of colonic obstruction with expandable metal stents: radiologic features. AJR Am J Roentgenol 1997;168(1):199–205.
[92] Davies RJ, D'Sa IB, Lucarotti ME, et al. Bowel function following insertion of self-expanding metallic stents for palliation of colorectal cancer. Colorectal Dis 2005;7(3): 251–3.
[93] Watson AJ, Shanmugam V, Mackay I, et al. Outcome after placement of colorectal stents. Colorectal Dis 2005;7(1):70–3.
[94] Law WL, Chu KW, Ho JW, et al. Self-expanding metallic stent in the treatment of colonic obstruction caused by advanced malignancies. Dis Colon Rectum 2000;43(11): 1522–7.
[95] Ptok H, Meyer F, Marusch F, et al. Palliative stent implantation in the treatment of malignant colorectal obstruction. Surg Endosc 2006;20(6):909–14.
[96] Dafnis G. Repeated coaxial colonic stenting in the palliative management of benign colonic obstruction. Eur J Gastroenterol Hepatol 2007;19(1):83–6.
[97] Jost RS, Jost R, Schoch E, et al. Colorectal stenting: an effective therapy for preoperative and palliative treatment. Cardiovasc Intervent Radiol 2007;30(3):433–40.

[98] Stone JM, Bloom RJ. Transendoscopic balloon dilatation of complete colonic obstruction. An adjunct in the treatment of colorectal cancer: report of three cases. Dis Colon Rectum 1989;32(5):429–31.
[99] Araki Y, Iosomoto H, Matsumoto A, et al. Endoscopic decompression procedure in acute obstructing colorectal cancer. Endoscopy 2000;32(8):641–3.
[100] Kiefhaber P, Kiefhaber K, Huber F. Preoperative neodymium-YAG laser treatment of obstructive colon cancer. Endoscopy 1986;18(Suppl):44–6.
[101] Arrigoni A, Pennazio M, Spandre M, et al. Emergency endoscopy: recanalization of intestinal obstruction caused by colorectal cancer. Gastrointest Endosc 1994;40(5):576–80.
[102] Courtney ED, Raja A, Leicester RJ. Eight years experience of high-powered endoscopic diode laser therapy for palliation of colorectal carcinoma. Dis Colon Rectum 2005;48(4): 845–50.
[103] Eckhauser ML, Mansour EG. Endoscopic laser therapy for obstructing and/or bleeding colorectal carcinoma. Am Surg 1992;58(6):358–63.
[104] Mangiante EC, Croce MA, Fabian TC, et al. Sigmoid volvulus: a four-decade experience. Am Surg 1989;55(1):41–4.
[105] Cowlam S, Watson C, Elltringham M, et al. Percutaneous endoscopic colostomy of the left side of the colon. Gastrointest Endosc 2007;65(7):1007–14.
[106] Rabinovici R, Simansky DA, Kaplan O, et al. Cecal volvulus. Dis Colon Rectum 1990; 33(9):765–9.
[107] Anderson JR, Welch GH. Acute volvulus of the right colon: an analysis of 69 patients. World J Surg 1986;10(2):336–42.

ELSEVIER
SAUNDERS

THE MEDICAL CLINICS OF NORTH AMERICA

Med Clin N Am 92 (2008) 599–625

# Gastrointestinal Perforation and the Acute Abdomen

John T. Langell, MD, PhD, MPH[a,*], Sean J. Mulvihill, MD[a,b]

[a]*Department of Surgery, University of Utah, 30 North 1900 East, SOM 3B115, Salt Lake City, UT 84132, USA*
[b]*Huntsman Cancer Institute, 2000 Circle of Hope, Salt Lake City, UT 84112, USA*

The acute abdomen accounts for up to 40% of all emergency-surgical hospital admissions and is considered in the differential in the more than 7 million visits to the emergency department annually for abdominal pain in the United States [1–3]. A large percentage of these cases are secondary to perforation or impending gastrointestinal perforation [1–3]. Gastrointestinal perforation causes considerable mortality and usually requires emergency surgery. Mortality of secondary peritonitis was as high as 90% in the early Twentieth century and is still 30% to 50% despite advances in antibiotics, surgical technique, radiographic imaging, and resuscitation therapy [4,5]. Rapid diagnosis and treatment of these conditions is essential to reduce the high morbidity and mortality of late-stage presentation. Successful treatment requires a thorough understanding of the anatomy, microbiology, and pathophysiology of this disease process and in-depth knowledge of the therapy, including resuscitation, antibiotics, source control, and physiologic support.

The gastrointestinal tract is a continuous luminal (hollow) viscera composed of named organs based on physiologic or anatomic variations that result in functional differences in ingestion, digestion, processing, absorption, and elimination of nutritional substances. Gastrointestinal organs are traditionally categorized according to their embryonic derivation: Structures proximal to the ligament of Treitz are derived from the embryonic foregut, structures from the ligament of Treitz to the hepatic flexure of the colon from the embryonic midgut, and structures distal to the hepatic flexure from the embryonic hindgut [6]. Although this classification is useful to understand the developmental anatomy, vascular anatomy, and pain

* Corresponding author.
*E-mail address:* john.langell@hsc.utah.edu (J.T. Langell).


doi:10.1016/j.mcna.2007.12.004 *medical.theclinics.com*

perception distribution of gastrointestinal organs, it is not useful to determine the severity and rapidity of disease progression in gastrointestinal perforation.

The relative proximal to distal location of an insult is useful to understand the clinical presentation and progression of disease. From proximal to distal, the gastrointestinal tract includes the stomach, duodenum, jejunum, ileum, appendix, colon, and peritonealized rectum. The gastrointestinal lumen serves as a space to contain, process, and selectively absorb from the extracorporeal environment. Breach of the gastrointestinal wall causes intra-abdominal contamination with peritonitis or abscess formation [4]. The type and degree of peritoneal contamination depends on the site, size, and duration of the perforation and on the physiologic state, including the time from the last meal, administration of a mechanical bowel preparation before the perforation, coexistent diseases, and the presence or absence of an ileus or bowel obstruction with accompanying bacterial overgrowth [7–13]. These factors affect the relative degree and type of bacterial and fungal contamination from perforation. The anatomic site of perforation significantly affects the type and burden of enteric contamination [8,9,12,13]. The degree and type of microbiologic colonization of the gastrointestinal tract varies for different gastrointestinal organs and depends upon the local microenvironment. Microbiological colonization increases from proximal to distal, with the stomach showing the lowest number of viable microorganisms per cubic centimeter of luminal contents. Despite individual variation, the microbiologic content of the normal, healthy stomach and duodenum is less than $10^3$ organisms per gram of luminal contents due to a hostile local milieu from acidic, biliary, and pancreatic secretions [12,13]. The microbiologic load progressively increases from approximately $10^4$ organisms per gram of luminal contents in the proximal jejunum to $10^7$ organisms per gram in the terminal ileum [12,13]. The colon has the highest microorganism burden, with loads as high as $10^{12}$ organisms per gram of luminal content [12,13]. The composition of the microflora of the gastrointestinal tract varies greatly. Gastric flora are composed of yeast, aerobic bacteria (predominantly *Staphylococci*, *Streptococci*, and *Hemophilus* species), and anaerobic bacteria (predominantly *Bacteroides*, *Veillonella*, and *Bifidobacterium* species). Gastric anaerobes outnumber aerobes by about 1000-fold. The relative frequency of aerobes progressively increases along the small bowel, with gram-negative aerobes becoming the predominant organisms in the terminal ileum. The microfloral load and composition dramatically and abruptly changes between the terminal ileum and the colon. Colonic anaerobes outnumber aerobes by up to 1000-fold, with the predominant genera consisting of *Bacteroides*, *Bifidobacterium*, *Eubacterium*, *Clostridium*, *Lactobacillus*, *Fusobacterium*, and a limited variety of gram-positive anaerobes [12,13]. Understanding the characteristic microflora of each gastrointestinal organ is clinically important in selecting antibiotics for secondary peritonitis and potential sepsis.

The microorganism load is inversely related to the relative toxicity of organ fluid composition. The stomach and duodenum contain acidic contents or erosive biliary and pancreatic fluid, whereas the distal small bowel and colon contain a relatively neutral environment [12]. Organ-specific fluid composition affects bacterial load and bacterial species composition, which can lead to different initial presenting symptoms from a perforated viscous that may be diagnostically helpful. Patients who have gastric and duodenal perforation tend to present with highly acute pain due to a rapid chemical peritonitis, often followed by a systemic inflammatory response syndrome (SIRS), which can lead to rapid clinical deterioration [5,14,15]. Patients often recall the exact time of symptom onset. The perforation may progress to an infected peritonitis and sepsis in untreated patients or in patients who have late-stage presentations [5]. Colonic perforations may present without immediate perforation-associated pain and tend to have a slower clinical progression, with the development of a secondary bacterial peritonitis or localized abscess formation [16,17] partly due to the relatively neutral and nonerosive nature of the chemical environment within the colon [12]. With some exceptions, peritoneal contamination from intraluminal colonic contents progressively leads to purulent or fecal peritonitis or to the development of an intra-abdominal abscess. Few of the more than 500 different microfloral species in the colon can survive outside their normal environment [12,18]. In fact, only 22 genera of bacteria were isolated from cultures of intra-abdominal fluid collected among 255 patients who had secondary bacterial peritonitis [5,19]. Over 70% of isolates were from the genera *Bacteroides*, *Streptococcus*, *Escherichia*, *Peptostreptococcus*, and *Fusobacterium* [5,18,19].

## Mechanisms of gastrointestinal perforation

All causes of gastrointestinal tract perforation involve loss of gastrointestinal wall integrity and the release of intraluminal contents into the normally sterile peritoneal cavity. The numerous underlying causes are categorized according to the initial pathophysiology as (1) penetrating foreign body perforation, (2) extrinsic bowel obstruction, (3) intrinsic bowel obstruction, (4) direct loss of bowel wall integrity without foreign body perforation, (5) gastrointestinal ischemia, and (6) infection (Table 1).

Gastrointestinal perforation secondary to a penetrating foreign body can result from the ingestion of sharp, pointed, or jagged objects [20,21], such as chicken bones, fish bones, nails, razor blades, and tooth picks [22–25]. Although these perforations can occur anywhere along the gastrointestinal tract, they more commonly occur in the small intestine and colon. More frequently, foreign body perforation involves external penetrating trauma from knife injuries, gunshot wounds, or falls onto sharp protruding objects [26]. Iatrogenic perforations have significantly increased recently due to the

Table 1
Classification of gastrointestinal perforations

| Mechanism | Examples |
|---|---|
| Foreign body perforation | Penetrating trauma |
| | Endoscopy/iatrogenic |
| | Ingestion of foreign objects |
| Extrinsic bowel obstruction | Gastrointestinal stromal tumors |
| | Lymphoma |
| | Surgical adhesions |
| | Hernia |
| | Volvulus |
| Intrinsic bowel obstruction | Phytobezoar |
| | Crohn's stricture |
| | Diverticulitis/appendicitis |
| | Intraluminal neoplasm |
| Loss of gastrointestinal wall integrity | Peptic ulcer |
| | Crohn's disease |
| | Tumor lysis syndrome |
| Gastrointestinal ischemia | Shock/hypotension |
| | Thromboembolic event |
| | Visceral arterial sclerosis |
| | Portal vein thrombosis |
| Infection | *Salmonella typhosa* |
| | *Clostridium difficile* |
| | Cytomegalovirus |

greater use of invasive diagnostic and therapeutic medical procedures [7,27,28], including upper endoscopy, colonoscopy, interventional radiologic guided tissue biopsy and fluid drainage, paracentesis, nasogastric tube insertion, laparoscopy, and laparotomy [7,27,28]. The risk of gastrointestinal perforation from colonoscopy or upper endoscopy markedly increases with therapeutic procedures and with diagnostic procedures that involve tissue sampling [27].

Gastrointestinal perforation from extrinsic obstruction may be caused by mass effect from benign or malignant neoplasms, including primary gastrointestinal wall neoplasms such as gastrointestinal stromal tumors, leiomyomas, leiomyosarcomas, lymphomas, and duplication cysts [29–31]. Extrinsic compression may also occur secondary to nongastrointestinal neoplasms located adjacent to the compressed segment of bowel or metastatic to the gastrointestinal tract and associated mesentery [32,33]. Other common causes include surgical adhesions, malrotation, volvulus, and intra-abdominal or fascial wall herniation [34–36]. These conditions can cause loss of gastrointestinal wall integrity via a single point of obstruction or a closed loop obstruction. Compression at a single point can produce complete bowel obstruction. In this case, the pathophysiology involves dilation of the proximal bowel and a progressive increase in venous congestion followed by arterial stasis, ischemia, necrosis, and loss of mural integrity leading to perforation [37]. With a single point of distal compression this series of events is not a certainty, but it is more likely with very distal obstruction. If a point of distal fixation or compression leads to a gastrointestinal twist or volvulus, this may cause a closed loop obstruction [34,36,37]. Closed loop obstruction can abruptly block vascular inflow to the compromised segment with rapid progression of tissue ischemia, necrosis, and perforation. Alternatively, a closed loop obstruction can evolve slowly through mucosal secretion into a closed luminal space, luminal distention and pressurization, venous congestion, arteriolar stasis, and thrombosis, followed by tissue ischemia, necrosis, and perforation [38]. The pathophysiology of the latter mechanism is similar to non–closed loop obstructions but occurs with greater certainty and more rapidity.

Intrinsic gastrointestinal obstruction results from intraluminal obstruction from neoplasms, phytobezoars, ischemic or radiation-induced strictures, and Crohn's disease–related strictures [39–41]. The most common causes of intraluminal obstruction with perforation is appendicitis and diverticulitis [38,42]. Congenital and acquired gastrointestinal diverticuli and the vermiform appendix are blind-end intestinal outpouchings [38,42–44]. The small lumens of these structures are subject to obstruction by fecal impaction, neoplastic obstruction, and lymphoid hyperplasia [38,42–44]. Intrinsic obstructions generally manifest the same pathophysiology as extrinsic nonclosed loop obstructions with progressive bowel distention, venous congestion, and arteriolar stasis followed by ischemia, necrosis, and loss of mural integrity [38]. As with nonclosed loop obstruction, perforation is unusual and more commonly occurs with distal obstructions. Obstruction of the blind loop segments of bowel with diverticulitis and appendicitis creates a closed loop bowel obstruction with secretion into a closed luminal space and a more certain and rapid onset of pathology [16,38,42].

Gastrointestinal wall integrity can be breached without distal obstruction or trauma from preexistent diseases or treatments for diseases involving the gastrointestinal wall. Common examples of the former mechanism include peptic ulcer disease and Crohn's disease [45–49]. Since the discovery of *Helicobacter pylori*, peptic ulcer perforations can be categorized as an infectious cause of gastrointestinal perforation, but up to 50% of patients who have duodenal and gastric ulcer perforations are *H pylori* negative [48–51]. These disease processes lead to local pathologic changes of the normal mural anatomy, including loss of normal mucosal integrity, local inflammation, and eventually focal perforation [52]. Focal loss of normal mucosal integrity may also result from neoplastic growth or from adjuvant or neoadjuvant therapy [53–57]. Perforation with a primary neoplasm is usually due to local tumor infiltration, replacement or displacement of the normal histology, tumor expansion, and overgrowth of the vascular blood supply, followed by ischemia, necrosis, and eventual perforation [54–57]. Malignant perforation can result from rapid tumor lysis from adjuvant or neoadjuvant therapy with loss of integrity of the involved gastrointestinal wall [54–57].

Ischemia is a relatively common cause of gastrointestinal necrosis and perforation in elderly and critically ill patients. The major direct mechanisms of ischemia are embolic occlusion, severe arterial stenosis, systemic hypotension, or venous outflow obstruction [58,59]. Underlying pathologic states that lead to proximal arterial thrombus formation can cause release of thrombotic debris to smaller-caliber distal vessels with embolic occlusion [58]. Common sources of emboli are thrombi located in the aorta or heart chambers. The site of thromboembolic occlusion is determined by the size of the embolus and the caliber of the vessel in which it becomes lodged [58,60]. Because emboli often are small fragments of a thrombus, they commonly obstruct distal arteries and cause relatively short segmental ischemia and necrosis. Large emboli or critical stenosis may occlude the celiac, superior mesenteric, or inferior mesenteric arteries or their major proximal branches [58,60]. This may produce extensive gastrointestinal ischemia, depending on the degree of coexistent vasculopathy or development of collateral circulatory flow. Ischemia rarely occurs in the stomach because of its highly redundant blood supply. Thromboembolic events may abruptly occlude arterial inflow and rapidly produce tissue ischemia, necrosis, and perforation [58,60].

Visceral arterial stenosis, usually of the celiac, superior mesenteric, or inferior mesenteric arteries, typically develops at or near their origin from the aorta. These vessels slowly and progressively stenose; this may cause complete obstruction [58]. Because the process slowly evolves, the body has time to develop a collateral blood supply derived from the other main visceral arteries. Due to vascular collaterals and redundancy, occlusive stenosis of at least two of the three main visceral vessels is usually required to cause bowel necrosis via this process. Severe multivessel stenosis frequently predisposes to obstructive flow through the stenotic region when a second event, such as hypotension or embolic occlusion, occurs that completely blocks or further reduces the already compromised blood flow [58,61,62]. The ensuing events are the same as described for thromboembolic occlusion of relatively normal vessels but tend to produce extensive bowel necrosis due to the proximal nature of the occlusion [58].

Gastrointestinal ischemia can develop from marked and prolonged hypotension secondary to sepsis, congestive heart failure, acute myocardial infarction, and hypovolemic shock [58–62]. These diverse insults can lead to intestinal ischemia, necrosis, and perforation [58–62].

Venous outflow can be obstructed, most commonly from thrombotic occlusion of the portal or superior mesenteric veins [58–60]. This obstruction can be well tolerated due to compensatory mechanisms or can produce severe venous congestion of a bowel segment, leading to arteriolar stasis and thrombosis followed by ischemic perforation, similar to the mechanism described for distal bowel obstruction [58–60].

Numerous microorganisms have been associated with gastrointestinal perforation, including *Clostridium difficile*, *Salmonella typhi*, *Mycobacterium tuberculosis*, and cytomegalovirus [63–69]. Although infection may lead to gastrointestinal perforation in any host, perforation is more common in immunocompromised patients, patients with poor nutritional states, and critically ill patients [64,65,69,70]. The injury varies in severity depending upon the virulence factors associated with the specific infectious agent. Many virulent bacterial organisms, including *C difficile* and *S typhi*, produce toxins that contribute to the pathologic insult to the gastrointestinal wall [63–65,69,70]. The pathophysiology of gastrointestinal perforation from infection includes a severe inflammatory reaction leading to ileus, bowel dilatation, and eventual loss of gastrointestinal wall integrity [63–70].

## Clinical evaluation

Suspected gastrointestinal perforation should be excluded in patients who have an acute abdomen. Although the term "acute abdomen" sometimes refers to conditions requiring urgent surgery, the term most often refers to any patient who develops abdominal pain over a relatively short time interval. There are many causes of acute abdominal pain, and many of them do not require surgery. It is important to rapidly differentiate between disease processes that require urgent or emergent surgery versus those that may be treated conservatively. A thorough history and physical examination is critical [14,71,72]. Although the history and physical examination may fail to identify the specific anatomic source of pathology with gastrointestinal perforation, they can rapidly determine the patient's acuity, differentiate likely surgical emergencies from benign disease processes, evaluate surgical risk, guide supplemental diagnostic testing and interventions, and tailor the therapeutic preoperative optimization to the individual patient. The history and physical examination may have to be abridged in patients who are obtunded or in extremis, but a limited history of key information should be obtained from the patient, family, or bystanders when possible.

The history should be detailed and complete and should focus on the history of the present condition, particularly the presenting symptoms, time course of events, and associated symptoms. When evaluating acute abdominal pain, inquiry into the antecedent events; the location, quality, duration, nature, and migration or extension of the pain; and modifiers of the pain is important for determining the diagnosis [71–73]. Other important points include symptoms of nausea, vomiting, anorexia, change in bowel habits, weight loss, syncope, dizziness, and dysuria. A complete medical history to include prior surgery, current medications and allergies, a family history, and a review of systems should be obtained to refine the differential diagnosis and guide diagnostic testing. Aspects of the history pertinent to the acute abdominal pain should be emphasized.

Pain is universal in patients who have an acute abdomen. It usually represents the reason for seeking medical attention [72,74]. Descriptions of the pain can help diagnose the etiology of the abdominal pain. Important descriptors include the time course of the pain (eg, When did it start? Is it recurrent? Has it progressed, diminished, or changed from the time of onset?). Hyperacute and immediately severe pain is consistent with gastrointestinal perforation but may occur with ureteral obstruction or biliary colic. What is the quality of the pain? Is it sharp, stabbing, dull, or colicky? Intermittent colicky pain is unusual in patients who have hollow viscous perforation or impending perforation [72,74]. Determine the severity of the pain based on a scale from 1 to 10. Determine radiation or migration of the pain. Where the pain started may help in determining the etiology. Foregut pathology tends to present with epigastric pain, midgut pathology tends to present with periumbilical pain, and hindgut pathology tends to present with infraumbilical pain. With time, the pain often migrates and localizes to the abdominal wall location juxtaposed to the offending organ due to localized peritoneal inflammation. Frank perforation usually causes severe, diffuse abdominal pain. Inquire as to what relieves or aggravates the pain [72,74]. Ask whether the pain is modified by position, eating, or movement. Pain that is exacerbated by movement is consistent with peritonitis, whereas pain that improves with meals is consistent with peptic ulceration [14,71,72,74].

The past medical history helps assess the surgical risk preoperatively. If the patient has undergone appendectomy, cholecystectomy, or total colectomy, then diseases of these organs would be excluded. Patients who have had prior abdominal operations are prone to bowel obstruction secondary to postsurgical adhesions [32,36]. Patients who have peptic ulcer disease, cancer, diverticulosis, or inflammatory bowel disease are at increased risk of gastrointestinal perforation from these diseases [16,47,50,75–77]. A review of recent medications is important. Patients on chronic high-dose nonsteroidal anti-inflammatory drugs or corticosteroids are at increased risk of gastrointestinal perforation. Patients who have had an acute onset of abdominal pain and diarrhea after recent antibiotic use should be suspected of having *C difficile* colitis [65].

The physical examination is important to help secure the diagnosis and to detect signs of coexistent diseases that can affect treatment options or can require specific preoperative interventions [71,72,74]. The initial focus should be on the overall appearance of the patient. Patients who are obtunded or in extremis should, like trauma patients, have an initial assessment of their airway, breathing, and circulatory status. These parameters can be assessed by conversation with the awake and alert patient. The vital signs provide clues regarding disease severity, volume status, pain severity, SIRS, and sepsis. Tachycardia, hypoxia, tachypnea, and hypotension suggest a compromised physiologic state consistent with shock [72,78]. Tachycardia with hypertension in an otherwise stable patient may be secondary to pain or anxiety.

For a suspected acute abdomen, thoroughly examine the abdomen, groin, and perineum and perform a digital rectal examination on all patients and a pelvic examination on female patients. Many practitioners find it useful to slightly bump the patient's bed or ask the patient to cough [79]. Patients who have peritonitis often wince in discomfort with these maneuvers. The rapid diaphragmatic excursion and resultant increased intra-abdominal pressure or the forced movement of the patient elicits peritoneal pain. The examination includes visual assessment, auscultation, palpation, and percussion of the abdominal wall. Inspect for previous surgical scars, open wounds, ostomies, masses, hernias, rashes, and ecchymoses indicative of trauma, past surgeries, or current disease. An ostomy provides a unique opportunity to partially evaluate bowel viability. Inspect the mucosa for edema, pallor, and necrosis and inspect the ostomy appliance for output quality and quantity.

Abdominal palpation is gently initiated in an area where the patient has reported the least pain, and then the entire abdomen is progressively and thoroughly examined. It is helpful to engage the patient in conversation during the examination to distract the patient from the palpation to more accurately assess the abdomen [72]. Percuss the abdomen and listen for tympany, which may be secondary to a diffuse pneumoperitoneum or bowel obstruction.

Diffuse peritonitis is a relatively straightforward clinical diagnosis. Aside from a history of severe pain exacerbated by movement, abdominal examination demonstrates exquisite tenderness and involuntary guarding manifested as a rigid abdomen [72,79] due to inflammation of the abdominal wall muscles. Patients who have gastrointestinal perforation do not necessarily present with diffuse peritonitis. They may exhibit local peritoneal irritation due to perforation contained by intra-abdominal defense mechanisms that results in abscess or phlegmon formation. Patients who have iatrogenic perforation may have extensive pneumoperitoneum with a distended and tympanitic abdomen without overt peritonitis. Classic signs of localized peritonitis include the obturator sign, Fothergill's sign, Rovsing's sign, psoas sign, and Murphy's sign [72].

Examination of the groin and perineum may reveal hernias; testicular, vulvar, anal, or perianal pathology; or trauma. In female patients, a bimanual pelvic examination may reveal adnexal tenderness or masses indicative of gynecologic pathology. A digital rectal examination may reveal rectal masses, perirectal abscesses, or prostatic pathology.

## Laboratory and radiographic testing

Supplemental laboratory studies are selectively ordered based on the pretest differential diagnoses to help secure the diagnosis. Laboratory testing for comorbid conditions is initiated if the results are needed to guide therapeutic intervention, for further diagnostic studies, or for preoperative optimization. Typically ordered tests include a complete blood cell count with differential, coagulation panel, electrolyte panel, liver function tests, urinalysis, lipase or amylase, arterial blood gas, and serum lactate level

[14,71,72,74,75]. Not all of these tests are indicated in every patient. The complete blood cell count is useful to evaluate the patient's white blood cell (WBC) count, which is a marker of inflammation or infection. Although the WBC may occasionally be normal in these patients, an elevation or significant depression helps in forming the differential diagnosis. The hematocrit is used to detect anemia due to concurrent disease or the presenting problem. It can help gauge the patient's volume status; an elevated hematocrit may be secondary to hypovolemia. Furthermore, assessing the hematocrit level and platelet count can help guide the type of fluid resuscitation (crystalloid versus blood transfusions) and the need for blood products for surgery.

An electrolyte panel, which usually includes serum sodium, potassium, chloride, bicarbonate, creatinine, blood urea nitrogen, and glucose and often includes a calcium level, is helpful. Although electrolyte panels are not necessarily diagnostically useful, they provide important data regarding the physiologic status and volume status that guide resuscitation efforts. The patient's renal function may affect the radiologic evaluation (eg, whether to use intravenous contrast agents). Liver function tests, amylase, and lipase are useful in patients who have suspected hepatobiliary or pancreatic disorders. Performing an arterial blood gas in patients who have some distress or with known pulmonary disease provides information regarding their respiratory status and acid–base balance [71,72,74,75]. These data are essential for initiating preoperative therapy, planning postoperative care, and evaluating for the onset of metabolic acidosis, which is a harbinger of shock. When ischemic bowel is suspected, a serum lactate level is useful. It is fairly sensitive but is not very specific for this diagnosis. The urinalysis, a relatively inexpensive test, helps diagnose urinary tract infection. Other potential tests include a beta-human chorionic gonadotropin for women of childbearing age and *C difficile* toxin analysis for patients suspected of having that form of infectious colitis.

Radiographic evaluation of the acute abdomen traditionally began with a three-view acute abdominal series consisting of an upright chest radiograph and upright and supine abdominal radiographs. Recent clinical studies have found this abdominal series to be a relatively poor instrument to evaluate the acute abdomen. In a study by MacKersie and colleagues [80], this three-view abdominal series had a sensitivity of 30%, an accuracy of 56%, and a negative predictive value of 51% in patients who had nontraumatic acute abdominal pain. Despite this poor performance, some authorities argue that it is an inexpensive and rapid test of patients who have a high pretest suspicion for hollow viscus perforation. Patients who have acute abdominal pain and pneumoperitoneum on a plain abdominal radiograph traditionally underwent urgent laparotomy without further diagnostic evaluation. This argument has been challenged by recent studies that have found plain radiographs to be insufficiently sensitive to evaluate pneumoperitoneum [80–85]. Others have reported that the sensitivity can be as high as 100% for large-volume pneumoperitoneum if the patient is placed in an upright or decubitus position for 5 to 10 minutes before an upright chest or lateral decubitus radiograph is performed [86]. However, nearly 50% of patients who had hollow viscus perforation at laparotomy failed to demonstrate pneumoperitoneum on plain abdominal radiographs [87]. Moreover, the finding of pneumoperitoneum on plain radiographs in patients who have acute abdominal pain is not always associated with the need for surgery for hollow viscus perforation. Roh and colleagues [88] reported that 14% of their patients who had abdominal pain and pneumoperitoneum on plain abdominal radiographs underwent an unnecessary laparotomy because the pneumoperitoneum was from sources other than a perforated viscus. They noted that the clinical presentation of their patients who had surgical versus nonsurgical causes of pneumoperitoneum was indistinguishable [88]. Others have reported similar conclusions, with about 10% of cases of pneumoperitoneum secondary to nonsurgical causes [89–92]. Numerous case series of nonsurgical causes of pneumoperitoneum have been reported [89–95]. Box 1 lists commonly reported causations.

**Box 1. Nonsurgical causes of pneumoperitoneum**

- Thoracic sources
  - Positive pressure ventilation
  - Pulmonary bleb rupture
  - Asthma
  - Coughing/retching/valsalva
  - Bronchoscopy
  - Cardiopulmonary resuscitation
- Abdominal sources
  - Endoscopic procedures
  - Recent laparoscopy
  - Recent laparotomy
  - Spontaneously sealed peptic ulcer perforation
  - Diverticulosis
  - Peritoneal dialysis
  - Blunt abdominal trauma
  - Spontaneous bacterial peritonitis
- Gynecologic sources
  - Pelvic inflammatory disease
  - Vaginal douching
  - Sexual intercourse
  - Vaginal insufflation
  - Pelvic examination
- Idiopathic

Helical CT has become the radiographic test of choice to evaluate the acute abdomen based on numerous retrospective and prospective studies. These studies have reported a diagnostic sensitivity of 95% to 98%, a specificity of 95.1% to 97%, and an accuracy of 95.6% [82–84,96–99]. It is also a rapid and cost-effective imaging modality [96–99]. Recent advances in helical CT scanners, improvements in contrast agents, and refinement of CT protocols have further enhanced the utility of this test. Its accuracy highly depends upon the CT protocol [99]. Communication between the ordering physician and the radiologist is vital, as is selection of the CT protocol based on the pretest differential diagnosis. The protocol variables include the use of contrast agents, acquisition phases, collimation parameters, pitch, and the reconstruction interval [99]. These variables can greatly affect the diagnostic accuracy of the CT scan for specific disease processes. Urban and Fishman [99] have published an excellent CT protocol for nonlocalized acute abdominal pain. They recommend 750 to 1000 mL of an oral contrast agent and 110 to 120 mL of a nonionic intravenous contrast agent delivered at 2 mL/s. A single portal venous phase CT is performed 70 to 90 seconds after intravenous contrast infusion from the diaphragm to the pubic symphysis with a 5-mm collimation, a pitch of 1.6, and a 5-mm reconstruction interval [99].

Helical CT is an excellent tool to assess suspected gastrointestinal perforation [98]. When feasible, oral and intravenous contrast agents are used to facilitate identification of perforation, peritonitis, ischemic bowel, and abscess formation [98,99]. Oral contrast helps accurately localize the site of perforation by visualization of extravasation of contrast outside the gastrointestinal lumen [98,99]. A water-soluble contrast agent is important in patients who have suspected hollow viscus perforation because extravasation of barium can cause severe peritonitis that carries a mortality of up to 50% [100,101]. CT is also excellent at detecting free intraperitoneal air, but the location of the free air does not necessarily correlate with the site of the perforation [98,99]. Other localized CT findings include inflammation and focal fluid or air collections [99].

Other helpful radiographic studies include ultrasonography and MRI [102–104]. Ultrasonography is an inexpensive, rapid, and nonradioactive test. Although it is only a fair diagnostic test, it is an excellent tool to rapidly evaluate pneumoperitoneum, free intra-abdominal fluid, and gynecologic pathology. It is frequently used to evaluate trauma patients. In prospective studies of suspected nontraumatic hollow viscus perforations, ultrasonography had a 93% to 100% sensitivity and 64% to 99% specificity for the detection of pneumoperitoneum [102,103]. It is not the diagnostic study of choice in stable patients because it fails to identify the source of perforation, perforation without pneumoperitoneum, or nonsurgical causes of pneumoperitoneum. In preliminary studies of MRI for acute abdominal pain, it has shown no significant benefit over CT [104]. MRI is also slow and frequently unavailable.

## Therapeutic intervention

The treatment of gastrointestinal perforation includes fluid resuscitation, antibiotics, source control, organ system support, and nutrition [4,5,15,105,106]. The overall clinical state of the patient dictates the treatment. Patients in extremis from gastrointestinal perforation and diffuse peritonitis require rapid resuscitation, initiation of antibiotics, and emergency surgery. Relatively stable patients undergo a similar therapeutic approach but with a greater focus on preoperative optimization of the patient's physiologic status with vigorous resuscitation and correction of any concurrent coagulopathy, acidosis, and electrolyte disturbances [5,105,106]. Concurrent comorbid conditions should be treated or prophylaxed as necessary, such as preoperative beta-blockade for normotensive and hypertensive patients at high risk for myocardial infarction or preoperative beta-agonists, ipratropium, or corticosteroids for patients who have significant pulmonary disease [107,108]. Patients who have documented adrenocortical insufficiency or chronic corticosteroid use should receive intravenous corticosteroids, whereas diabetic and septic patients should have serum glucose levels monitored and insulin therapy administered as needed [109].

Antibiotics are standard treatment for gastrointestinal perforation [4,5,15,105,106,110]. The antibiotic is selected according to the specific site of perforation [5,105,110]. Broad-spectrum antimicrobial coverage is instituted in the preoperative period, and the therapy is then tailored based on operative findings of source and degree of contamination. Excellent broad-spectrum coverage is provided by various agents or a combination of agents [5,105,106,110,111]. The choice of antimicrobials is based on adequacy of microbial coverage, patient allergies, hospital-specific resistance patterns, patient comorbidities, cost-effectiveness, and practitioner comfort with the drug. Many efficacious regimens have been described, and no single agent or combination of agents has been found to be superior to the others [110,112,113]. A recent Cochrane database meta-analysis of 40 randomized and quasi-randomized controlled studies including 5094 patients treated for secondary peritonitis of gastrointestinal origin found no significant difference in patient outcomes based on the antibiotic coverage [112]. The antibiotic regimens included 16 different single or combination antimicrobial agents, including aminoglycosides with antianaerobes or with broad-spectrum penicillins coupled with a beta-lactamase inhibitor, broad-spectrum penicillins alone or with a beta-lactamase inhibitor, aminoglycosides plus a broad-spectrum penicillin and an anti-anaerobe, carbapenems, cephalosporins with or without a beta-lactamase inhibitor alone or with an antianaerobe, clindamycin, fluoroquinolones with or with out an antianaerobe, monobactams plus an antianaerobe, or imipenam/cilastatin [112]. Most authorities recommend initiation of a regimen that broadly covers gram-negative, gram-positive, and anaerobic organisms [4,5,15,105,106,110]. An important issue is coverage for Candidal or Enterococcal infections [105].

The current data suggest that Enterococcal coverage is unnecessary for community-acquired peritonitis but should be considered for hospital-acquired peritonitis, immunosuppressed patients, patients who have prosthetic heart valves, or patients who have recurrent intra-abdominal infections accompanied by septic shock [105]. The need for anti-Candidal coverage in secondary peritonitis is debatable due to the variably reported frequency of Candidal species in the peritoneal fluid of patients who have gastrointestinal perforations. Some authors reported Candida to be the first or second most frequently isolated species from peritoneal fluid cultures, whereas others reported isolation of Candida in only 12% of patients [13]. In a placebo-controlled trial of patients who had gastrointestinal perforations, Eggimann and colleagues [114] showed that administration of fluconazole significantly reduced the rate of intra-abdominal candidiasis in high-risk patients. Most authorities consider the addition of anti-Candidal therapy only for immunosuppressed patients, septic patients, and patients who have positive fungal cultures. When used, anti-Candidial therapy should be continued for 2 to 3 weeks [105,115].

Antimicrobial therapy is an adjunctive treatment of secondary peritonitis to prevent local spread of infections, bacteremia, and sepsis and to reduce late complications [4,5,15,105,106,110]. The dosage and length of antimicrobial therapy is unclear in a particular patient. Despite many years of antibiotic use for secondary peritonitis, a unified consensus statement based on scientific evidence from randomized controlled trials is unavailable. Blot and De Waele [105] recommended, based on the 2002 Surgical Infection Society guidelines, that the type and time course of antimicrobial management should be based on (1) whether the source has been adequately controlled by appropriate drainage and correction of the underlying process [105,116], (2) whether therapy is required beyond 24 hours (they advocate no more than 24 hours of antibiotics for uncomplicated gastroduodenal perforations or for traumatic or iatrogenic small and large bowel perforations operated on within 24 hours of onset), (3) whether anti-fungal or enterococcal coverage is needed [105,116], and (4) whether coverage of resistant pathogens is needed for hospital-acquired perforations. The duration of antibiotic coverage is controversial [105,116]. Some authors advocate a standard treatment of 7 to 14 days, whereas others recommend continuing antibiotics until the WBC count has normalized and the patient is afebrile [105,110]. Current general consensus advocates antimicrobial therapy for 5 to 7 days if the clinical signs of infection have resolved [105,116]. If the patient fails to improve or worsens during this period, the adequacy of source control or appropriateness of antibiotic coverage must be questioned [105].

The most important therapy for gastrointestinal perforation is source control [5,15,105,106]. Traditionally, source control is acquired by surgery, but selected conditions are increasingly treated conservatively by radiologic or endoscopic intervention. The principles of source control dictate direct containment and control of the site of perforation, evacuation of intraperitoneal contamination, drainage of abscesses, debridement of necrotic tissue and foreign matter, and re-establishment of functional anatomy [5,15,105,106]. An exploratory laparotomy is usually performed via a midline incision and provides excellent visualization and easy access to the entire abdomen. The exploration is performed in a standard and regimented fashion to evaluate all gastrointestinal structures from the gastroesophageal junction to the peritoneal reflection of the rectum. Obvious sources of perforation are isolated and controlled. The remainder of the gastrointestinal tract is then explored. This exploration is important to find concurrent pathology or an underlying cause for the perforation, such as distal obstruction. When an obvious site of perforation is identified, exploration can be limited to an evaluation that does not unnecessarily disrupt intact anatomic structures, such as the gastrocolic ligament. Visceral exploration should include examination of the anterior stomach, the jejunum from the ligament of Treitz to the terminal ileum, the entire colon, and the peritonealized rectum. If a perforation is not identified, then the lesser sac should be entered through the gastrocolic ligament to evaluate the posterior stomach and anterior duodenum. If the source of contamination is still not evident, a Kocher maneuver can be performed to inspect the posterior and posterolateral duodenum. Most surgeons use open exploration, but a minimally invasive laparoscopic approach is an effective means of surgical exploration and source control in experienced hands [3,117–121].

Operative containment and control of the perforation is achieved by resection or repair of the anatomic site of damage. The chosen method depends on the underlying pathologic process and the size and duration of the perforation [5,15,105,106]. Small perforations can be repaired primarily by simple interrupted sutures if the following two criteria are met: (1) The lesion must not be malignant. If malignancy is possible, this question can be resolved by intraoperative biopsy with frozen section (FS) pathologic evaluation. If FS evaluation is nondiagnostic or unavailable, perforations from possible malignant processes should be resected. (2) The tissue surrounding the perforation must be healthy, wellperfused, and viable. All foreign material or necrotic debris must be removed from the perforated lumen, and only healthy, well perfused tissue must remain. The repair may be buttressed with an omental patch or with an adjacent segment of healthy bowel, such as an ileal patch, if the area is markedly inflamed [122]. Primary repair can sometimes be safely performed laparoscopically. Recently, minimally invasive repair of relatively clean colonic perforations have been successfully performed using surgical clips instead of the traditional suture repair. The initial data, consisting of scattered case reports, are promising.

Primary repair of perforated bowel is preferable to resection and anastomosis because it carries a lower complication rate [123]. This better outcome may reflect the limited tissue injury in these patients [123]. Primary repair should not be performed in patients who have malignant lesions, necrotic bowel, perforations associated with mesenteric vascular injuries, lesions involving more than 50% of the bowel circumference, or multiple contiguous perforations. When resection is required, the entire diseased segment is resected, leaving healthy, well perfused ends for anastomosis. The technique for the enteroenterostomy, whether stapled or hand-sewn, seems to have little impact on the anastomotic complication rate [123]. Primary bowel anastomosis must be considered cautiously in the setting of gross purulent or feculent peritonitis because of a high rate of serious complications [123,124]. Traditionally, a damage control operation was performed with resection of the injured bowel and peritoneal toilet [5,15,106], followed by a washout and reanastomosis if the conditions were favorable. It was recently shown that the functional anatomy may be safely restored during the first operation, but lumen patency and bowel wall viability should be monitored by planned relaparotomy [124]. The principles of colonic resection are similar to those for small bowel, with resection of the diseased segment and adequate peritoneal toilet [4,105]. Restoration of functional anatomy is approached differently in the setting of generalized peritonitis. Primary colocolonic anastomosis is avoided because of a high complication rate [16,125–127]. The standard approach for middle and distal colonic perforations in the presence of generalized peritonitis has been a Hartmann's procedure, with creation of a proximal end-colostomy and a distal colonic pouch with or without a mucous fistula [42]. Take-down of a Hartmann's pouch with restoration of colorectal continuity can be performed subsequently for most benign diseases, but this operation can be challenging. Some surgeons advocate a primary colocolonic anastomosis with a diverting loop ileostomy to avoid the complications and technical difficulties of a Hartmann's take-down. Ileal diversion seems to be a safe and promising alternative to the traditional Hartmann's procedure, but a randomized controlled trial comparing the two techniques has not been performed.

Perforation from ischemic bowel follows the treatment principles discussed previously. A critical difference involves determination of viable versus nonviable bowel. It is important to preserve as much viable bowel as possible to prevent the short gut syndrome, especially when long segments of bowel are ischemic. At surgery all clearly nonviable bowel is resected. When nonviable bowel is flanked by segments of questionable viability, clearly necrotic bowel is removed, and areas of uncertain viability are left in situ and in discontinuity. Re-exploration is performed to resect any newly demarcated bowel followed by functional anatomic restoration [105]. Alternatively, bowel viability is determined intraoperatively by clinical judgment, ultrasonography, electromyography, fluorescein viability testing, or laser Doppler flowmetry [128–130]. Clinical judgment based on bowel color, motility, pulsation, and mucosal bleeding has a sensitivity of 91% and a specificity of 82%. It is the most used and least cumbersome approach [58]. Several papers have been published on the other techniques, with mixed results [58,128,129]. Superior Mesenteric Artery (SMA) blood flow must be assessed [58]. If SMA flow is severely compromised due to arterial thrombosis or embolism, patency must be restored by embolectomy or bypass grafting [58]. Once viability has been determined, resection is performed, leaving viable ends for primary anastomosis. If concern still exists, a second-look operation is performed to assess anastomotic integrity and intestinal viability.

Gastric and duodenal perforations are common causes of free intra-abdominal hollow viscus perforation [50], most commonly secondary to peptic ulcer disease (PUD) [48–51,131]. Treatment of PUD has changed dramatically over the last several decades since the identification of *H pylori* as a major etiologic factor. The mainstay of PUD therapy is *H pylori* eradication and proton pump inhibitors (PPIs) [48–51,132]. This approach has almost eliminated the need for elective surgery for PUD. However, the incidence of perforated PUD may be increasing [50]. These and other data have led to speculation that perforated PUD may have a different etiology than non-perforated PUD. Although 95% of patients who have duodenal ulcers (DU) and 60% of patients who have gastric ulcers (GU) have *H pylori*, as few as 50% of patients who have perforated GU and DU have *H pylori* [48]. Regardless of this debate, the surgical approach to perforated PUD has dramatically changed from extensive resections and acid-suppressing procedures to simple closures, with or without omental patching [48,50,57,132]. Simple closure for a perforated DU, coupled with temporary acid suppression with PPI and *H pylori* eradication, entails a less than 5% recurrence rate at 1 year, which rises to 38% when *H pylori* therapy is not instituted [50,132]. In a series of 88 consecutive patients who had perforated DU treated by this approach, Rodriguez-Sanjuan and colleagues [51] noted no ulcer relapse during a mean follow-up 22.3 months (range, 1–80 months) [50]. This study and other studies have established that simple closure, acid-suppression medication, and *H pylori* eradication for *H pylori*–positive patients is the standard therapy for perforated DU [50,132]. The treatment for perforated GU is debatable partly due to the 10% to 30% risk of cancer in these gastric ulcers [133,134]. The current practice is to resect the GU, including an adequate margin, and obtain FS analysis. If the lesion is benign, then simple closure with an omental patch coupled with PPI therapy and *H pylori* eradication for *H pylori*–positive patients is the standard approach. This approach is somewhat controversial due to a rate of GU recurrence as high as 75% and the risk of repeated perforation [51]. A dilemma arises when FS evaluation is unavailable or nondiagnostic; some authorities advocate simple closure with reoperation if the final pathologic review demonstrates cancer, whereas others argue for a distal gastric resection incorporating the perforation according to established oncologic principles, followed by lymph node dissection at a separate surgery if the final pathologic analysis indicates cancer. This latter policy is based on the relatively high incidence of gastric cancer in perforated GU and the high long-term mortality from simple closure of a perforated gastric cancer [51,135,136]. The correct approach is uncertain and is in the hands of the individual surgeon.

The approach to gastric cancer perforation, documented by the patient history or FS evaluation, is fairly well established. It was previously believed that perforation represented late-stage cancer with tumor dissemination into the peritoneal cavity [136]. Based on this belief, simple closure was believed to provide the appropriate palliation while minimizing the surgical stress in a critically ill patient [136]. Recent surgical data show significantly increased perioperative and long-term mortality with simple closure compared with gastric resection [135–138]. Therefore, patients who have perforated gastric cancer should undergo appropriate gastric resection in spite of concurrent peritonitis unless the patient is hemodynamically unstable or has unresectable cancer [135–138].

Many patients who have gastrointestinal perforations develop SIRS or sepsis with accompanying hemodynamic compromise, hypothermia, acidosis, and a coagulopathy [4,139–141]. These patients require rapid resuscitation and rapid surgery. The challenge is to provide life-saving surgery without causing further physiologic compromise from the stress of surgery in these already compromised patients. The standard approach is known as "damage control" or "salvage" surgery. The goal is to rapidly obtain source control and peritoneal toilet without prolonging the surgery to restore functional anatomy or extensively mobilize tissues [105]. This surgery may simply involve suture control of perforations or rapid resection of frankly necrotic bowel [4]. Frequently, the bowel is left in discontinuity, the abdomen is cleared of gross debris, and a temporary abdominal closure is performed. The patient is then returned to the intensive care unit for appropriate resuscitative measures [142]. After stabilization, the patient can undergo a more deliberate and definitive surgery. Management of the open abdomen is greatly facilitated by the "vacuum-pack" procedure [142–144], which involves placement of a perforated, nonadherent polyethylene sheet over the exposed viscera and under the anterior borders of the opened abdominal fascia. A layer of compressible, absorbable material (surgical sponge or towel) is placed over the polyethylene sheet along with two silastic drains. A sheet of self-adhesive polyester (or equivalent) is placed across the skin of the outer abdominal wall, fully encompassing the other components of the vacuum device. The drains are connected to a continuous suction device set at 100 to 150 mm Hg negative pressure [142]. The vacuum pack effectively isolates the intra-abdominal cavity from the environment, provides drainage of abdominal fluids, provides for internal expansion to avoid the abdominal compartment syndrome, and facilitates emergency access and reoperation of the abdomen [142–144].

Iatrogenic gastrointestinal perforations from endoscopic instrumentation can provide a unique opportunity for conservative management. Endoscopic perforations often occur in a prepared and relatively clean intestinal tract [7,27,28]. The perforation may also be identified immediately or within minutes of its occurrence. If the perforation is recognized quickly and the patient has a relatively clean preparation, nonsurgical management is often successful [7,27,28]. Nonsurgical management highly depends on the time of diagnosis, location and size of the perforation, degree of contamination, and condition of the patient. Nonsurgical management can be successful in stable patients who have minimal signs and symptoms of peritonitis and who have small injuries to the stomach, duodenum, and retroperitoneal portions of the colon [7]. These locations offer possible anatomic containment of the perforation by the retroperitoneal space or omentum. Perforations of the intraperitoneal small bowel and colon usually require surgery, except for microperforations. Microperforations often cause minimal peritoneal contamination and can seal spontaneously [7,145]. Treatment of endoscopic perforations is rapidly evolving. Numerous case reports and case series have demonstrated the efficacy of endoscopic repair of injuries at the time of occurrence by approximating the two ends of a perforated segment via endoluminal clips [146–155]. Although these clinical reports are limited to small perforations, experimental studies of large endoscopic perforations in laboratory animals have produced similar results [156]. In one study, animals were randomized to open repair with interrupted sutures versus endoscopic repair with vascular clips for standardized iatrogenic injuries. The authors reported no difference in clinical outcome, repair burst strength, or hydroxylproline levels between the two groups. Iatrogenic gastric perforations have also been successfully repaired endoscopically by pulling extramural omentum into the gastric defect and tacking it to the muscularis propria with clips to endoscopically create an omental patch [7]. These endoscopic therapies are in their infancy but may become a standard therapeutic approach for iatrogenic perforations in stable patients.

Nonosurgical management can be occasionally applied to nonendoscopic perforations of the stomach, duodenum, and colon. These perforations are usually small and have been contained by local tissue, omentum, or the retroperitoneum [7]. These include small gastric and duodenal perforations caused by benign diseases, such as PUD. In these cases, the perforation may be spontaneously sealed by the greater or lesser omentum. The resultant omental patch is similar to a surgically created patch and may be sufficient therapy [145]. It is difficult to determine whether a perforation has spontaneously sealed, but a CT scan with oral contrast may be helpful [157]. Nonsurgical management of spontaneously sealed perforations should be considered only in stable patients who do not have overt signs of peritonitis [7]. These patients must undergo endoscopy after recovery from the acute process to ensure appropriate healing and to exclude cancer. Selected colonic perforations, such as certain iatrogenic injuries or perforation secondary to diverticulitis, may also be managed nonoperatively [42]. Not all diverticular perforations can be managed nonoperatively. Spontaneously sealed perforations and perforations that are contained with the development of an associated abscess cavity can often be successfully managed without surgery [42]. An excellent and clinically useful classification system for diverticular perforations was developed by Hinchey and colleagues [16] and modified by others. In short, Hinchey stage 1 (pericolic or mesenteric abscess) and stage 2 (walled-off or pelvic abscess) disease is usually treated conservatively with antibiotics, radiologically guided abscess drainage, and parenteral nutritional support. Hinchey stage 3 (generalized purulent peritonitis without colonic communication) or stage 4 (generalized fecal peritonitis with colonic communication) requires emergency surgery, following the treatment principles for gastrointestinal perforation discussed previously [16,42].

## Postoperative care

The medical management of patients treated surgically or conservatively for gastrointestinal perforation is partly based on the physiologic state of the patient and the clinician's perceived risk of further deterioration. The level of required care is individually assessed based upon the general underlying principles of management. Emphasis is placed on continued resuscitation, antibiotics, physiologic support of compromised organ systems, nutrition, and pain management [4,5,15,72,105]. Fluid management is usually the key resuscitative measure. Peritonitis directly causes loss of intravascular fluid volume [4]. The peritoneum is composed of a basement membrane with an inner single-cell layer of mesothelial cells. This lining permits free bidirectional exchange of fluids across an average surface area of 1.7 $m^2$ [2,4]. Gastrointestinal perforation with generalized peritoneal inflammation results in hyperemia and exudation of large amounts of fluid containing WBC and opsonins into the peritoneal cavity [4]. A massive fluid shift from the intravascular compartment into the peritoneal cavity can lead to the development of hypovolemia and shock. The degree of hypovolemia is partially determined by the size, location, and duration of the perforation [4,5,105]. Fluid loss during open abdominal surgery and postoperative open abdominal management can aggravate the fluid deficit. Crystalloid fluid resuscitation is usually indicated, but transfusion of blood products should be considered in patients who are coagulopathic, have ongoing bleeding, or have profound anemia that is insufficient to meet the patient's oxygen delivery requirements. Determination of the adequacy of resuscitation is controversial, and there are no universally accepted criteria. Restoration of normal hemodynamic parameters, normalization of urine output (0.5–1.0 mL/kg/h), and correction of acidosis are considered reasonable clinical indicators of adequate resuscitation [4], but these parameters can be complicated by acute or pre-existent organ system failures, especially of the heart, kidneys, or liver.

When gastrointestinal perforation results in SIRS or sepsis, patients often develop shock accompanied by multiorgan failure, coagulopathy, hypothermia, and acidosis [141]. Ongoing resuscitative and supportive measures focus on vigorous warming of the patient, correction of the coagulopathy, and acid–base management through ventilator and fluid manipulation [4,5,105,141]. These patients often require mechanical ventilation, hemofiltration, and mechanical cardiac augmentation, which can provide a lifesaving bridge while the underlying disease process is treated. Invasive monitoring can provide instantaneous, accurate clinical data to guide the administration of pharmacologic hemodynamic support. The most important treatment of gastrointestinal perforation is source control. All other therapies, including antibiotics, are adjunctive or supportive measures [4,5,15,105].

## Summary

Perforation of the gastrointestinal tract remains a considerable cause of morbidity and mortality. The treatment relies on a thorough understanding of the anatomy, microbiology, and pathophysiology of the underlying disease and resultant acute processes. Optimal patient care depends upon early diagnosis and rapid therapy.

The diagnosis is founded on a well conducted history and physical examination, supplemented by appropriate laboratory and radiologic studies. Once gastrointestinal perforation has been diagnosed, strict adherence to the principles of management is essential, including resuscitation, antibiotics, source control, and physiologic support. Source control is the most important step in the definitive management of these patients and must be rapidly achieved. The other supportive or adjunctive therapies help to supplement adequate source control.

## References

[1] McCaig L, Burt CW. National ambulatory medical care survey: 2002 emergency department summary. Adv Data 2004;340:1–34.

[2] Court-Brown CM, McQueen MM, Patterson-Brown S, et al. Emergency surgical care in Scotland. Surgeon 2007;5(2):72–5.

[3] Schietroma M, Cappelli S, Carlei F, et al. Acute abdomen: early laparoscopy or active laparotomic-laparoscopic observation? Hepatogastroenterology 2007;54(76):1137–41.

[4] Ordonez CA, Puyana JC. Management of peritonitis in the critically ill patient. Surg Clin North Am 2006;86:1323–49.

[5] Wittman DH, Schein M, Condon RE. Management of secondary peritonitis. Ann Surg 1996;224(1):10–8.

[6] Glasgow RE, Mulvihill SJ. Abdominal pain. In: Friedman M, Friedman LS, Sleisenger MH, editors. Sleisenger and Fordtran's gastrointestinal and liver disease: pathophysiology, diagnosis, management. 7th edition. Philadelphia: WB Saunders; 2002. p. 71–82.

[7] Putcha R, Burdick JS. Management of iatrogenic perforation. Gastroenterol Clin North Am 2003;32:1289–309.

[8] Sjöstedt S, Kager L, Heimdahl A, et al. Microbial colonization of tumors in relation to the upper gastrointestinal tract in patients with gastric carcinoma. Ann Surg 1998;207:341–6.

[9] Sjöstedt S, Heimdahl A, Kager L, et al. Microbial colonization of the oropharynx, esophagus, and stomach in patients with gastric diseases. Eur J Clin Microbiol 1985;4:49–51.

[10] Corrodi P. Jejunoileal bypass: change in the flora of the small intestine and its clinical impact. Rev Infect Dis 1984;6(Suppl 1):S80–4.
[11] Guarner F. The intestinal flora in inflammatory bowel disease: normal or abnormal? Curr Opin Gastroenterol 2005;21:414–9.
[12] Guarner F. Enteric flora in health and disease. Digestion 2006;73(Suppl 1):5–12.
[13] Guarner F, Malageleda JR. Gut flora in health and disease. Lancet 2003;361:512–9.
[14] Lyon C, Clark DC. Diagnosis of acute abdominal pain in older patients. Am Fam Physician 2006;74(9):1537–44.
[15] Nathens AB, Rotstein OD. Therapeutic options in peritonitis. Surg Clin North Am 1994; 74(3):677–92.
[16] Hinchey EJ, Schaal PG, Richards GK. Treatment of perforated diverticular disease of the colon. Adv Surg 1978;12:85–109.
[17] Mai V, Morris JG. Colonic bacterial flora: changing understandings in the molecular age. J Nutr 2004;134:459–64.
[18] Condon RE. Microbiology of intra-abdominal infection and contamination. Eur J Surg Suppl 1996;576:9–12.
[19] Krepel CJ, Gohr CM, Edmiston CE, et al. Surgical sepsis: constancy of antibiotic susceptibility of causative organisms. Surgery 1995;117:505–9.
[20] Huttunen R, Kairaluoma MI, Mokka RE, et al. Nontraumatic peroforation of the small intestine. Surgery 1977;81(2):184–8.
[21] Goh BK, Chow PK, Quah HM, et al. Penetration of the gastrointestinal tract secondary to ingestion of foreign bodies. World J Surg 2006;30(3):372–7.
[22] Ozel H, Topaloglu S, Yuksel BC, et al. Jejunal perforation in mentally retarded patient due to an ingested chicken bone. Hepatogastroenterology 2003;50(Suppl 2):ccxxxviii–ccxxxix.
[23] Glasson R, Haghighi KS, Richardson G. Chicken bone perforation of a sigmoid diverticulum. ANZ J Surg 2002;72(6):448–9.
[24] Nigri GR, Giulio E, Di Nardo R, et al. Duodenal perforation and right hydronephrosis due to toothpick ingestion. J Emerg Med 2008 Jan;34(1):55–7.
[25] Steenvoorde P, Moues CM, Viersma JH. Gastric perforation due to ingestion of a hollow toothpick: report of a case. Surg Today 2002;32(8):731–3.
[26] Espinoza R, Rodriguez A. Traumatic and non-traumatic perforation of hollow viscera. Surg Clin North Am 1997;77(6):1291–304.
[27] Cobb WS, Heniford BT, Sigmon LB, et al. Colonoscopic perforations: incidence, management, and outcomes. Am Surg 2004;70:750–7.
[28] Luning TH, Keemers-Gels ME, Barendregt WB, et al. Colonoscopic perforations: a review of 33,366 patients. Surg Endosc 2007;21:994–7.
[29] Sunamak O, Karabicak I, Avdemir I, et al. An intraluminal leiomyoma of the small intestine causing invagination and obstruction: a case report. Mt Sinai J Med 2006;73(8):1079–81.
[30] Yildirgan MI, Bosoglu M, Atamanalp SS, et al. Duodenal stromal tumor: report of a case. Surg Today 2007;37(5):426–9.
[31] Yokota T, Meguro K, Yamada Y, et al. Diffuse peritonitis caused by perforation of ileal lymphoma: two case reports and clinicopathological features of 81 cases in Japan. Leuk Lymphoma 2006;47(6):1157–9.
[32] Garwood RA, Sawyer MD, Ledesma EJ, et al. A case and review of bowel perforation secondary to metastatic lung cancer. Am Surg 2005;71(2):110–6.
[33] O'Hanlan KA, Kargas S, Schreiber M, et al. Ovarian carcinoma metastases to gastrointestinal tract appear to spread like colon carcinoma: implication for surgical resection. Gynecol Oncol 1995;59(2):200–6.
[34] Gurleyik E, Gurleyik G. Small bowel volvulus: a common cause of mechanical intestinal obstruction in our region. Eur J Surg 1998;164(1):51–5.
[35] Kimchi NA, Broide E, Shapiro M, et al. Non-traumatic perforation of the small intestine: report of 13 cases and a review of the literature. Hepatogastroenterology 2002;49(46): 1017–22.

[36] Moran BJ. Adhesion-related small bowel obstruction. Colorectal Dis 2007;9(Suppl 2): 39–44.
[37] Attard JA, MacLean AR. Adhesive small bowel obstruction: epidemiology, biology, and prevention. Can J Surg 2001;50(4):291–300.
[38] Graffeo CS, Counselman FS. Appendicitis. Emerg Med Clin North Am 1996;14(4):653–71.
[39] Hatoum OA, Binion DG, Phillips SA, et al. Radiation induced small bowel "web" formation is associated with acquired microvascular dysfunction. Gut 2005;54(12):1797–800.
[40] Oktar SO, Erbas G, Yucel C, et al. Closed perforation of the small bowel secondary to a phytobezoar: imaging findings. Diagn Interv Radiol 2007;13:19–22.
[41] Wig JD, Malik AK, Suri S, et al. Acute segmental enteritis. J Diarrhoeal Dis Res 1984;2(1): 37–40.
[42] Rafferty J, Shellito P, Hyman NH, et al. Practice parameters for sigmoid diverticulitis. Dis Colon Rectum 2006;49:939–44.
[43] Lempinen M, Salmela K, Kemppainen E. Jejunal diverticulosis: a potentially dangerous entity. Scand J Gastroenterol 2004;39(9):905–9.
[44] Hildebrand P, Kropp M, Stellmacher F, et al. Surgery for right-sided colonic diverticulitis: results of a 10-year-observation period. Langenbecks Arch Surg 2007;392:143–7.
[45] Greenstein AJ, Aufses AH Jr. Differences in pathogenesis, incidence, and outcomes of perforation in inflammatory bowel disease. Surg Gynecol Obstet 1985;160(1):63–9.
[46] Itte VN, Mallick IH, Kaur G. An interesting case of acute abdomen: Crohn's disease with perforation. J Gastrointestin Liver Dis 2007;16(2):192, 220.
[47] Ferraro V, Hunt PS. Perforation in Crohn's disease of the small bowel. Med J Aust 1984; 140(2):101–2.
[48] Smith BR, Stabile BE. Emerging trends in peptic ulcer disease and damage control surgery. Am Surg 2005;71:797–801.
[49] Behrman SW. Management of complicated peptic ulcer disease. Arch Surg 2005;140:201–8.
[50] Sarosi GA, Jaiswal KR, Nwariaku FE, et al. Surgical therapy of peptic ulcers in the 21st century: more common than you think. Am J Surg 2005;190:775–9.
[51] Rodriguez-Sanjuan JC, Fernandez-Santiago R, Garcia RA, et al. Perforated peptic ulcer treated by simple closure and helicobacter pylori eradication. World J Surg 2005;29: 849–52.
[52] Okabe S, Amagase K. An overview of acetic acid ulcer models: the history and state of the art of peptic ulcer research. Biol Pharm Bull 2005;28(8):1321–41.
[53] Kashakura Y, Ajani JA, Fugii M, et al. Management of perforated gastric carcinoma: a report of 16 cases and review of world literature. Am Surg 2002;68:434–40.
[54] Ara C, Coban S, Kayaalp C, et al. Spontaneous intestinal perforation due to non-Hodgkin's lymphoma: evaluation of eight cases. Dig Dis Sci 2007;52(8):1752–6.
[55] Yabuki K, Tamasaki Y, Satoh K, et al. Primary gastric lymphoma with spontaneous perforation: report of a case. Surg Today 2000;30(11):1030–3.
[56] de Haan D, van den Berg M. Colonic perforation secondary to taxol therapy: an unusual presentation. Onkologie 2006;29:541–2.
[57] Carter J, Durfee J. A case of bowel perforation after neoadjuvant chemotherapy for advanced epithelial ovarian cancer. Gynecol Oncol 2007;107(3):586–9.
[58] Clevland TJ, Nawaz S, Gaines PA. Mesenteric arterial ischaemia: diagnosis and therapeutic options. Vasc Med 2002;7:311–21.
[59] Bayraktar Y, Harmanci O. Etiology and consequences of thrombosis in abdominal vessels. World J Gastroenterol 2006;12(8):1165–74.
[60] Menon NJ, Amin AM, Mohammed A, et al. Acute mesenteric ischemia. Acta Chir Belg 2005;105(4):344–54.
[61] Ludwig KA, Quebbeman EJ, Bergstein JM, et al. Shock-associated right colon ischemia and necrosis. J Trauma 1995;35(6):1171–4.
[62] Levandoski G, Deitrick JE, Brotman S. Necrosis of the colon as a complication of shock. Am Surg 1998;54(10):621–6.

[63] Hayetian FD, Read TE, Brozovich M, et al. Ileal perforation secondary to Clostridium difficile enteritis. Arch Surg 2006;141:97–9.
[64] Hosoglu S, Aldemir M, Akalin S, et al. Risk factors for enteric perforation in patients with typhoid fever. Am J Epidemiol 2004;160:46–50.
[65] Koss K, Clark A, Sanders DSA, et al. The outcome of surgery in fulminant Clostridium difficile colitis. Colorectal Dis 2005;8:149–54.
[66] Nishii T, Rno Y, Ando K, et al. Successful treatment of multiple small- bowel perforations caused by cytomegalovirus in a patient with malignant lymphoma: report of a case. Surg Today 2006;36(10):930–3.
[67] Ara C, Sogutlu G, Yildiz R, et al. Spontaneous small bowel perforation due to intestinal tuberculosis should not be repaired by simple closure. J Gastrointest Surg 2005;9(4):514–7.
[68] Megarbane B, Resiere D, Ferrand J, et al. Difficulties in assessing cytomegalovirus-associated gastric perforation in an HIV-infected patient. BMC Infect Dis 2005;5(1):28.
[69] Kouame J, Kouadio L, Turquin HT. Typhoid ileal perforation: surgical experience of 64 cases. Acta Chir Belg 2004;104(4):445–7.
[70] Chamberlain RS, Atkins S, Saini N, et al. Ileal perforation caused by cytomegalovirus infection in a critically ill adult. J Clin Gastroenterol 2000;30(4):432–5.
[71] Gerhardt RT, Nelson BK, Keenan S, et al. Derivation of a clinical guideline for the assessment of nonspecific abdominal pain: the guideline for abdominal pain in the ED setting (GAPEDS) phase 1 study. Am J Emerg Med 2005;23:709–17.
[72] Martin RF, Rossi RL. The acute abdomen and overview and algorithms. Surg Clin North Am 1997;77(6):1227–43.
[73] Ramakrishnan K, Salinas RC. Peptic ulcer disease. Am Fam Physician 2007;76(7):1005–12.
[74] Flasar MH, Goldberg E. Acute abdominal pain. Med Clin North Am 2006;90:481–503.
[75] Janes SEJ, Meagher A, Frizelle FA. Management of diverticulitis. BMJ 2006;332:271–5.
[76] Higam J, Kang JY, Majeed A. Recent trends in admissions and mortality due to peptic ulcer in England: increasing frequency of haemorrhage among older subjects. Gut 2002;50: 460–4.
[77] Greenstein AJ, Mann D, Sachar DB, et al. Free perforation in Crohn's disease: 1. A survey of 99 cases. Am J Gastroenterol 1985;80(9):682–9.
[78] Sihler KC, Nathens AB. Management of severe sepsis in surgical patients. Surg Clin North Am 2006;86(6):1457–81.
[79] Taylor S, Watt M. Emergency department assessment of abdominal pain: clinical indicator tests for detecting peritonitis. Eur J Emerg Med 2005;12(6):275–7.
[80] MacKersie AB, Lane MJ, Gerhardt RT, et al. Nontraumatic acute abdominal pain: unenhanced helical CT compared with three-view acute abdominal series. Radiology 2005;239: 114–22.
[81] Butler J. Detection of pneumoperitoneum on erect chest radiograph. Emerg Med J 2002;19: 46–50.
[82] Gupta H, Dupuy D. Advances in imaging of the acute abdomen. Surg Clin North Am 1997; 77(6):1245–63.
[83] Billittier AJ, Abrams BJ, Brunetto A. Radiographic imaging modalities for the patient in the emergency department with abdominal complaints. Emerg Med Clin North Am 1996;14(4):789–850.
[84] Ahn SH, Mayo-Smith WW, Murphy BL, et al. Acute nontraumatic abdominal pain in adult patients: abdominal radiography compared with CT evaluation. Radiology 2002; 225(1):159–64.
[85] Stapakis JP, Thickman D. Diagnosis of pneumoperitoneum: abdominal CT vs. upright chest films. J Comput Assist Tomogr 1992;16(5):713–6.
[86] Miller RE, Nelson SW. The roentgenologic demonstration of tiny amounts of free intraperitoneal gas: experimental and clinical studies. Am J Roentgenol Radium Ther Nucl Med 1971;112(3):574–85.

[87] Winek TG, Mosely HS, Grout G, et al. Pneumoperitoneum and its association with ruptured abdominal viscus. Arch Surg 1988;123:709–12.
[88] Roh JJ, Thompson JS, Harned RK, et al. Value of pneumoperitoneum in the diagnosis of visceral perforation. Am J Surg 1983;146(6):830–3.
[89] Mularski RA, Ciccolo ML, Rappaport WD. Nonsurgical causes of pneumoperitoneum. West J Med 1999;170:41–6.
[90] McGlone FB, Vivion CG, Meir L. Spontaneous pneumoperitoneum. Gastroenterology 1966;51:393–8.
[91] Rowe NM, Kahn FB, Acinapura AJ, et al. Nonsurgical pneumoperitoneum: a case report and a review. Am Surg 1998;64(4):313–22.
[92] Mularski RA, Sippel JM, Osborne ML. Pneumoperitoneum: a review on nonsurgical causes. Crit Care Med 2000;28(7):2638–44.
[93] Schauer PR, Page CP, Ghiatas AA, et al. Incidence and significance of subdiaphragmatic air following laparoscopic cholecystectomy. Am Surg 1997;63(2):132–6.
[94] Mezghebe HM, Leffall LD Jr, Siram SM, et al. Asymptomatic pneumoperitoneum diagnostic and therapeutic dilemma. Am Surg 1994;60(9):691–4.
[95] Johnson EK, Choi YU, Jarrard SW, et al. Pneumoperitoneum after rough sexual intercourse. Am Surg 2002;68:430–3.
[96] Tsushima Y, Yamada S, Aoki J, et al. Effect of contrast-enhanced computed tomography on diagnosis and management of acute abdomen in adults. Clin Radiol 2002;57(6):507–13.
[97] Fishman EK. Spiral CT: applications in the emergency patient. Radiographics 1996;16: 943–8.
[98] Fultz PJ, Skucas J, Weiss SL. CT in upper gastrointestinal tract perforations secondary to peptic ulcer disease. Gastrointest Radiol 1992;17:5–8.
[99] Urban BA, Fishman EK. Tailored helical ct evaluation of acute abdomen. Radiographics 2000;20(3):725–49.
[100] Grobmeyer AJ 3rd, Kerlan RA, Peterson CM, et al. Barium peritonitis. Am Surg 1984; 50(2):116–20.
[101] de Feiter PW, Soeters PB, Dejong CHC. Rectal perforations after barium enema: a review. Dis Colon Rectum 2005;49:261–71.
[102] Chen S, Wang H, Chen W, et al. Selective use of ultrasonography for the detection of pneumoperitoneum. Acad Emerg Med 2002;9:643–5.
[103] Asrani A. Sonographic diagnosis of pneumoperitoneum using the 'enhancement of the peritoneal stripe sign': a prospective study. Emerg Radiol 2007;14:29–39.
[104] Oto A, Ernst RD, Shah R, et al. Right-lower-quadrant pain and suspected appendicitis in pregnant women: evaluation with MR imaging-initial experience. Radiology 2005;234: 445–51.
[105] Blot S, De Waele JJ. Critical issues in the clinical management of complicated intra-abdominal infections. Drugs 2005;65(12):1611–20.
[106] Chong AJ, Dellinger EP. Current treatment of intraabdominal infections. Surg Technol Int 2005;14:29–33.
[107] Auerbach AD, Goldman L. beta-Blockers and the reduction of cardiac events in noncardiac surgery: scientific review. JAMA 2002;287(11):1434–44.
[108] Doyle RL. Assessing and modifying the risk of postoperative pulmonary complications. Chest 1999;115(5 Suppl):77S–81S.
[109] Jenkins I. Evidence-based sepsis therapy: a hospitalist perspective. J Hosp Med 2006;1(5): 285–9.
[110] Farber MS, Abrams JH. Antibiotics for the acute abdomen. Surg Clin North Am 1997; 77(6):1395–417.
[111] Berger D, Buttenschoen K. Management of abdominal sepsis. Arch Surg 1998;383:35–43.
[112] Wong PF, Gilliam AD, Kumar S, et al. Antibiotic regimens for secondary peritonitis of gastrointestinal origin in adults [review]. The Cochrane Library 2007;2:CD004539.

[113] Sotto A, Lefrant JY, Fabbro-Peray P, et al. Evaluation of antimicrobial therapy management of 120 consecutive patients with secondary peritonitis. J Antimicrob Chemother 2002; 50:569–76.
[114] Eggimann P, Francioli P, Bille J, et al. Fluconazole prophylaxis prevents intra-abdominal candidiasis in high-risk surgical patients. Crit Care Med 1999;27:1066–72.
[115] Blot S, Vandewoude K. Management of invasive candidiasis in critically ill patients. Drugs 2004;64:2159–75.
[116] Mazuski JE, Sawyer RG, Mathens AB, et al. The Surgical Infection Society guidelines on antimicrobial therapy for intra-abdominal infections: an executive summary. Surg Infect (Larchmt) 2002;3:161–73.
[117] Memon MA, Fitztgibbons RJ. The role of minimal access surgery in the acute abdomen. Surg Clin North Am 1997;77(6):1333–53.
[118] Golash V, Willson PD. Early laparoscopy as a routine procedure in the management of acute abdominal pain. Surg Endosc 2005;19:882–5.
[119] Navez B, Tassetti V, Scohy JJ, et al. Laparoscopic management of acute peritonitis. Br J Surg 1998;85:32–6.
[120] Mattei P, Alonso M, Justinich C. Laparoscopic repair of colon perforation after colonoscopy in children: report of 2 cases and a review of the literature. J Pediatr Surg 2005; 40(10):1651–3.
[121] Robertson GS, Wemyss-Holden SA, Maddern GJ. Laparoscopic repair of perforated peptic ulcers: the role of laparoscopy in generalized peritonitis. Ann R Coll Surg Engl 2000; 82(1):6–10.
[122] Abbasi HR, Bolandparvaz S, Yarmohammadi H, et al. Experimental evaluation of ileal patch in delayed primary repair of penetrating colon injuries. Asian J Surg 2006;29(4): 223–6.
[123] Kirkpatrick AW, Baxter KA, Simons RK, et al. Intra-abdominal complications after surgical repair of small bowel injuries: an international review. J Trauma 2003;55(3):399–406.
[124] de Graff JS, Van Goor H, Bleichrodt RP. Primary small bowel anastomosis in generalized peritonitis. Eur J Surg 1996;162:55–8.
[125] Nespoli A, Ravazzini C, Trivella M. The choice of surgical procedure for peritonitis due to colonic perforation. Arch Surg 1993;128:814–8.
[126] Wyrzykowski AD, Feliciano DV, George TA, et al. Emergent right hemicolectomies. Am Surg 2005;71(8):653–6.
[127] Kriwanek S, Armbruster C, Beckerhinn P, et al. Prognostic factors for survival in colonic perforation. Int J Colorectal Dis 1994;9:158–62.
[128] Bulkley GB, Zuidema GD, Hamilton SR, et al. Intraoperative determination of small intestinal viability following ischemic injury. Ann Surg 1981;193:628–37.
[129] Redaelli CA, Schilling MK, Buchler MW. Intraoperative laser Doppler flowmetry: a predictor of ischemic injury in acute mesenteric infarction. Dig Surg 1998;15:55–9.
[130] Orland PJ, Cazi GI, Semmlow JL, et al. Determination of small bowel viability using quantitative myoelectrical and color analysis. J Surg Res 1993;55(6):581–7.
[131] Hobsley M, Tovey FI, Holton J. Precise role of H pylori in duodenal ulceration. World J Gastroenterol 2006;12(40):6413–9.
[132] Ng EK, Lam MY, Sung JJ, et al. Eradication of Helicobacter pylori prevents recurrence of ulcer after simple closure of duodenal ulcer perforation: randomized controlled trial. Ann Surg 2000;231:153–8.
[133] Gugler R. Current diagnosis and selection of patients for treatment of peptic ulcer disease. Dig Dis Sci 1985;30(11 Suppl):30S–5S.
[134] Cameron JL. Current surgical therapy. 7th edition. St. Louis: Mosby; 2001.
[135] Roviello F, Simone R, Marrelli D, et al. Perforated gastric carcinoma: a report of 10 cases and review of the literature. World J Surg Oncol 2006;4:19–24.
[136] Jwo S, Chien R, Chao T, et al. Clinicopathalogical features, surgical management, and disease outcome of perforated gastric cancer. J Surg Oncol 2005;91:219–25.

[137] Adachi Y, Mori M, Maehara Y, et al. Surgical results of perforated gastric carcinoma: an analysis of 155 Japanese patients. Am J Gastroenterol 1997;92:516–8.
[138] Lehnert T, Buhl K, Dueck M, et al. Two-stage radical gastrectomy for perforated gastric cancer. Eur J Surg Oncol 2000;26:780–4.
[139] Pine RW, Wertz MJ, Lennard ES, et al. Determinants of organ malfunction or death in patients with intra-abdominal sepsis: a discriminant analysis. Arch Surg 1983;118:242–9.
[140] Dellinger RP, Carlet JM, Masur H, et al. Surviving sepsis and septic shock. Intensive Care Med 2004;30:536–55.
[141] Talmor M, Hydo L, Barie PS. Relationship of systemic inflammatory response syndrome to organ dysfunction, length of stay, and mortality in critical surgical illness. Arch Surg 1999; 134:81–7.
[142] Barker DE, Green JM, Maxwell RA, et al. Experience with vacuum-pack temporary abdominal wound closure in 258 trauma and general and vascular surgical patients. J Am Coll Surg 2007;204:784–93.
[143] De Costa A. Making a virtue of necessity: managing the open abdomen. ANZ J Surg 2006; 76:356–63.
[144] Barker DE, Kaufman HJ, Smith LA, et al. Vacuum pack technique of temporary abdominal closure: a 7-year experience with 112 patients. J Trauma 2000;48(2):201–6.
[145] Jeong G, Lee JH, Yu MK, et al. Non-surgical management of microperforation induced by EMR of the stomach. Dig Liver Dis 2006;38(8):605–8.
[146] Amodio PM, Faggiani R, Pastorelli A, et al. Selected treatments for duodenal perforation after ERCP: a report of three cases. Chir Ital 2007;59(3):343–6.
[147] Sebastian S, Byrne AT, Torreggiani WC, et al. Endoscopic closure of iatrogenic duodenal perforation during endoscopic ultrasound. Endoscopy 2004;36(3):245.
[148] Roses LL, Ramirez AG, Seco AL, et al. Clip closure of a duodenal perforation secondary to a biliary stent. Gastrointest Endosc 2000;51:487–9.
[149] Seibert DG. Use of an endoscopic clipping device to repair a duodenal perforation. Endoscopy 2003;35(2):189.
[150] Kaneko T, Akamatsu T, Shimodaira K, et al. Nonsurgical treatment of duodenal perforation by endoscopic repair using a clipping device. Gastrointest Endosc 1999;50(3):410–3.
[151] Yoshikane H, Hidano H, Sakakibara A, et al. Endoscopic repair by clipping of iatrogenic colonic perforation. Gastrointest Endosc 1997;46(5):464–6.
[152] Altinli E, Saribeyoglu K, Karahasanoglu T, et al. Are clips useful in the surgical repair of colonic perforations? Acta Chir Belg 2005;105(4):410–2.
[153] Matsushita M, Takakuwa H, Nishio A. Endoscopic removal techniques and clipping for closure of chicken bones wedged transversely in the colon. Dis Colon Rectum 2001; 44(5):749–50.
[154] Gleichmann D, Stienecker K, Glaser J. Endoscopic clipping of a gastric perforation after GIST resection. Med Klin (Munich) 2004;99(9):537–9 [in German].
[155] Barbagallo F, Castello G, Latteri S, et al. Successful endoscopic repair of an unusual colonic perforation following polypectomy using an endoclip device. World J Gastroenterol 2007;13(20):2889–91.
[156] Raju GS, Ahmed I, Brining D, et al. Endoluminal closure of large perforations of colon with clips in a porcine model [with video]. Gastrointest Endosc 2006;64(4):640–6.
[157] Hainaux B, Agneessens E, Bertinotti R, et al. Accuracy of MDCT in predicting site of gastrointestinal tract perforation. AJR Am J Roentgenol 2006;187:1179–83.

ELSEVIER
SAUNDERS

Med Clin N Am 92 (2008) 627–647

THE MEDICAL CLINICS OF NORTH AMERICA

# Acute Abdominal Vascular Emergencies

Charles J. Shanley, MD, FACS*,
Jeffrey B. Weinberger, MD

*Department of Surgery, William Beaumont Hospital, 3601 West Thirteen Mile Road, Royal Oak, MI 48073, USA*

Abdominal vascular emergencies are relatively uncommon, frequently catastrophic, and highly lethal. Despite improved understanding of the pathophysiology and natural history of these disorders, delays in diagnosis and treatment remain the most important factors contributing to the observed high mortality. Although diagnostic imaging may confirm the diagnosis or help plan the surgery, it is important to remain clinically vigilant because an initially stable patient can rapidly deteriorate. Despite the complexities of clinical management, preoperative decision making is generally straightforward. For a suspected abdominal vascular emergency, the advantage of delaying intervention to obtain confirmatory diagnostic tests and for extensive preoperative resuscitation is outweighed by the risk for fatal massive intestinal necrosis or exsanguination. When an abdominal vascular catastrophe is clinically suspected, therefore, the presence of a competent surgeon and an available suitably equipped operating room are generally the only prerequisites to proceed with intervention. In these situations, the consequence of further delays in treatment perforce outweighs the probability of finding new, clinically useful information through additional diagnostic tests or the benefits of further emergency resuscitation. Treatment delays are also generally more costly in patients who have multiple comorbidities and poor physiologic reserve. Any delay should be undertaken in consultation with the surgeon who is ultimately responsible for the care of the patient. More patients die of not receiving an emergency operation to stop hemorrhage or to restore intestinal perfusion, than die of a negative laparotomy. A high index of clinical suspicion together with a sound understanding of the clinical presentation, natural history, and management of these disorders are critical to improving outcomes. This

* Corresponding author.
*E-mail address:* cshanley@beaumont.edu (C.J. Shanley).


doi:10.1016/j.mcna.2008.01.004 *medical.theclinics.com*

article focuses on abdominal vascular emergencies presenting with acute visceral ischemia or catastrophic intra-abdominal hemorrhage (Table 1).

## Abdominal vascular emergencies: acute visceral ischemia

### *Acute embolic mesenteric ischemia*

Acute embolic occlusion of the superior mesenteric artery (SMA) remains a catastrophic vascular disorder with a mortality exceeding 50% [1–6]. Delayed diagnosis and treatment leading to intestinal necrosis and infarction is responsible for this high mortality. The classic presentation is the sudden onset of severe abdominal pain out of proportion to the physical findings and often accompanied by abrupt emptying of the gut with vomiting or diarrhea. Bloody diarrhea, peritonitis, and sepsis are late findings associated with transmural intestinal ischemia and infarction; they portend a poor outcome.

Cardiogenic emboli underlie most cases. Risk factors include atrial fibrillation, recent myocardial infarction, ventricular aneurysm, prosthetic heart valve, and rheumatic heart disease. Synchronous emboli to the brain or extremities are not uncommon. A complete neurologic and peripheral vascular examination is imperative in these patients. Although many patients have prior cardiac or atherosclerotic diseases, few patients have antecedent symptoms of chronic mesenteric ischemia, such as postprandial abdominal pain or weight loss.

The differential diagnosis of the acute onset of severe abdominal pain includes perforated ulcer, intestinal obstruction, acute pancreatitis, acute cholecystitis, and nephrolithiasis. Laboratory findings are nonspecific but may include hemoconcentration, leukocytosis, hyperamylasemia, metabolic acidosis, hyperkalemia, and azotemia. The most common finding on plain abdominal radiography is adynamic ileus; however, plain radiography may help exclude other causes of acute abdominal pain, such as intestinal obstruction, perforation, or volvulus. Pneumoperitoneum, pneumatosis intestinalis, and portal venous gas are suggestive of bowel infarction. Gastrointestinal endoscopy and barium radiography are of limited diagnostic usefulness and are potentially deleterious for suspected acute embolic mesenteric ischemia. Diagnostic testing in these patients is generally nonspecific and should not delay operative intervention when acute embolic mesenteric ischemia is strongly suspected.

Biplanar mesenteric arteriography remains the gold standard when the diagnosis is unclear. The ubiquity of helical CT has, however, led to increased focus on this modality [7,8]. The oblique origin of the SMA from the aorta helps explain the predilection of emboli for this vessel. Most emboli lodge distal to the proximal jejunal and middle colic branches. The classic angiographic finding is an abrupt cut-off of the SMA (meniscus sign) several centimeters beyond its origin from the abdominal aorta and just distal to the origin of the middle colic artery. Emboli less commonly lodge at the ostium of the SMA or in the distal mesenteric arterial arcades.

Optimal outcomes depend on a high index of clinical suspicion and on prompt revascularization. Once the diagnosis is considered, initial management is centered on fluid resuscitation and systemic anticoagulation to prevent thrombus propagation. In addition to placement of a urinary catheter to continuously monitor urine output, central venous and peripheral arterial access should be considered for hemodynamic monitoring and blood sampling. Broad-spectrum antibiotics with activity against enteric Gram-negative and anaerobic bacteria are standardly administered. Severe acidosis, unresponsive to adequate fluid resuscitation, may require administration of sodium bicarbonate.

The primary goal of therapy is rapid restoration of mesenteric blood flow to prevent intestinal infarction. The treatment of choice is exploratory laparotomy with open surgical embolectomy [3,5,6,9]. Although endovascular techniques and pharmacologic agents are undoubtedly helpful in selected circumstances, these therapies must be considered supportive until more prospective evidence is available [10,11]. Depending on the delay from symptom onset to surgical exploration, findings at laparotomy include variable degrees of midgut ischemia potentially extending distally to the ascending and proximal transverse colon. Sparing of the proximal jejunum is common owing to the typical location of the embolus beyond the proximal jejunal branches of the SMA. At surgery, the SMA is isolated at the base of the transverse mesocolon as it emerges from beneath the pancreas to cross the third portion of the duodenum. A standard surgical embolectomy is performed and mesenteric blood flow is assessed at the antimesenteric intestinal border using continuous-wave Doppler ultrasonography. Only clearly nonviable, necrotic intestine is resected at the initial laparotomy. If intestinal viability remains questionable following restoration of mesenteric blood flow, a second-look laparotomy is performed 24 to 48 hours after the embolectomy and as often as necessary thereafter until all nonviable intestine is resected.

### *Acute thrombotic mesenteric ischemia*

Acute mesenteric arterial thrombosis from severe atherosclerosis is another uncommon but potentially lethal abdominal vascular emergency. Despite the high frequency of asymptomatic chronic visceral artery atherosclerosis, progression to symptomatic acute mesenteric ischemia is relatively uncommon [12,13]. The typical patient is a woman who has a history of heavy tobacco use and hypertension. Most patients have postprandial abdominal pain (abdominal angina) and weight loss. The pain characteristically begins within one hour after eating and lasts for several hours. The associated weight loss may exceed 20 pounds.

Thrombotic occlusion of the SMA in the patient who has chronic mesenteric ischemia from atherosclerosis is frequently caused by intravascular

Table 1
Acute abdominal vascular emergencies

| Disease | Risk factors | Clinical presentation | Diagnosis | Treatment |
|---|---|---|---|---|
| Acute embolic mesenteric ischemia | Atrial fibrillation, recent myocardial infarction, ventricular aneurysm, valvular heart disease | Abdominal pain out of proportion to physical findings, evacuation of GI tract (vomiting, diarrhea), peritonitis late (infarction, perforation) | Clinical suspicion, arteriography | Systemic anticoagulation, supportive care, emergent laparotomy, surgical embolectomy, limited bowel resection (nonviable, perforated), second-look laparotomy, thrombolysis/endovascular treatments rare |
| Acute thrombotic mesenteric ischemia | Chronic mesenteric ischemia, smoking, hypertension, hyperlipidemia | Chronic postprandial abdominal pain and weight loss, acute pain out of proportion to physical findings, peritonitis late (infarction, perforation) | Clinical suspicion, arteriography | Systemic anticoagulation, supportive care, emergent laparotomy with revascularization, limited bowel resection (nonviable, perforated), second-look laparotomy, thrombolysis/endovascular treatments rare |
| Mesenteric venous thrombosis | Primary (idiopathic); secondary: polycythemia vera, hypercoagulable states, malignancy, intra-abdominal inflammation, history of VTE, alcoholism, cirrhosis | Vague abdominal pain, anorexia, nausea, vomiting, distention, ascites, peritonitis late (infarction, perforation) | Clinical suspicion, CT, MRI, duplex ultrasound | Systemic anticoagulation, supportive care, laparotomy only if peritonitis (infarction, perforation); limited bowel resection (nonviable, perforated), second-look laparotomy, rarely surgical thrombectomy, thrombolysis |

| | | | | |
|---|---|---|---|---|
| Nonocclusive mesenteric ischemia (NOMI) | Low cardiac output states (MI, cardiogenic shock, severe CHF), dehydration, digitalis glycosides, high-dose vasopressors | Variable abdominal pain, progressive acidosis, abdominal distention, oliguria, hypotension | Clinical suspicion, arteriography, echocardiography | Systemic anticoagulation, supportive care, direct arterial vasodilators, laparotomy only if peritonitis (infarction, perforation) |
| Abdominal aortic dissection | Smoking, hypertension, atherosclerosis, hyperlipidemia, connective tissue disorders, cocaine or amphetamine abuse, pregnancy, iatrogenic aortic manipulation | Variable abdominal pain, progressive acidosis, abdominal distention, oliguria | Clinical suspicion, CT, MRI, duplex/intravascular ultrasound, arteriography | Aortic reconstruction (Type I, II), endovascular fenestration, stenting |
| Ruptured AAA | Age, male gender, smoking, hypertension, hyperlipidemia, family history, known AAA | Back or abdominal pain, pulsatile abdominal mass, hypotension, diminished pulses | Clinical suspicion, rarely CT, ultrasound | Emergency laparotomy with aortic reconstruction, EVAR (protocol only) |
| Ruptured visceral artery aneurysm | Female gender, pregnancy, medial fibrodysplasia (splenic, renal), male gender (hepatic, celiac, mesenteric), necrotizing pancreatitis (splenic, gastroduodenal, pancreaticoduodenal) | Abdominal pain, abdominal apoplexy (hypovolemic shock), massive gastrointestinal hemorrhage (hemobilia, hemosuccus pancreaticus) | Clinical suspicion, female gender/pregnancy, arteriography, CT, MRI, ultrasound | Abdominal apoplexy (emergency laparotomy with ligation, exclusion and revascularization if needed); may require hepatectomy (hepatic), pancreatectomy (splenic, pancreatic, pancreaticoduodenal), bowel resection (mesenteric), splenectomy (distal splenic), possible endovascular embolization/exclusion (if stable) |

*Abbreviations:* AAA, abdominal aortic aneurysm; CHF, congestive heart failure; EVAR, endovascular aneurysm repair; GI, gastrointestinal; MI, myocardial infarction; VTE, venous thromboembolism.

volume depletion from dehydration. This dehydration can occur from diarrhea or vomiting from benign or malignant gastrointestinal diseases, postoperative fluid losses, or intra-abdominal inflammatory processes, such as acute pancreatitis. Hypotension from a low flow state, such as congestive heart failure or myocardial infarction, can also precipitate thrombosis of a stenotic visceral artery. Failure to consider acute thrombosis in a patient presenting with chronic abdominal pain from mesenteric ischemia often leads to delayed diagnosis with resultant intestinal necrosis leading to a progressive increase in fluid requirements, abdominal distention, oliguria, and metabolic acidosis.

Because of the exceedingly high mortality of visceral infarction, patients who have a history of postprandial pain and weight loss who present with an acute exacerbation of abdominal pain should undergo prompt biplanar aortography [13–19]. Duplex ultrasound, despite a clear diagnostic role in the evaluation of chronic mesenteric ischemia, has limited usefulness in suspected acute thrombosis [20,21]. Arteriography is useful to confirm the diagnosis and to provide the anatomic details to plan for surgery. Arteriography frequently demonstrates extensive atherosclerosis or occlusion of the celiac and superior mesenteric arteries near their origins from the aorta, and the presence of well-developed collaterals [12,13]. The inferior mesenteric artery may be chronically occluded or provide significant mesenteric collateral flow by way of central anastomotic arcades. Despite these advantages, arteriography should not delay surgery when impending intestinal infarction is clinically suspected.

Many of these patients are nutritionally debilitated, volume contracted, and anemic, with markedly reduced physiologic reserve. An aggressive approach to resuscitation and hemodynamic monitoring is strongly encouraged, but should not delay surgery. Arterial and pulmonary artery catheters are used liberally to guide fluid resuscitation and perioperative management. Patients who have a delayed presentation should undergo surgery expeditiously because of a high risk for intestinal infarction.

Open surgical revascularization is generally the treatment of choice [13–19]. The goals of surgical therapy are to restore mesenteric blood flow, assess intestinal viability, and resect nonviable or necrotic intestine. Endarterectomy or antegrade multivessel bypass using a prosthetic conduit are the revascularization procedures of choice in the absence of enteric contamination. When overt intestinal necrosis or perforation is present, a retrograde, single-vessel revascularization of the SMA with an autogenous saphenous vein conduit is expeditious and lifesaving.

Endovascular treatments, such as thrombolysis, are generally avoided owing to the urgent need to restore intestinal perfusion and prevent intestinal infarction. Thrombolysis has been successfully used in this setting, however [22–26]. Intra-arterial administration of thrombolytic agents has effectively restored mesenteric blood flow in selected patients when administered within hours of symptom onset [10,11]. Successful thrombolysis facilitates identification of the underlying occlusive process, and can guide operative revascularization or balloon angioplasty and stent placement. Potential drawbacks include the inability to assess intestinal viability and the time delay for catheter-based thrombolysis and revascularization. Delaying definitive revascularization may predispose to death from massive midgut infarction in these patients. Catheter-directed thrombolysis and endovascular therapy should thus be undertaken by experienced interventionalists in highly selected patients only under a well-established protocol.

*Acute mesenteric venous thrombosis*

Mesenteric venous thrombosis is another uncommon abdominal vascular emergency that can cause acute visceral ischemia. Acute, fulminant mesenteric venous thrombosis has a mortality of up to 50% [27–32]. Mesenteric venous thrombosis is distinctly uncommon, comprising less than 15% of all cases of mesenteric ischemia. Most cases of mesenteric venous thrombosis involve the superior mesenteric vein. The portal or splenic veins are much less frequently involved. Mesenteric venous thrombosis is described as primary or idiopathic when it occurs spontaneously [33]. Mesenteric venous thrombosis is secondary to a known hypercoagulable disorder in up to 50% of cases [33–39]. Commonly associated conditions include polycythemia vera, neoplasms, and heparin-induced thrombocytopenia.

The onset of mesenteric venous thrombosis is often subacute and manifested by dull abdominal pain, anorexia, distention, vomiting, and diarrhea. Patients infrequently present with gastrointestinal bleeding or ascites. Although the presentation is frequently insidious, patients occasionally have an acute and fulminant course that mimics acute arterial mesenteric ischemia. Acute peritonitis is a poor prognostic sign that signifies transmural intestinal necrosis and infarction.

Plain radiography and routine laboratory studies are nonspecific for the diagnosis. Computed tomography is the diagnostic procedure of choice, with a near 100% sensitivity [40–42]. The most common finding is the presence of a hypodense thrombus in the superior mesenteric vein (target sign); other findings include bowel wall edema, pneumatosis intestinalis, and stranding of the mesentery. Portal venous gas suggests bowel infarction. Mesenteric venous duplex has a reported sensitivity of 80% when performed early, and may become a useful screening technique. MRI has similar sensitivity and specificity to CT, without the risk for contrast-induced nephropathy.

Nonoperative management is the mainstay of therapy for most patients [27–32]. Prompt fluid resuscitation, administration of broad-spectrum antibiotics, and immediate systemic anticoagulation to prevent propagation of the existing thrombus along with close clinical observation for signs of peritonitis are generally the most appropriate management. Exploratory laparotomy is reserved for patients who have acute peritonitis or clinical deterioration suggestive of intestinal necrosis or perforation. At exploration, determination of bowel viability can be difficult. Only clearly nonviable or perforated intestine should be resected at the initial laparotomy. One or more second-look laparotomies are frequently necessary to preserve as much viable intestine as possible [43]. Thrombectomy of the superior mesenteric vein and thrombolytic therapy entail high rates of failure and complications [27–32,44]. Reports of success are presently anecdotal. In the absence of prospective data demonstrating efficacy, these modalities should be limited to highly selected cases at experienced centers. Despite anticoagulation and supportive therapy, the in-hospital mortality for acute mesenteric venous thrombosis approaches 50% related to the high rate of recurrence despite anticoagulation.

### *Acute nonocclusive mesenteric ischemia*

Acute nonocclusive mesenteric ischemia (NOMI) is characterized by a low flow state resulting in arterial insufficiency from mesenteric arterial vasospasm. NOMI most commonly occurs in elderly patients who have a history of severe congestive heart failure; myocardial infarction with cardiogenic shock; severe hypovolemic, septic, or hemorrhagic shock; and necrotizing pancreatitis [45–50]. Administration of digitalis glycosides and high-dose alpha agonists has also been associated with NOMI [11,46,48,49,51]. Patients who have NOMI do not universally present with acute abdominal pain. When present, abdominal pain may be variable in character, intensity, and location, further confounding the clinical diagnosis. Abdominal distention, progressive systemic acidosis, and peritonitis may therefore be the only clinical signs of intestinal infarction necessitating a high index of clinical suspicion for NOMI in high-risk patients.

Laboratory evaluation and plain abdominal radiography are relatively nonspecific. Pneumoperitoneum, pneumatosis intestinalis, and portal vein gas are suggestive of intestinal infarction. Mesenteric angiography is usually highly important for the diagnosis and therapy. Arteriographic findings include segmental vasospasm (pruning) in the peripheral distribution of the SMA, whereas the proximal SMA is relatively normal in appearance.

Optimal outcomes depend on a high index of suspicion, adequate resuscitation, and prompt arteriography. Treatment of NOMI is largely supportive and nonoperative. Catheter-based directed arterial infusion of papaverine at 30 to 60 mg/h is initiated, vasoconstrictor agents are discontinued, and broad-spectrum antibiotics are administered [3,11,46–50]. Systemic anticoagulation to prevent thrombosis of the proximal SMA at the site of cannulation and in the distal mesenteric arcades is immediately initiated. The patient is returned to the ICU for hemodynamic monitoring and supportive therapy to correct the underlying low cardiac output. The patient is monitored closely for symptomatic improvement. Serial arteriography can be obtained to monitor resolution of the vasospasm. Laparotomy with resection of nonviable intestine is performed if the patient develops signs of peritonitis or worsening sepsis suggestive of intestinal necrosis or perforation. At laparotomy, the principles of surgery are identical to those described for other forms of mesenteric ischemia. Until recently, the mortality of NOMI approached 100% owing to the advanced age of the patients and the number and severity of the underlying comorbidities causing the low flow state; however, the mortality has recently declined with use of afterload-reducing agents and vasodilators [11]. A high index of suspicion coupled with prompt diagnosis and aggressive supportive therapy provide the best outcomes.

### *Acute aortic dissection*

The mortality of acute aortic dissection, complicated by visceral ischemia, exceeds 50% [52,53]. The classic pathophysiology of aortic dissection is acute hemorrhage within the aortic media originating from a tear in the intima (entry tear) originating somewhere between the aortic root and the proximal one third of the descending thoracic aorta. The medial hemorrhage (dissection) extends both circumferentially and distally. In classic aortic dissection, the native aortic lumen (true lumen) collapses and the channel created within the outer media by the dissecting hemorrhage (false lumen) expands. Circumferential and distal extension of the medial hemorrhage creates the intervening septum (intimal flap) and the classic "double barrel" appearance of the acutely dissected aorta on cross-sectional imaging. Obstruction of major branch arteries with acute visceral ischemia can occur by way of the following mechanisms [53–55]: (1) Direct or "static" obstruction caused by extension of the intimal flap into the origin of a major branch artery, compromising or completely obstructing blood flow and possibly leading to thrombosis. (2) Indirect or "dynamic" obstruction caused by collapse (or prolapse) of the intimal flap during the cardiac cycle. Collapse of the proximal aortic lumen by the intimal flap can cause visceral ischemia by reducing aortic perfusion distally or by prolapse of an intimal flap across the origin of a major visceral branch artery.

Acute visceral ischemia from aortic dissection is difficult to recognize clinically. A high index of suspicion is necessary to avoid visceral infarction. The diagnosis is often confirmed by a combination of dynamic cross-sectional imaging with CT or MRI, and conventional contrast arteriography, along with measurement of pressure gradients between the branch arteries and the true and false lumens of the aortic dissection.

Fortunately, in type I/II aortic dissections, where the entry tear or the medial dissection involves the ascending aorta, static and dynamic obstructions of the visceral branch arteries usually disappear after direct aortic reconstruction. Various catheter-based endovascular treatments are employed to restore visceral perfusion in patients who have visceral ischemia from type III aortic dissection, where the entry tear and dissection is confined to the descending thoracic and abdominal aorta; in patients who have type I/II aortic dissection where branch artery obstruction persists after successful aortic reconstruction; or in patients where aortic reconstruction is contraindicated [52–55]. Static or fixed (stenotic) obstructions usually require placement of a stent. Dynamic obstructions may involve aortic fenestration to equalize pressures between the true and false lumen together with stent placement to restore visceral perfusion. The surgical management of visceral ischemic complications of intestinal infarction or perforation is identical to that described for acute mesenteric ischemia.

## Abdominal vascular emergencies presenting with catastrophic hemorrhage

### *Ruptured abdominal aortic aneurysm*

Rupture of an abdominal aortic aneurysm is the 10th leading cause of death in the United States, making this entity the most common, highly lethal hemorrhagic abdominal vascular emergency. Moreover, the prevalence of abdominal aortic aneurysm will increase in the coming decades because of the aging population of the United States [56–58]. Despite significant advances in perioperative care during the past 4 decades, the mortality of this rupture continues to range from 40% to 70% [59–61]. Moreover, the mortality of an aneurysm that ruptures out-of-hospital is substantially higher. Without an effective preventive or medical treatment of this disease, population-based screening and elective surgical repair remain the most effective strategies to reduce the overall mortality. A high index of clinical suspicion and prompt surgery remain the only effective strategies to improve clinical outcomes for the foreseeable future.

Ninety-five percent of abdominal aortic aneurysms are infrarenal, with a smaller percentage extending proximally to involve the renal and visceral vessels. Degenerative abdominal aortic aneurysms were classically associated with severe atherosclerosis of the aorta and iliac vessels, with approximately 5% classified as inflammatory or infected [56–62]. Age, tobacco use, male gender, hypertension, hyperlipidemia, peripheral vascular disease, myocardial infarction, and family history of abdominal aortic aneurysm are risk factors. Recent data suggest that the cause of abdominal aortic aneurysm is multifactorial, with contributions from a constellation of genetic, metabolic, extracellular matrix, and inflammatory mechanisms [62–69].

The risk for rupture of an abdominal aortic aneurysm strongly correlates with aneurysm diameter [70–73]. For example, the risk for rupture is less than 1% annually for aneurysms less than 4 cm in maximal diameter, but increases to approximately 5% annually if the diameter exceeds 5 cm, and may be as high as 30% to 40% annually for aneurysms exceeding 8 cm in diameter. Although aneurysms on average slowly expand at 0.2 to 0.3 cm per annum, aneurysm growth in individuals is rarely linear. The presence of symptoms, such as abdominal or back pain, or the presence of risk factors, such as female gender, diastolic hypertension, and chronic obstructive pulmonary disease, increase the risk for rupture even for small aneurysms

[70–73]. Irrespective of aneurysm diameter, a high index of suspicion of aneurysm rupture is thus highly important.

The most common presenting symptom of a symptomatic or ruptured abdominal aortic aneurysm is the acute onset of persistent abdominal or back pain. The pain is quite variable in character, and it may radiate to the flank, groin, or genitalia. The pain is occasionally associated with syncope or near syncope. The classic clinical triad of abdominal or back pain, an expansile abdominal mass, and hypotension, although highly variable, is pathognomonic. A pulsatile abdominal mass can be difficult to appreciate in an obese patient or in a patient who has significant abdominal distension from hemoperitoneum. The extremities may be warm and well perfused or may be cool and cyanotic with absent pulses depending on the degree of hemorrhage. Hypotension and tachycardia with a suspected ruptured abdominal aortic aneurysm suggest major blood loss and mandate emergency surgery to prevent fatal exsanguinating hemorrhage.

The differential diagnosis of severe abdominal or back pain includes a wide spectrum of intra-abdominal pathology. Unfortunately, diagnostic investigation is often nonspecific and may result in unnecessary and potentially fatal treatment delays in patients who have symptomatic or ruptured abdominal aortic aneurysm.

Emergent surgical repair is the only effective treatment. Exploratory laparotomy with aortic cross-clamping to control hemorrhage and prosthetic graft reconstruction has been performed for more than 50 years with an operative mortality of 40% to 60% [57,59–61]. In contrast, emergency repair of symptomatic, but intact, abdominal aortic aneurysm carries a mortality of 15% to 20%, and elective repair of abdominal aortic aneurysm carries a mortality of 1% to 4% at high-volume centers.

Endovascular aneurysm repair has revolutionized the elective treatment of abdominal aortic aneurysm and markedly decreased the early morbidity from laparotomy. Early studies on endovascular repair in selected patients have suggested improved morbidity and mortality, including reductions in pulmonary, renal, and bleeding complications, and reductions in hospital length of stay [74–78]. Endovascular treatment is appropriate for only highly selected, hemodynamically stable patients, however. The single most important management principle is prompt control of intra-abdominal hemorrhage. For this reason, the adverse consequences of delay in patients presenting with exsanguinating hemorrhage attributable to ruptured abdominal aortic aneurysm applies to endovascular treatment. Until more prospective data are available, endovascular aneurysm repair for aneurysm rupture should be limited to highly experienced centers with well-established imaging and treatment protocols.

### *Visceral artery aneurysms*

Compared with ruptured abdominal aortic aneurysms, visceral artery aneurysms are extremely uncommon abdominal vascular emergencies. The ubiquity of advanced diagnostic imaging suggests a recent trend toward increasing detection of asymptomatic visceral artery aneurysms [79–81] This trend is a positive development because previously reported series of visceral aneurysms reported a mortality of up to 70% [82–88] The rarity of these aneurysms is underscored by the prevalence in the literature of small single-institution series and isolated case reports, suggesting a bias in the reported literature toward extraordinary clinical presentations and positive clinical outcomes. The risk for catastrophic bleeding from a ruptured visceral artery aneurysm mandates clinical vigilance and an aggressive approach to their diagnosis and treatment.

The senior author has published several reviews on this subject, which form the basis of the following review [82–84]. The traditionally reported distribution of visceral artery aneurysms are: splenic (60%), hepatic (20%), superior mesenteric (5.5%), celiac (4%), gastric and gastroepiploic (4%), jejunal and ileocolic (3%), pancreaticoduodenal and pancreatic (2%), gastroduodenal (1.5%), and inferior mesenteric (<1%) [85–87]. Although the epidemiology and natural history of these aneurysms have probably not recently changed, a series of recent reviews by the senior author suggested that false aneurysms of the hepatic arteries may be the most frequently currently reported visceral artery aneurysm [82–88]. This frequency of reporting relates to increased percutaneous diagnostic and therapeutic biliary procedures and ubiquitous use of CT and MRI that has led to increased detection of posttraumatic false aneurysms of intrahepatic arterial branches.

### *Splenic artery aneurysm*

Traditionally, the most commonly reported visceral artery aneurysms involved the splenic artery (60% of cases). Splenic artery aneurysms are much more common in women. They typically present in the sixth decade. Risk factors include multiple pregnancies, medial fibrodysplasia, portal hypertension, splenomegaly, and previous liver transplantation. Most are small (<2.0 cm) and saccular. More than 80% are located in the middle or distal splenic artery. Calcific atherosclerosis and inflammation are prominent pathologic features of longstanding splenic artery aneurysms. Atherosclerotic changes are usually limited to the region of the aneurysm and are believed to be a secondary feature. Calcification is no longer believed to portend a higher risk for rupture. Perivascular inflammation from pancreatitis and pseudocyst formation may result in a splenic artery pseudoaneurysm in up to 10% of patients who have necrotizing pancreatitis. Inflammation and infection attributable to bacterial endocarditis and inflammation attributable to vasculitis are other causes.

Most patients are asymptomatic, and most aneurysms are detected incidentally on diagnostic studies undertaken for other indications. A classic presentation in an asymptomatic patient is the appearance of curvilinear or signet ring–shaped calcifications in the left upper quadrant of an abdominal radiograph. Up to 20% of patients in a large series had symptoms, usually of epigastric or left upper quadrant abdominal pain.

The risk for aneurysm rupture has been reported as 10%, but the risk is probably much lower in the population at large. Mortality after aneurysm rupture is as high as 33%. Rupture may cause severe abdominal pain and hemorrhagic shock. Bleeding may be confined to the lesser sac initially, resulting in a period of clinical stabilization and an opportunity for intervention. Eventually the hemorrhage escapes from the lesser sac into the free peritoneal cavity either through the foramen of Winslow or rupture of the pars flaccida, the so-called "double-rupture" phenomenon. Rarely, the aneurysm may erode into the pancreatic duct, leading to hematobilia or hemosuccus pancreaticus. Occasionally, splenic artery aneurysms erode into the adjacent splenic vein resulting in an arteriovenous fistula [82,84–89].

Treatment of asymptomatic splenic artery aneurysms is recommended for all good-risk patients who have relatively large aneurysms (>2.0 cm). Poor-risk asymptomatic patients, particularly those who have small aneurysms (<2.0 cm), can be managed expectantly. Stanley and colleagues recommend elective operation for asymptomatic patients if the predicted surgical mortality is less than 0.5%. A splenic artery aneurysm in a woman of childbearing age is an exception. Most splenic artery aneurysms discovered during pregnancy are ruptured (95%) with concomitant maternal mortality of 70% and fetal mortality of 95% [90,91].

Increasingly, endovascular approaches, including catheter-based embolization or covered stent placement, are becoming the dominant approach to the elective management of these lesions, especially in high-risk elderly patients and those who have portal hypertension [92].

Urgent treatment is recommended for symptomatic patients, pregnant women, or women of childbearing age and for patients who have pseudoaneurysms associated with inflammatory processes. Standard surgical treatment includes aneurysm resection or ligation/exclusion. Distal or hilar splenic artery aneurysms may require splenectomy.

### *Hepatic artery aneurysm*

Intrahepatic false aneurysms now account for nearly 50% of reported hepatic artery aneurysms. Historically, medial degeneration, trauma, and mycotic aneurysms were the most commonly reported causes of hepatic artery aneurysms, with approximately equal frequencies. Uncommon causes include vasculitides, such as polyarteritis nodosa, or periarterial inflammation caused by cholecystitis or pancreatitis. Atherosclerosis is present in up to 30% of such lesions, but is believed to be a secondary process. Traditionally, more than 80% of spontaneous hepatic artery aneurysms were extrahepatic. Most of these aneurysms were solitary and were located in the common hepatic or right hepatic arteries. Increased reporting of intrahepatic false aneurysms after trauma or iatrogenic injury has recently changed the relative frequencies of intrahepatic and extrahepatic aneurysms [82,84–88].

Hepatic artery aneurysms are more common in men. Most are asymptomatic at presentation, noted incidentally on a diagnostic study undertaken for a different reason. Large aneurysms may present with a pulsatile mass or an abdominal bruit, but usually the physical examination is unrevealing. In symptomatic patients, right upper quadrant or epigastric abdominal pain is the most common symptom [93,94]. Up to 10% have obstructive jaundice from extrinsic compression of the bile duct by the aneurysm. Gastrointestinal hemorrhage or hematobilia occur in nearly 50% of symptomatic patients.

Rupture occurs in less than 20% of patients. It often presents with hypovolemic shock secondary to free intraperitoneal hemorrhage or massive gastrointestinal bleeding. Extrahepatic artery aneurysms may rupture into the peritoneal cavity and cause exsanguinating hemorrhage. Intrahepatic and occasionally extrahepatic aneurysms may rupture into the hepatobiliary system leading to the classic triad of biliary colic, hematobilia, and jaundice. Ruptured hepatic artery aneurysms have an approximately 35% mortality [82,84–88].

Surgical treatment depends on the aneurysm location and the regional vascular anatomy. Intrahepatic aneurysms require individualized treatment. Large proximal aneurysms may require liver resection. For an extrahepatic aneurysm, restoration of arterial continuity can be achieved by aneurysmorrhaphy or by resection and interposition or bypass grafting. Catheter-based endovascular approaches, including embolization and endograft exclusion, are increasingly common and frequently preferable to open surgical intervention for complex hepatic artery aneurysms [93–96].

### *Superior mesenteric artery aneurysm*

SMA aneurysms account for 5.5% of visceral artery aneurysms. Up to one third of reported aneurysms involving the SMA are mycotic. Other causes include medial degeneration associated with atherosclerosis (25%), aortic dissection, and false aneurysms associated with trauma or inflammatory processes, such as pancreatitis or biliary tract disease (12%). Most cases occur in males younger than 50 years of age.

More than 90% of patients have symptoms, usually moderate to severe abdominal pain and a palpable mass. These aneurysms often present as abdominal vascular emergencies from either mesenteric ischemia in the case of thrombosis or from exsanguinating intra-abdominal hemorrhage in the case of rupture. The mortality of aneurysm rupture approaches 30%. In the presence of extensive infection or inflammation, simple ligation or exclusion may be indicated assuming that adequate collateral flow is demonstrated. When the aneurysm is not infected and there is no intestinal ischemia, a synthetic bypass graft can be safely performed. In the presence of an infected aneurysm or intestinal ischemia, a saphenous vein bypass graft or reimplantation into the infrarenal abdominal aorta may be necessary. Endovascular approaches, including embolization and exclusion with stent graft devices, are appealing because of the formidable technical challenges of surgery for these lesions. Extensive local inflammation and infection increase the likelihood of technical failure of endovascular approaches [4,82–88,93–97].

*Celiac artery aneurysm*

Celiac artery aneurysms represent approximately 4% of visceral artery aneurysms. They present most frequently in the sixth decade, and are more common in men. The most common pathologic finding is medial degeneration and atherosclerosis. False aneurysms caused by penetrating trauma, aortic dissection, and mycotic aneurysms have also been reported. In up to 40% of cases an abdominal aortic, visceral, or peripheral artery aneurysm is also present.

Most celiac artery aneurysms are asymptomatic or incidental findings on diagnostic imaging undertaken for other purposes. Symptomatic aneurysms may present with epigastric abdominal pain, a pulsatile mass, or an abdominal bruit. The acute onset of worsening abdominal pain can indicate acute aneurysm expansion. Gastrointestinal hemorrhage, jaundice, and hemoptysis have also been reported. The risk for rupture has been estimated at 13%, with an exceedingly high associated mortality. Surgical options include ligation, aneurysmorrhaphy, or resection with or without revascularization. Endovascular approaches are less common because of the need to occlude the branch hepatic, splenic, and left gastric arteries, but can be considered in selected high-risk patients [4,82,84–88,95,96,98,99].

*Pancreaticoduodenal and gastroduodenal artery aneurysms*

Aneurysms of the pancreaticoduodenal and gastroduodenal arteries are extremely uncommon, accounting for approximately 3% of visceral artery aneurysms. These aneurysms typically occur as a complication of acute necrotizing pancreatitis or from erosion by an expanding pancreatic pseudocyst. Owing to the association with acute and chronic pancreatitis, they are most commonly reported in men in the fifth decade, and most are symptomatic at the time of diagnosis. Abdominal pain is the most common symptom. It is often difficult to determine whether the pain is secondary to acute or chronic pancreatitis versus the aneurysm. Aneurysm rupture or erosion into the adjacent gastrointestinal tract is present at the time of diagnosis in more than 50% of cases, whereas free intraperitoneal bleeding is present in approximately 15%. The mortality with rupture ranges from 25% to 50%. Whenever possible, both arteriography and abdominal CT help in planning operative therapy [83–88].

Aggressive surgery is recommended for these lesions because of the high risk for rupture. Open surgical techniques include ligation, aneurysmectomy, or aneurysmorrhaphy. Aneurysms involving the middle or distal pancreas may require partial pancreatic resection or splenectomy. Endovascular catheter-based approaches, including embolization and exclusion, are frequently considered owing to the intimate relationship of these lesions to the pancreas and other adjacent viscera and the severity of the underlying disease. There have been reports of catheter-based therapies resulting in rupture or recurrent bleeding and foregut ischemia in patients who have concomitant celiac artery stenosis or occlusion [95,96].

### *Jejunal, ileal, colic, and branch mesenteric artery aneurysms*

Aneurysms of the jejunal, ileal, colic, and intestinal branch arteries account for less than 2% of visceral artery aneurysms. The causes are diverse and include arteriosclerosis, inflammation, and infection. These aneurysms are usually isolated and small (diameter <1 cm). Most are symptomatic. Up to 50% present with rupture causing either intraperitoneal hemorrhage or gastrointestinal bleeding [60,96]. Aggressive surgical therapy is indicated. The precise surgical approach depends on the location of the aneurysm. Endovascular strategies, including embolization, are undertaken with caution owing to the risk for acute intestinal ischemia with necrosis or perforation and of chronic ischemia with an intestinal stricture. Surgical ligation and exclusion may obligate segmental intestinal resection if collateral flow is insufficient to maintain intestinal viability or if the aneurysm is intramural. Extensive mesenteric hematomas during laparotomy may make the aneurysm difficult to identify [83–88,95–97].

### *Renal artery aneurysm*

Renal artery aneurysms are another uncommon abdominal vascular emergency that presents as hemorrhage. Most are saccular and extrarenal, frequently occurring at primary and secondary renal artery branch points. Renal artery aneurysms are more common in women who have arterial fibrodysplasia [100]. Arteriosclerotic changes frequently occur, but they are believed to be a secondary phenomenon. Most patients are asymptomatic at presentation, but some may have abdominal, flank, or back pain because of aneurysm expansion or rupture. Associated stenoses of branch renal arteries, compression or distortion of these branches by the aneurysm, and embolization of mural debris in the wall of the aneurysm all contribute to the common association with renin-mediated hypertension.

Overt rupture is rare (<3%) and mortality is uncommon (<10%). Loss of the affected kidney is almost universal in the event of rupture, supporting an aggressive approach to surgical repair [101].

Symptomatic aneurysms, aneurysms during pregnancy or in women of childbearing age, and aneurysms with concomitant branch renal artery stenoses, mural thrombus, or documented renovascular hypertension should generally be treated surgically. As with a splenic artery aneurysm, a renal artery aneurysm in a woman of childbearing age is serious and potentially lethal. Rupture during pregnancy is common with a maternal mortality in excess of 50%, and a fetal mortality in excess of 80%. In good-risk patients, asymptomatic aneurysms greater than 1.5 cm in diameter are considered for elective repair. Open surgical reconstruction for renal artery aneurysms is technically demanding; the surgeon must have extensive experience with various renal revascularization techniques to ensure optimal results. Catheter-based endovascular interventions have greatest usefulness for proximal lesions and arterial dissections that are amenable to covered stent therapy, and for intraparenchymal lesions. Although primary nephrectomy is often the only viable therapy for aneurysm rupture, it should almost never be considered as the primary therapeutic strategy for intact aneurysms of the main renal artery or branch vessels. Partial nephrectomy is occasionally useful for localized intraparenchymal aneurysms [100–103].

## Acknowledgments

A special acknowledgment is made to Rose Callahan, MS, who was invaluable in preparation of this manuscript.

## References

[1] Vicente DC, Kazmers A. Acute mesenteric ischemia. Curr Opin Cardiol 1999;14(5):453–8.
[2] Chang JB, Stein TA. Mesenteric ischemia: acute and chronic. Ann Vasc Surg 2003;17(3): 323–8.
[3] Schoots IG, Koffeman GI, Legemate DA, et al. Systematic review of survival after acute mesenteric ischemia according to disease etiology. Br J Surg 2004;91(1):17–27.
[4] Oldenburg WA, Lau LL, Rodenberg TJ, et al. Acute mesenteric ischemia: a clinical review. Arch Intern Med 2004;164(10):1054–62.
[5] Park WM, Gloviczki, Cherry KJ Jr, et al. Contemporary management of acute mesenteric ischemia: factors associated with survival. J Vasc Surg 2002;35(3):445–52.
[6] Kibbe MR, Hassoun HT. 6 vascular system, 4 acute mesenteric ischemia: diagnosis and management of acute bowel ischemia. In ACS Surgery Online. In: Souba WN, editor. New York: WebMD, Inc.; 2005. Available at: http://www/acssurgery.com. Accessed February 18, 2008.
[7] Rubin GD, Walker PJ, Dake MD, et al. Three-dimensional spiral computed tomographic angiography: an alternative imaging modality for the abdominal aorta and its branches. J Vasc Surg 1993;18(4):656–64 [discussion: 665].
[8] McLeod R, Lindsay T, O'Malley M. Canadian Association of General Surgeons and American College of Surgeons evidence based reviews in surgery. 15. Biphasic CT with mesenteric CT angiography in the evaluation of acute mesenteric ischemia: initial experience. Can J Surg 2005;48(6):491–3.
[9] Kazmers A. Operative management of acute mesenteric ischemia. Ann Vasc Surg 1998; 12(2):187–97.
[10] Schoots IG, Levi MM, Reekers JA, et al. Thrombolytic therapy for acute superior mesenteric artery occlusion. J Vasc Interv Radiol 2005;16(3):317–29.
[11] Kozuch PL, Brandt LJ. Review article: diagnosis and management of mesenteric ischaemia with an emphasis on pharmacotherapy. Aliment Pharmacol Ther 2005;21(3):201–15.
[12] Derrick JR, Pollard HS, Moore RM. The pattern of arteriosclerotic narrowing of the celiac and superior mesenteric arteries. Ann Surg 1959;149(5):684–9.
[13] Thomas JH, Blake K, Pierce GE, et al. The clinical course of asymptomatic mesenteric arterial stenosis. J Vasc Surg 1998;27(5):840–4.

[14] Park WM, Cherry KJ Jr, Chua HK, et al. Current results of open revascularization for chronic mesenteric ischemia: a standard for comparison. J Vasc Surg 2002;35(5):853–9.
[15] Calderon M, Reul GJ, Gregoric ID, et al. Long-term results of the surgical management of symptomatic chronic intestinal ischemia. J Cardiovasc Surg (Torino) 1992;33(6):723–8.
[16] Cunningham CG, Reilly LM, Rapp JH, et al. Chronic visceral ischemia. Three decades of progress. Ann Surg 1991;214(3):276–87 [discussion: 287–8].
[17] Shanley CJ, Ozaki K, Zelenock GB. Bypass grafting for chronic mesenteric ischemia. Surg Clin North Am 1997;77(2):381–95.
[18] Geelkerken RH, van Bockel JH, de Roos WK, et al. Chronic mesenteric vascular syndrome. Results of reconstructive surgery. Arch Surg 1991;126(9):1101–6.
[19] Johnston KW, Lindsay TF, Walker PM, et al. Mesenteric arterial bypass grafts: early and late results and suggested surgical approach for chronic and acute mesenteric ischemia. Surgery 1995;118(1):1–7.
[20] Moneta GL, Yeager RA, Dalman R, et al. Duplex ultrasound criteria for diagnosis of splanchnic artery stenosis or occlusion. J Vasc Surg 1991;14(4):511–8 [discussion: 518–20].
[21] Moneta GL, Lee RW, Yeager RA, et al. Mesenteric duplex scanning: a blinded prospective study. J Vasc Surg 1993;17(1):79–84 [discussion: 85–6].
[22] Matsumoto AH, Angle JF, Spinosa DJ, et al. Percutaneous transluminal angioplasty and stenting in the treatment of chronic mesenteric ischemia: results and longterm followup. J Am Coll Surg 2002;194(1 Suppl):S22–31.
[23] Sharafuddin MJ, Olson CH, Sun S, et al. Endovascular treatment of celiac and mesenteric arteries stenoses: applications and results. J Vasc Surg 2003;38(4):692–8.
[24] Landis MS, Rajan DK, Simons ME, et al. Percutaneous management of chronic mesenteric ischemia: outcomes after intervention. J Vasc Interv Radiol 2005;16(10):1319–25.
[25] Atkins MD, Kwolek CJ, LaMuraglia GM, et al. Surgical revascularization versus endovascular therapy for chronic mesenteric ischemia: a comparative experience. J Vasc Surg 2007; 45(6):1162–71.
[26] Piffaretti G, Tozzi M, Lomazzi C, et al. Endovascular therapy for chronic mesenteric ischemia. World J Surg 2007;31(12):2416–21.
[27] Sack J, Aldrete JS. Primary mesenteric venous thrombosis. Surg Gynecol Obstet 1982; 154(2):205–8.
[28] Abdu RA, Zakhour BJ, Dallis DJ. Mesenteric venous thrombosis—1911 to 1984. Surgery 1987;101(4):383–8.
[29] Harward TR, Green D, Bergan JJ, et al. Mesenteric venous thrombosis. J Vasc Surg 1989; 9(2):328–33.
[30] Boley SJ, Kaleya RN, Brandt LJ. Mesenteric venous thrombosis. Surg Clin North Am 1992;72(1):183–201.
[31] Rhee RY, Gloviczki P, Mendonca CT, et al. Mesenteric venous thrombosis: still a lethal disease in the 1990s. J Vasc Surg 1994;20(5):688–97.
[32] Bayraktar Y, Harmanci O. Etiology and consequences of thrombosis in abdominal vessels. World J Gastroenterol 2006;12(8):1165–74.
[33] Kitchens CS. Evolution of our understanding of the pathophysiology of primary mesenteric venous thrombosis. Am J Surg 1992;163(3):346–8.
[34] Morasch MD, Ebaugh JL, Chiou AC, et al. Mesenteric venous thrombosis: a changing clinical entity. J Vasc Surg 2001;34(4):680–4.
[35] Bontempo FA, Hassett AC, Faruki H, et al. The factor V Leiden mutation: spectrum of thrombotic events and laboratory evaluation. J Vasc Surg 1997;25(2):271–5 [discussion: 276].
[36] Inagaki H, Sakakibara O, Miyaike H, et al. Mesenteric venous thrombosis in familial free protein S deficiency. Am J Gastroenterol 1993;88(1):134–8.
[37] Ostermiller W Jr, Carter R. Mesenteric venous thrombosis secondary to polycythemia vera. Am Surg 1969;35(6):407–9.

[38] Tollefson DF, Friedman KD, Marlar RA, et al. Protein C deficiency. A cause of unusual or unexplained thrombosis. Arch Surg 1988;123(7):881–4.

[39] Wilson C, Walker ID, Davidson JF, et al. Mesenteric venous thrombosis and antithrombin III deficiency. J Clin Pathol 1987;40(8):906–8.

[40] Vogelzang RL, Gore RM, Anschuetz SL, et al. Thrombosis of the splanchnic veins: CT diagnosis. AJR Am J Roentgenol 1988;150(1):93–6.

[41] Rahmouni A, Mathieu D, Golli M, et al. Value of CT and sonography in the conservative management of acute splenoportal and superior mesenteric venous thrombosis. Gastrointest Radiol 1992;17(2):135–40.

[42] Miller VE, Berland LL. Pulsed Doppler duplex sonography and CT of portal vein thrombosis. AJR Am J Roentgenol 1985;145(1):73–6.

[43] Levy PJ, Krausz MM, Manny J. The role of second-look procedure in improving survival time for patients with mesenteric venous thrombosis. Surg Gynecol Obstet 1990;170(4):287–91.

[44] Inahara T. Acute superior mesenteric venous thrombosis: treatment by thrombectomy. Ann Surg 1971;174(6):956–61.

[45] Ende N. Infarction of the bowel in cardiac failure. N Engl J Med 1958;258(18):879–81.

[46] Bailey RW, Bulkley GB, Hamilton SR, et al. Protection of the small bowel from nonocclusive mesenteric ischemia injury due to cardiogenic shock. Am J Surg 1987;153(1):108–16.

[47] Brandt LJ, Boley SJ. Nonocclusive mesenteric ischemia. Annu Rev Med 1991;42:107–17.

[48] Ward D, Vernava AM, Kaminski DL, et al. Improved outcome by identification of high risk nonocclusive mesenteric ischemia, aggressive re-exploration, and delayed anastomosis. Am J Surg 1995;170(6):577–80 [discussion: 580–1].

[49] Trompeter M, Brazda T, Remy CT, et al. Non-occlusive mesenteric ischemia: etiology, diagnosis, and interventional therapy. Eur Radiol 2002;12(5):1179–87.

[50] Kolkman JJ, Mensink PB. Non-occlusive mesenteric ischaemia: a common disorder in gastroenterology and intensive care. Best Pract Res Clin Gastroenterol 2003;17(3):457–73.

[51] Gazes PC, Holmes CR, Moseley V, et al. Acute hemorrhage and necrosis of the intestines associated with digitalization. Circulation 1961;23:358–64.

[52] Fann JJ, Sarris GE, Mitcell RS. Treatment of patients with aortic dissection presenting with peripheral vascular complications. Ann Surg 1990;212(6):705–13.

[53] Williams DM, Lee DY, Hamilton B, et al. The dissected aorta: percutaneous treatment of ischemic complications—principles and results. J Vasc Interv Radiol 1997;8(4):605–25.

[54] Slonim SM, Nyman U, Semba CP, et al. Aortic dissection: percutaneous management with endovascular stents and balloon fenestration. J Vasc Surg 1996;23(2):241–51 [discussion: 251–3].

[55] Williams DM, Lee DY, Hamilton BH, et al. The dissected aorta. Part III, Anatomy and radiologic diagnosis of branch-vessel compromise. Radiology 1997;203(1):37–44.

[56] Lederle FA, Johnson GR, Wilson SE, et al. Prevalence and associations of abdominal aortic aneurysm detected through screening. Aneurysm Detection and Management (ADAM) Veterans Affairs Cooperative Study Group. Ann Intern Med 1997;126(6):441–9.

[57] Brewster DC, Croenwett JL, Hallett JW Jr, et al. Guidelines for the treatment of abdominal aortic aneurysms. Report of a subcommittee of the Joint Council of the American Association for Vascular Surgery and Society for Vascular Surgery. J Vasc Surg 2003;37(5):1106–17.

[58] Johnston KW, Rutherford RB, Tilson MD, et al. Suggested standards for reporting on arterial aneurysms. Subcommittee on Reporting Standards for Arterial Aneurysms, Ad Hoc Committee on Reporting Standards, Society for Vascular Surgery and North American Chapter, International Society for Cardiovascular Surgery. J Vasc Surg 1991;13(3):452–8.

[59] Halpern VJ, Kline RG, D'Angelo AJ, et al. Factors that affect the survival rate of patients with ruptured abdominal aortic aneurysms. J Vasc Surg 1997;26(6):939–45 [discussion: 945–8].

[60] Harris JR, Forbes TL, Steiner SH, et al. Risk-adjusted analysis of early mortality after ruptured abdominal aortic aneurysm repair. J Vasc Surg 2005;42(3):387–91.
[61] Heller JA, Weinberg A, Arons R, et al. Two decades of abdominal aortic aneurysm repair: have we made any progress? J Vasc Surg 2000;32(6):1091–100.
[62] Reddy DJ, Shepard AD, Evans JR, et al. Management of infected aortoiliac aneurysms. Arch Surg 1991;126(7):873–8 [discussion: 878–9].
[63] Sho E, Sho M, Hoshina K, et al. Hemodynamic forces regulate mural macrophage infiltration in experimental aortic aneurysms. Exp Mol Pathol 2004;76(2):108–16.
[64] Busuttil RW, Abou-Zamzam AM, Machleder HI. Collagenase activity of the human aorta. A comparison of patients with and without abdominal aortic aneurysms. Arch Surg 1980; 115(11):1373–8.
[65] Baxter BT, McGee GS, Shively VP, et al. Elastin content, cross-links, and mRNA in normal and aneurysmal human aorta. J Vasc Surg 1992;16(2):192–200.
[66] Lindholt JS, Jorgensen B, Klitgaard NA, et al. Systemic levels of cotinine and elastase, but not pulmonary function, are associated with the progression of small abdominal aortic aneurysms. Eur J Vasc Endovasc Surg 2003;26(4):418–22.
[67] Newman KM, Ogata Y, Malon AM, et al. Identification of matrix metalloproteinases 3 (stromelysin-1) and 9 (gelatinase B) in abdominal aortic aneurysm. Arterioscler Thromb 1994;14(8):1315–20.
[68] Newman KM, Jean-Claude J, Li H, et al. Cytokines that activate proteolysis are increased in abdominal aortic aneurysms. Circulation 1994;90(5 Pt 2):II224–7.
[69] Eliason JL, Hannawa KK, Ailawadi G, et al. Neutrophil depletion inhibits experimental abdominal aortic aneurysm formation. Circulation 2005;112(2):232–40.
[70] Cornuz J, Sidoti Pinto C, Tevaearai H, et al. Risk factors for asymptomatic abdominal aortic aneurysm: systematic review and meta-analysis of population-based screening studies. Eur J Public Health 2004;14(4):343–9.
[71] Brady AR, Thompson SG, Fowkes FG, et al. Abdominal aortic aneurysm expansion: risk factors and time intervals for surveillance. Circulation 2004;110(1):16–21.
[72] Collin J, Araujo L, Walton J. How fast do very small abdominal aortic aneurysms grow? Eur J Vasc Surg 1989;3(1):15–7.
[73] Solberg S, Singh K, Wilsgaard T, et al. Increased growth rate of abdominal aortic aneurysms in women. The Tromso study. Eur J Vasc Endovasc Surg 2005;29(2):145–9.
[74] Alsac JM, Desgranges P, Kobeiter H, et al. Emergency endovascular repair for ruptured abdominal aortic aneurysms: feasibility and comparison of early results with conventional open repair. Eur J Vasc Endovasc Surg 2005;30(6):632–9.
[75] Alsac JM, Kobeiter H, Becquemin JP, et al. Endovascular repair for ruptured AAA: a literature review. Acta Chir Belg 2005;105(2):134–9.
[76] Brandt M, Walluscheck KP, Jahnke T, et al. Endovascular repair of ruptured abdominal aortic aneurysm: feasibility and impact on early outcome. J Vasc Interv Radiol 2005; 16(10):1309–12.
[77] Franks S, Lloyd G, Fishwick G, et al. Endovascular treatment of ruptured and symptomatic abdominal aortic aneurysms. Eur J Vasc Endovasc Surg 2006;31(4):345–50.
[78] Greco G, Egorova N, Anderson PL, et al. Outcomes of endovascular treatment of ruptured abdominal aortic aneurysms. J Vasc Surg 2006;43(3):453–9.
[79] Grierson C, Uthappa MC, Uberoi R, et al. Multidetector CT appearances of splanchnic arterial pathology. Clin Radiol 2007;62(8):717–23.
[80] Horton KM, Smith C, Fishman EK. MDCT and 3D CT angiography of splanchnic artery aneurysms. AJR Am J Roentgenol 2007;189(3):641–7.
[81] Pilleul F, Beuf O. Diagnosis of splanchnic artery aneurysms and pseudoaneurysms, with special reference to contrast enhanced 3D magnetic resonance angiography: a review. Acta Radiol 2004;45(7):702–8.
[82] Shanley CJ, Shah NL, Messina LM. Common splanchnic artery aneurysms: splenic, hepatic and celiac. Ann Vasc Surg 1996;10(3):315–22.

[83] Shanley CJ, Shah NL, Messina LM. Uncommon splanchnic artery aneurysms: pancreaticoduodenal, gastroduodenal, superior mesenteric, inferior mesenteric and colic. Ann Vasc Surg 1996;10(5):506–15.
[84] Messina LM, Shanley CJ. Visceral artery aneurysms. Surg Clin North Am 1997;77(2): 425–42.
[85] Stanley JC, Thompson NW, Fry WJ. Splanchnic artery aneurysms. Arch Surg 1970;101(6): 689–97.
[86] Busuttil RW, Brin BJ. The diagnosis and management of visceral artery aneurysms. Surgery 1980;88(5):619–24.
[87] Pasha SF, Gloviczki P, Stanson AW, et al. Splanchnic artery aneurysms. Mayo Clin Proc 2007;82(4):472–9.
[88] Salo JA, Salmenkivi K, Tenhunen A, et al. Rupture of splanchnic artery aneurysms. World J Surg 1986;10(1):123–7.
[89] Stanley JC, Fry WJ. Pathogenesis and clinical significance of splenic artery aneurysms. Surgery 1974;76(6):898–909.
[90] English JD. Spontaneous rupture of a splenic artery aneurysm in the third trimester. Ir J Med Sci 1993;162(5):169–70.
[91] Lowry SM, O'Dea TP, Gallagher DI, et al. Splenic artery aneurysm rupture: the seventh instance of maternal and fetal survival. Obstet Gynecol 1986;67(2):291–2.
[92] McDermott VG, Shlansky-Goldberg R, Cope C. Endovascular management of splenic artery aneurysms and pseudoaneurysms. Cardiovasc Intervent Radiol 1961;17(4):179–84.
[93] Jeans PL. Hepatic artery aneurysms and biliary surgery: two cases and a literature review. Aust N Z J Surg 1988;58(11):889–94.
[94] Psathakis D, Muller G, Noah M, et al. Present management of hepatic artery aneurysms. Symptomatic left hepatic artery aneurysm; right hepatic artery aneurysm with erosion into the gallbladder and simultaneous colocholecystic fistula - a report of two unusual cases and the current state of etiology, diagnosis, histology and treatment. Vasa 1992;21(2):210–5.
[95] Rossi M, Rebonato A, Greco L, et al. Endovascular exclusion of visceral artery aneurysms with stent-grafts: technique and long-term follow-up. Cardiovasc Intervent Radiol 2008; 31(1):36–42.
[96] Carroccio A, Jacobs TS, Faries P, et al. Endovascular treatment of visceral artery aneurysms. Vasc Endovascular Surg 2007;41(5):373–82.
[97] Reuter SR, Fry WJ, Bookstein JJ. Mesenteric artery branch aneurysms. Arch Surg 1968; 97(3):497–9.
[98] Graham LM, Stanley JC, Whitehouse WM Jr, et al. Celiac artery aneurysms: historic (1745–1949) versus contemporary (1950–1984) differences in etiology and clinical importance. J Vasc Surg 1985;2(5):757–64.
[99] Risher WH, Hollier LH, Bolton JS, et al. Celiac artery aneurysm. Ann Vasc Surg 1991;5(4): 392–5.
[100] Stanley JC, Rhodes EL, Gewertz BL, et al. Renal artery aneurysms: significance of macroaneurysms exclusive of dissections and fibrodysplatic mural dilations. Arch Surg 1975;110(11):1327–33.
[101] Lumsden AB, Salam TA, Walton KG. Renal artery aneurysm: a report of 28 cases. Cardiovasc Surg 1996;4(2):185–9.
[102] Hupp T, Allenberg JR, Post K, et al. Renal artery aneurysm: surgical indications and results. Eur J Vasc Surg 1992;6(5):477–86.
[103] Henke PK, Cardeau JD, Welling TH III, et al. Renal artery aneurysms: a 35 year clinical experience with 252 aneurysms in 168 patients. Ann Surg 2001;234(4):454–62 [discussion: 462–3].

ELSEVIER
SAUNDERS

Med Clin N Am 92 (2008) 649–670

THE MEDICAL CLINICS OF NORTH AMERICA

# Adynamic Ileus and Acute Colonic Pseudo-Obstruction

Mihaela Batke, MD*, Mitchell S. Cappell, MD, PhD

*Division of Gastroenterology, Department of Medicine, William Beaumont Hospital, MOB 233, 3601 West Thirteen Mile Road, Royal Oak, MI 48073, USA*

A clinical review of adynamic ileus and acute colonic pseudo-obstruction (ACPO) is important and timely. First, these clinical entities have a significant clinical and social impact. For example, postoperative ileus directly costs more than one billion dollars annually in the United States, because of prolonged hospitalization, and causes substantial postoperative morbidity, while ACPO contributes to many thousands of deaths annually in the United States [1]. Second, delayed diagnosis and inappropriate therapy for colonic pseudo-obstruction frequently occurs and results in markedly increased morbidity and mortality [2]. For example, in a relatively recent retrospective analysis from the Mayo Clinic, nearly half of the eligible patients did not receive the standard medical therapy of neostigmine for colonic pseudo-obstruction [3]. Third, clinicians have to be familiar with the new diagnostic modalities and the recent pharmacologic and colonoscopic therapies for these conditions. This article reviews the etiology, diagnosis, and therapy of ileus and ACPO, with attention to the role of the internist, gastroenterologist, radiologist, and surgeon in the clinical management, and with a focus on the newest therapies.

## Terminology

Impaired transit of intestinal contents can be caused by either mechanical obstruction or functionally deficient enteric propulsion from attenuated or uncoordinated intestinal muscle contractions. The definition and nosology of these entities is confusing because of an incomplete understanding of the pathophysiology and application of different meanings to the same term. For example, "gallstone ileus" is a misnomer, as it actually represents

* Corresponding author.
*E-mail address:* michidus@yahoo.com (M. Batke).


doi:10.1016/j.mcna.2008.01.002 ***medical.theclinics.com***

mechanical obstruction by an impacted gallstone and not a functional ileus. The commonly accepted definitions are described in Box 1 and the disorders are summarized in Table 1. ACPO, or Ogilvie's syndrome, is a variant of ileus, characterized by massive colonic dilatation [4].

Megacolon denotes an extremely dilated colon, defined as a luminal diameter of more than 12 cm for the cecum, 8 cm for the transverse colon, or 6.5 cm for the descending and sigmoid colon, as determined by a radiologic study [5]. Multiple criteria are necessary because air can accumulate in different colonic segments, depending on the patient's position and local colonic conditions.

Chronic intestinal pseudo-obstruction predominantly affects the small bowel, but may affect other parts of the gastrointestinal tract. It has a broad spectrum of clinical manifestations, from asymptomatic to recurrent episodes of severe abdominal distention. A similar clinical disorder without bowel dilatation is denoted as chronic intestinal dysmotility. These two rare disorders are outside the scope of this issue that deals with acute gastrointestinal emergencies.

## Ileus

### *Pathophysiology*

Abdominal incision, intraoperative spillage of irritating gastrointestinal contents (such as hydrocholoric acid or feculent material) within the peritoneum, and intestinal manipulation activate neuronal pathways and release inflammatory mediators that inhibit enteral transit. Putative neuronal pathways include adrenergic nerves [6], inhibitory motor neurons that release nitric oxide [7–9], and perhaps activation of vasoactive intestinal polypeptide, and $\mu$ or $\kappa$ opioid receptors [6,10]. Inflammatory mediators activate local macrophages and release proinflammatory cytokines, which recruit

**Box 1. Definitions of disorders with impaired transit of intestinal contents**

**Mechanical obstruction:** severely impaired transit of intestinal contents because of intrinsic luminal obstruction or extrinsic compression.

**Ileus:** severe functionally impaired transit of intestinal contents because of decreased peristaltic activity of the gastrointestinal tract in the absence of mechanical obstruction.

**Colonic pseudo-obstruction:** severe functionally impaired transit of colonic contents and massive dilatation of the colon, in the absence of mechanical obstruction, because of uncoordinated, nonperistaltic, or attenuated colonic muscle contractions.

Table 1
Differentiation between mechanical and functional intestinal obstruction

| Parameter | Mechanical obstruction | Ileus | Acute colonic pseudo-obstruction | Chronic intestinal pseudo-obstruction |
|---|---|---|---|---|
| Motility | Initially increased, later decreased proximal to obstruction | Decreased | Decreased or uncoordinated | Decreased |
| Obliterated lumen | Yes | No | No | No |
| Cut-off point on abdominal radiograph | Typical | Sometimes | Sometimes | No |
| Duration | Acute | Acute | Acute | Chronic |
| Dilatation | Yes, proximal to the obstruction | Sometimes | Yes, massive in colon | Yes |
| Predominant involvement | Bowel up to site of obstruction | Small bowel | Colon | Small bowel, colon |
| Air-fluid levels | Yes | No | Sometimes | No |
| Disease progression | Rapid without surgery in total mechanical obstruction | Typically slow, gradual recovery after postoperative ileus | Usually responds to nonoperative therapy, occasional major complications | Variable |
| Treatment | Usually surgery | Usually conservative (medical) therapy | Conservative therapy, then neostigmine, then decompressive colonoscopy | Variable |

circulating leukocytes and mast cells to intestinal muscle and inhibit bowel motility. Local effects on injured bowel are propagated to adjacent uninjured bowel segments by neuronal, cellular, and molecular mechanisms [9].

Corticotropin releasing-factor (CRF) may play a role in ileus via central and peripheral pathways. Stress causes central release of CRF from Barrington's nucleus that results in autonomic inhibition of gastric and small bowel motility. In an animal model, postoperative ileus did not occur in genetically altered mice lacking $CRF_1$ receptors or when a selective $CRF_1$ receptor antagonist was administered preoperatively. Additionally, peripheral administration of CRF induces changes in gut motility, resembling an ileus pattern through activation of CRF receptors within myenteric plexus neurons [11].

### *Etiology*

Ileus most commonly occurs in the postoperative period, where it is recognized as an obligatory physiologic response to abdominal surgery [12]. The duration of the ileus is related to the operative site. The duration is longest after colonic surgery. Gastrointestinal function returns after surgery in an orderly and predictable manner, with small intestine motility recovering after 0 to 24 hours, gastric motility recovering at 24 to 48 hours, and colonic motility recovering at 48 to 72 hours [13]. Some experts distinguish postoperative ileus, which reflects moderate inhibition of colonic motility that resolves spontaneously after 2 to 3 days, from paralytic ileus, which reflects severe inhibition of small bowel motility that lasts longer [14].

Opiates administered for postoperative analgesia are common contributing factors [15]. Opiates profoundly inhibit gastrointestinal motility and delay recovery from postoperative ileus [16]. Other implicated medications include anticholinergic drugs, calcium-channel antagonists, antihistamines, and various psychotropic agents, such as phenothiazines and tricyclic antidepressants [17]. Anesthetics do not significantly contribute to an ileus, as evidenced by prolonged administration of general anesthesia for nonabdominal operations without postoperative ileus [12].

Other contributing factors include critical illnesses, metabolic derangements, neurologic disorders, intraabdominal or retroperitoneal inflammation, thoracic diseases, and severe infections, such as pneumonia [5]. Metabolic derangements include electrolyte disturbances, such as hypokalemia, hyponatremia, hypomagnesemia, hypermagnesemia, hypocalcemia, or hypercalcemia; uremia; diabetic ketoacidosis or diabetic hyperosmolar coma; and hypoparathyroidism.

### *Clinical presentation*

Ileus presents with abdominal distention and with abdominal pain that is typically mild and poorly localized. Variable features include hypoactive or absent bowel sounds, lack of passage of flatus and stool, intolerance of oral intake, and nausea and emesis. Physical examination reveals a distended, tympanitic abdomen; hypoactive bowel sounds; and mild, diffuse abdominal tenderness. The patient may exhibit signs of dehydration, such as tachycardia, orthostatic hypotension, poor skin turgor, and dry mucous membranes.

### *Diagnosis and differential diagnosis*

Laboratory tests should include routine serum electrolytes, creatinine, blood urea nitrogen, complete blood count, liver function tests, amylase, lipase, and magnesium levels. Postoperative ileus must be differentiated from small bowel obstruction (SBO), which occurs in up to 1% of patients within 30 days after abdominal surgery [18]. This differentiation is frequently problematic; the differentiation is usually not possible based solely on the clinical presentation. Patients with ileus tend to have gastrointestinal symptoms immediately after surgery, while patients with postoperative SBO develop increasing gastrointestinal symptoms after a variable postoperative interval without symptoms. Patients with SBO tend to be sicker, have more severe gastrointestinal symptoms, and tend to progress more rapidly. For example, the abdominal pain in SBO tends to be more severe, more colicky, and more periumbilical. Obstipation progressively develops with total SBO. Bowel sounds tend to be hyperactive and tinkling initially with total SBO, but progressively become hypoactive and then disappear with progressive intestinal muscle fatigue. Differences between mechanical obstruction and functional obstruction are summarized in Table 1.

Patients with SBO have distended small bowel loops, air-fluid levels within these loops, and no colonic distention on plain abdominal roentgenograms. Plain abdominal roentgenograms in ileus reveal pronounced small bowel dilatation, but may reveal less pronounced large bowel dilatation. Additional imaging, such as abdominal CT or barium studies, may be necessary to exclude SBO, as described in the accompanying article by Cappell and Batke in this issue. Abdominal CT is up to 90% specific and sensitive in excluding SBO. Passage of orally administered contrast into the colon is delayed but not blocked in ileus, but is completely blocked in total SBO.

### *Treatment*

#### *General measures*

The treatment is largely supportive, including intravenous fluid resuscitation and correction of electrolyte abnormalities. Underlying conditions should be identified and aggressively treated: antibiotics for sepsis, and discontinuation of drugs that promote an ileus. Patients traditionally received nothing by mouth until resolution of the ileus, recognized by passage of flatus or stool, but this treatment harms the nutritional status, thereby potentially decreasing postoperative wound healing and immunologic function [19]. Recent studies suggest that early enteral feeding is safe, decreases the duration of postoperative ileus, and decreases the hospital stay [19–23]. Gum chewing is an inexpensive and safe method to promote gut motility and resolve a postoperative ileus through vagal and enteric hormonal stimulation (sham feeding), but randomized studies have shown variable efficacy [24–27]. Early ambulation does not reduce the duration of postoperative ileus, but does decrease complications from prolonged immobility [28].

Postoperative nasogastric decompression is no longer routinely recommended because of numerous negative clinical trials and the increased risks of pulmonary atelectasis, pneumonia, or pyrexia with a nasogastric tube [29]. A nasogastric tube is, however, selectively recommended for severe gastric dilatation or protracted vomiting [30].

#### *Pharmacotherapy*

Drug studies on reducing the duration of ileus tend to be small, retrospective, and have variable end-points [31]. Despite stimulation of the motilin receptor and the migrating motor complex, erythromycin failed to improve postoperative bowel motility in multiple placebo-controlled, randomized studies [32–34]. Metoclopramide, a dopamine antagonist, also failed to improve postoperative bowel function in multiple trials [12]. Randomized studies have yielded contradictory results on the effects of propranol on postoperative ileus [35,36].

Among nine studies of cisapride, four studies showed that cisapride significantly reduced postoperative ileus, one study noted an increase in the percentage of subjects passing flatus at 4 hours after surgery, and four studies were negative. Three of the four positive studies used intravenous cisapride, whereas three of the four negative studies used intrarectal cisapride. The effect of cisapride on ileus may therefore depend on the route of administration [12]. Cisapride was, however, recently withdrawn from the market in the United States because of rare, but severe, cardiac toxicity.

Neostigmine, an acetylcholinesterase inhibitor, is beneficial in ACPO as described below. Several studies have suggested that is also beneficial in ileus [37]. In uncontrolled studies, administration of laxatives resulted in early return of bowel motility and early discharge after gynecologic surgery [38]. These effects were confirmed in a randomized, double-blind, placebo-controlled study [39]. The data on homeopathic remedies for postoperative ileus are inconclusive [40,41].

Peripheral opiate antagonists are promising therapies for postoperative ileus [42]. Alvimopan, a selective peripheral mu-receptor opiate antagonist, antagonizes the gastrointestinal effects of nonselective opiates without affecting their central analgesic effects. In a recent meta-analysis, alvimopan more rapidly restored gastrointestinal function and reduced the time to discharge following major surgery when compared with placebo [43]. Development of this drug was, however, recently suspended because of cardiovascular and neoplastic side effects. Methylnaltrexone is a peripherally acting selective opioid antagonist that may promote intestinal motility in patients receiving nonselective opiate analgesics [44].

*Prevention*

Minimization of surgical invasiveness, laparotomy incisions, and intraoperative bowel manipulation decreases the risk of ileus. Laparoscopic surgical techniques decrease the rate of postoperative ileus because of reduced intraoperative gut manipulation [45–47]. Avoiding narcotics postoperatively, with replacement by nonsteroidal anti-inflammatory medications (NSAIDs) or selective cyclo-oxygenase-2 inhibitors, significantly decreases the duration of postoperative ileus [48–51]. In a meta-analysis, administration of epidural local anesthetics during and after laparotomy provided pain relief comparable to that of systemic opiates, but reduced the duration of ileus [52]. For effective pain relief, epidural anesthetics should be administered at the thoracic level [31] for up to 72 hours postoperatively [53].

*Summary*

Ileus is the functional inhibition of propulsive bowel activity. Postoperative ileus follows any abdominal operation, and usually resolves spontaneously within 2 to 3 days. Other conditions that can contribute to an ileus include metabolic derangements, drugs, infections, and inflammatory conditions. Ileus presents with abdominal distention and nonspecific abdominal pain. Abdominal roentgenograms reveal dilatation of the small and large bowel. Differentiation from SBO may require further radiologic studies.

The treatment is mainly supportive: treatment of the underlying conditions, intravenous fluid replacement, correction of electrolyte disorders, and nasogastric aspiration in selected patients. The incidence and duration of postoperative ileus is reduced by laparoscopy, postoperative thoracic epidural anesthesia, NSAIDs, and selective peripheral opiate antagonists. Relatively safe and possibly beneficial treatments include early refeeding, postoperative gum chewing, early ambulation, laxatives, and neostigmine. Agents with no demonstrable benefit include metoclopramide, cisapride, erythromycin, and alpha-receptor or beta-receptor adrenergic antagonists.

## Acute colonic pseudo-obstruction

Ogilvie [54] first described this syndrome in 1948 in association with retroperitoneal malignancy infiltrating the celiac plexus. Dudley and colleagues [55] named the syndrome acute colonic pseudo-obstruction in 1958, to recognize that the obstruction is functional rather than mechanical. ACPO has also been called colonic ileus, but this term is discouraged because ileus suggests motor inactivity, whereas ACPO can present with motor activity that is uncoordinated and nonperistaltic [56].

### *Pathophysiology*

The mechanism is poorly understood and likely multifactorial. The main theories involve an imbalance of autonomic influences that produces a hypotonic bowel, either through increased sympathetic activity or decreased parasympathetic activity [5]. In animals, stimulation of splachnic nerves diminishes intestinal muscle tone, reduces intestinal movements, and produces intestinal dilatation, whereas splanchniectomy prevents postoperative ileus [56]. Neostigmine improves bowel motility in patients with ileus, suggesting that sacral parasympathetic deficiency, with unopposed sympathetic activity, causes colonic hypotonia [57,58]. Local segmental bowel hypotonia from local bowel injury can induce hypotonia of adjacent bowel segments via the colocolonic inhibitory reflex mediated by prevertebral ganglia [59]. Colonic hypotonia produces luminal stasis and colonic dilatation by inefficient expulsion of intraluminal gas and stool.

### *Etiology*

ACPO usually presents in association with underlying medical or surgical disorders (Table 2). In a review of 1,027 cases of ACPO from 1948 to 1987, 93% of cases had underlying disorders, including: postoperative status in

Table 2
Conditions associated with acute colonic pseudo-obstruction

| | | |
|---|---|---|
| Drugs | Postoperative | Metabolic disturbance |
| Opiates | Cardiac surgery | Severe electrolyte imbalance |
| Calcium channel blockers | Renal transplantation | Renal failure |
| Antidepressants | Cesarean section | Hepatic failure |
| Phenothiazines | Gynecologic surgery | Diabetes mellitus |
| AntiParkinsonian medications | Orthopedic surgery | Alcohol abuse |
| Clonidine | Spine surgery | |
| Theophylline | Urologic surgery | |
| Baclofen | | |
| Chemotherapy | | |
| Corticosteroids | | |
| Trauma | Infection | Cardiovascular disease |
| Pelvic trauma | Acute cholecystitis | Acute myocardial infarction |
| Thoracic trauma | Meningitis | Congestive heart failure |
| Spinal cord trauma | Pelvic abscess | Cerebrovascular attack |
| Long bones fracture | Herpes zoster | |
| | Pneumonia | |
| | Cytomegalovirus | |
| | Lyme disease | |
| Neoplasm | Neurologic disease | Miscellaneous |
| Hematologic malignancy | Parkinson disease | Mechanical ventilation |
| Retroperitoneal malignancy | Alzheimer dementia | Pulmonary disease |
| Pelvic radiation therapy | Multiple sclerosis | Acute pancreatitis |
| Paraneoplastic syndrome | Lower spinal cord disease | Retroperitoneal hemorrhage |
| Multiple myeloma | Guillan-Barrè syndrome | Pregnancy |
| Connective tissue disease | Meningioma | Renal transplantation |
| Scleroderma | Diabetic neuropathy | Intoxication (drug overdose, *Amanita phalloides* ingestion, pesticides) |
| Systemic lupus erythematosus | Neurofibromatosis | |
| Vasculitis | Familial visceral neuropathy | |
| | | Thyrotoxic periodic paralysis |
| | | Sickle cell disease |
| | | Postcolonoscopy |
| | | Renal transplant malfunction |
| | | Familial visceral myopathy |

23.1%, cardiopulmonary disease in 17.5%, nonoperative trauma in 11.2%, neurologic disease in 8%, malignancy in 5.4%, intra-abdominal pathology in 4.6%, obstetric disorders in 4.4%, and retroperitoneal pathology in 3.5% [60]. Other large reviews reported similar rates of underlying diseases, ranging from 88% to 94% [57,61]. Narcotics and electrolyte disorders are frequent contributing factors [2].

ACPO is relatively uncommon. For example, it occurred in only 0.05% of cases of cardiac surgery in a review of 5,438 patients [62], and in only 0.29% of cases of severe burn injury in a review of 2,703 patients [63].

## *Clinical presentation*

ACPO can occur at any age but occurs more frequently in the elderly. Males have a 50% higher incidence than females [57]. It most commonly occurs in hospitalized or institutionalized patients who are frequently debilitated [2]. Obesity is another epidemiologic risk factor. Symptoms typically develop slowly over several days [64]. Patients typically present with massive abdominal distention and mild, diffuse, abdominal discomfort, with minimal systemic toxicity. Passage of stool or gas is absent in 50% [5], but patients occasionally, paradoxically, have diarrhea. Other symptoms include abdominal pain in 83%, nausea in 63%, and emesis in 57% [57]. Fever occurs frequently (78%) in patients with bowel ischemia or perforation, but occurs relatively infrequently (31%) in patients without complications.

Physical examination reveals abdominal distention and tympanism. Bowel sounds are hypoactive in 31%, high-pitched in 17%, and absent in 12%, but are sometimes normoactive because the small bowel is functional. Abdominal tenderness tends to be mild and relatively infrequent with moderate colonic distention, but tends to become progressively more frequent and severe with increasing colonic distention because of progressive colonic ischemia. Rectal examination generally reveals no fecal occult blood. The nasogastric aspirate typically reveals scant, clear fluid [65].

### *Differential diagnosis*

Colonic pseudo-obstruction is diagnosed only after excluding mechanical large bowel obstruction (LBO). Obstructed patients tend to be more acutely ill and have more severe abdominal symptoms and signs than patients with pseudo-obstruction. The pain with mechanical obstruction tends to be severe, midabdominal, and colicky. Obstipation favors the diagnosis of LBO. Feculant vomiting suggests mechanical obstruction. Patients with LBO may initially have hyperactive bowel sounds, but the bowel sounds become progressively hyopactive as the intestinal muscle fatigues. Patients with colonic pseudo-obstruction tend to have hypoactive bowel sounds because of decreased colonic motility, but may have some bowel sounds from preserved small intestinal motility. The abdominal findings generally progress more rapidly with total LBO than with pseudo-obstruction.

The differential diagnosis also includes toxic megacolon and ischemic colitis. Patients with toxic megacolon are generally acutely ill with pyrexia, tachycardia, and abdominal tenderness, while patients with colonic pseudo-obstruction tend to be only mild to moderately ill with minimal systemic toxicity unless they have a severe underlying medical disorder or experience complications of colonic ischemia or sepsis. Toxic megacolon tends to present with diarrhea that is often bloody, while ACPO tends to present with constipation rather than diarrhea and rarely causes bloody stools. Toxic megacolon is often associated with inflammatory bowel disease or with stool studies indicative of acute colonic infection. For example, *Clostridium difficile* colitis is diagnosed by the presence of toxin A in the stool. With toxic megacolon, flexible sigmoidoscopy or colonoscopy may reveal the characteristic pseudomembranes of *Clostridium difficile* consisting of 2-mm to 8-mm wide yellowish nodules composed of an adherent exudate overlying mucosa; or they may reveal mucosal erythema, friability, exudate, and ulceration characteristic of ulcerative colitis. Patients with ischemic colitis generally have abdominal pain that is more intense and more sudden in onset. Ischemic colitis is often associated with bloody diarrhea. Abdominal roentgenograms may reveal thumbprinting with ischemic colitis. Characteristic colonoscopic findings with ischemic colitis include: a de novo segmental colitis that typically spares the rectum; hemorrhagic nodules caused by intramural hemorrhage and edema; friable and ulcerated mucosa; and gray or dusky mucosa.

### *Diagnosis*

Initial laboratory tests should include a hemogram; routine metabolic tests for sodium, potassium, calcium, magnesium, phosphorus, blood urea nitrogen, and creatinine; liver function tests; and thyroid function tests. Blood or bodily fluid cultures are indicated if sepsis is clinically suspected. Leukocytosis is present in 100% of patients with colonic ischemia or perforation, but is present in only 25% of patients with uncomplicated ACPO [57].

Plain abdominal roentgenograms reveal massive colonic dilatation. Dilated colon is differentiated from dilated small bowel by a typically larger caliber, by a centrifugal distribution of the dilated bowel loops, and by incomplete intraluminal partitions created by the haustral folds, as compared with the complete partitions created by the valvulae conniventes in the small bowel. An air-filled dilated colon extending distally to the rectosigmoid strongly favors the diagnosis of ACPO rather than LBO, but this sign is insensitive. Differentiation of ACPO from LBO is challenging; the dilatation in both disorders is often greater in the right colon than the left colon [57,60,61]. Although a colonic cut-off point favors the diagnosis of LBO, 40% of patients with ACPO appear to have a cut-off point of colonic distention, most often at the splenic flexure, descending, or sigmoid colon [66]. Up to 80% of patients with ACPO have simultaneous dilatation of small bowel, although this dilatation is less pronounced [57]. In comparing ACPO with LBO, air-fluid levels are an unreliable marker (42% versus 60% rate) [57,66]; therefore contrast enemas, abdominopelvic computerized tomography, or colonoscopy are frequently necessary for the diagnosis.

Contrast enemas, with either barium or water-soluble contrast, are routinely performed to exclude LBO. They occasionally are therapeutic. Barium enema for ACPO entails a 1% risk of colonic perforation [57]. Up to 20% of patients fail to retain the enema [67]. Water-soluble contrast can potentially dehydrate patients because of contrast hyperosmolarity [66,68].

Abdominal CT, magnetic resonance imaging, or ultrasound can help differentiate ACPO from LBO and help detect potential complications. Abdominal CT has a sensitivity of 96% and specificity of 93% in the diagnosis of ACPO. Fast helical multidetector CT facilitates rapid acquisition of images during one breath-hold in frail and uncooperative patients without the need for rectal contrast or air insufflation [68].

Colonoscopy is an excellent diagnostic (and therapeutic) alternative. Colonoscopy is frequently performed at the bedside in an unprepped colon to avoid the risks from colonic preparation. Thick, viscous stool, which is difficult to aspirate, renders colonoscopy more difficult and dangerous because of limited visibility. Low-pressure normal saline enemas are sometimes administered before colonoscopy to improve colonoscopic visualization [57]. Colonoscopy is contraindicated in the presence of clinical or radiologic signs of peritonitis, and should be aborted if it reveals significant colonic ischemia. Colonoscopy reveals an extremely dilated, amotile, and highly compliant colon with no point of obstruction and no intrinsic colonic lesion.

### *Treatment*

#### *General measures*

Supportive care includes nothing by mouth, intravenous hydration, and discontinuation of narcotic, sedative, or anticholinergic medications. Precipitating conditions should be identified and treated. Electrolyte abnormalities, particularly hypokalemia, hypomagnesemia, and hypercalcemia, should be corrected to promote colonic motility. Antibiotics are administered if sepsis is clinically suspected. Heart failure is aggressively treated if present. Hypothyroidism occasionally presents with colonic pseudo-obstruction that responds to thyroid replacement. Although often inserted, a nasogastic tube has limited efficacy in decompressing the dilated colon. A rectal tube attached to gravity drainage may help decompress an air-filled sigmoid colon, but has limited efficacy in decompressing the proximal colon. Ambulation, if possible, or frequent patient repositioning, if ambulation is impossible, may help move intestinal gas toward the anus. Laxatives are generally avoided because ingested fluid tends to accumulate in the sluggish bowel.

Conservative management is maintained for 72 hours, provided the cecal diameter is less than 12 cm and there are no signs of bowel ischemia, bowel perforation, or peritonitis [69]. The abdomen is frequently monitored to exclude missed diagnoses of severe colonic conditions, such as LBO, that rapidly progress, and to exclude disease complications of colonic ischemia or perforation. Supine and dependent abdominal roentgenograms are obtained every 12 to 24 hours to monitor the cecal diameter and to exclude pneumoperitoneum [57]. Serum electrolytes and the leukocyte count are checked daily. Continued colonic dilatation beyond 12 cm in diameter despite supportive therapy or development of pyrexia, leukocytosis, metabolic acidosis, or significant abdominal signs, is worrisome. Tap water enemas are not recommended because of a risk of colonic perforation [57].

About 75% of cases spontaneously resolve with conservative therapy in a median of 4 days. For example, in a series of 25 patients with cancer managed by conservative measures, 92% had clinical resolution, with a mean time among responders of 3 days. Resolvers are less likely to have postoperative ileus and less likely to have been administered narcotics [3].

*Pharmacotherapy*

About 80% of patients with pseudo-obstruction respond to 2-mg neostigmine rapidly infused intravenously, with a mean response time of 4 minutes (range 3–30 minutes (Table 3); [70–78]). The dose may be reduced if side effects, particularly bronchospasm or bradycardia, are a concern. Glycopyrrolate, a cholinergic antagonist with limited activity on muscarinic colonic receptors, is sometimes coadministered to minimize systemic cholinergic side effects [79]. Favorable response to neostigmine occurs more frequently in females, the elderly, and postoperative patients; and less frequently in patients with electrolyte abnormalities or previously administered antimotility agents [3,71]. Contraindications to neostigmine include bradycardia, severe cardiac disease, hypotension, active bronchospasm requiring medication, renal insufficiency, and pregnancy. Neostigmine is not administered when LBO is suspected because the induced colonic muscular contractions may cause colonic perforation. Continuous cardiac monitoring is required during and immediately after the infusion. The patient should be supine during and briefly after the infusion because of the potential for bradycardia. Bradycardia is treated with infusion discontinuation, but sometimes requires atropine therapy. Other side effects, such as excessive salivation, hyperhidrosis, crampy abdominal pain, emesis, and bronchoconstriction, tend to be mild and transient. There are only two reported fatalities from neostigmine administration [80,81]. About 35% of responders relapse [73]. Relapsers receive a second infusion of neostigmine 4 hours later, with a 40% to 90% success rate [3,56,72–74,78].

Cisapride, a 5-HT4 receptor agonist, produced contradictory results in several patients with ACPO [82,83], possibly because of partial 5-HT3 antagonism that decreases bowel motility [84]. A literature search failed to reveal any reports regarding treatment with other approved or investigational 5-HT4 receptor agonists, including tegaserod, prucalopride, renzapride, norcisapride, or mosapride. The prokinetic agent erythromycin has been reported to be beneficial in ACPO in several case reports [85–87]. Clinical application of erythromycin is hampered by its short half-life and the rapid development of tachyphylaxis [84]. Metoclopramide primarily affects upper gastrointestinal motility and is not recommended for ACPO [64]. Mu receptor opioid antagonists, such as alvimopan and methylnaltrexone, and κ-receptor opioid antagonists, such as asimadoline, are promising investigational prokinetic agents. They have produced clinical improvement in patients with postoperative ileus and constipation-predominant irritable bowel syndrome in several trials [88–90]. Their clinical utility for ACPO is currently unproven. Epidural anesthesia resolved ACPO in several case reports with rare complications [84,91]. In one study, five of eight subjects

Table 3
Selected clinical trials of neostigmine for acute colonic pseudo-obstruction

| Study characteristics | Abeyta et al, [70] | Loftus et al, [3] | Mehta et al, [71] | Paran et al, [72] | Ponec et al, [73] | Sgouros et al, [74] | Stephenson et al, [75] | Trevisani et al, [76] | Turegano-Fuentes et al, [77] | Van der Spoel et al, [78] |
|---|---|---|---|---|---|---|---|---|---|---|
| Prospective | No | No | Yes | Yes | Yes | Yes | Yes | No | Yes | Yes |
| Randomized | No | No | No | No | Yes | No[a] | No | No | No | Yes |
| Double blind | No | No | No | No | Yes | No[a] | No | No | No | Yes |
| Number of patients | 10[b] | 18 | 19 | 11 | 11 (10 controls) | 25 | 12 | 28 | 16 | 13 (11 controls) |
| Dose (infusion duration) | 2 mg (bolus) | 2 mg (3–5 min) | 2 mg (15 min) | 2.5 mg (1 hr) | 2 mg (3–5 min) | 2 mg (3–5 min) | 2.5 mg (1–3 min) | 2.5 mg (3 min) | 2.5 mg (60 min) | 0.4–0.8 mg/hr drip |
| Rate of success of first dose | 60% | 89% | 84% | 64% | 91% | 88% | 93% | 93% | 75% | 85% |
| Recurrence rate | 0% | 31% | 38% | 22% | 27% | 23% | 17% | 8% | — | 0% |
| Rate of success of second dose | 75% | — | 83% | 100% | — | 40% | 100% | 100% | — | — |
| Overall long-term response rate | 90% | 61% | 79% | 82% | 64% | 88% | 100% | 93% | 81% | 85% |
| Bradycardia requiring atropine | 10% | 11% | 11% | 0% | 22% | 8% | — | 0% | 6% | 0% |

[a] Patients were not randomized and patients and physicians were not blinded with regards to neostigmine administration.
[b] Eight patients with 10 separate admissions for colonic pseudo-obstruction.

(62.5%) had colonic decompression within 2 hours of sympathetic blockade by continuous $T_{11\text{-}12}$ epidural anesthesia with bupivacaine [92]. The response rate was similar to that of colonoscopy but with fewer complications.

*Colonoscopic therapy*

Colonoscopy successfully decompresses the colon in up to 80% of cases [57,60,93–95]. For example, in a review of 292 reported patients, Rex [94] reported 69% had successful initial colonoscopic decompression. During colonoscopic intubation the colon is minimally insufflated with air, while during colonoscopic extubation air is almost continuously aspirated. Colonoscopic decompression is not required to the cecum. Adequate decompression is obtained if the hepatic flexure is intubated [57]. Decompressive colonoscopy can significantly reduce intraluminal colonic pressure without reducing the cecal diameter on abdominal roentgenograms [96], possibly because of initial colonic shortening subsequently followed by a decrease in luminal diameter [97]. In one study, the cecal diameter decreased by only 2 cm 1 day after colonoscopic decompression, despite clinical improvement [97]. In a retrospective analysis, the colonoscopy-related mortality was 3.4%, and the morbidity was 1.7% [60]. Severe colonscopic complications include colonic perforation or ischemia.

One-third of patients require repeat colonoscopic decompression because of recurrent colonic distention [93]. Insertion of a long decompression tube during colonoscopy decreases the recurrence rate [98,99]. A guidewire is passed through the colonoscopic channel and left in place as the colonoscope is withdrawn. A decompression tube is then passed over the guidewire into the right colon. Although expelled several days later by colonic peristalsis, this tube maintains colonic decompression during the first few critical days until normal colonic motility recovers.

Administration of polyethylene glycol after acute colonic decompression may help prevent relapse, possibly because of reduced nitric oxide production [6,100]. In one study, no subject receiving daily polyethylene glycol relapsed, while 33.3% of controls receiving placebo relapsed [74]. Polyethylene glycol produced only minor side effects of mild nausea or abdominal pain.

*Invasive therapy*

Persistent colonic dilatation in patients with multiple comorbidities who are poor surgical candidates can be treated by percutaneous transperitoneal cecostomy under either fluoroscopic, colonoscopic, or laparoscopic guidance [101]. These procedures were initially used to treat chronic colonic pseudo-obstruction or chronic constipation from neurogenic bowel [102,103]. Successful colonic decompression was achieved with aspiration using a 22-gauge needle or by insertion of an 8 to 12 French catheter in several small clinical series [104–106]. Complications of radiologic cecostomy include catheter leakage, abdominal wall cellulitis, and sepsis [104,107]. Percutaneous endoscopic cecostomy is modeled after percutaneous endoscopic gastrostomy using the pull technique [108]. Complications include pressure necrosis from the external bumper, profuse granulation tissue formation, abdominal wall cellulitis, abdominal sepsis, and peritonitis [103,109].

Surgical cecostomy or colostomy is associated with high morbidity and significant mortality [60]. In a series of 179 subjects undergoing surgery, the morbidity was 30% and the mortality was 6% [57]. It is reserved for very sick patients who do not respond to medical or colonoscopic therapy. Colonic perforation usually requires total colectomy with an ileostomy because anastomosis of a dilated and thin-walled colon to a nondilated terminal ileum is technically difficult and prone to leakage. Fig. 1 provides an algorithm for the diagnosis and therapy of colonic pseudo-obstruction in patients presenting with acute abdominal distention and failure to pass stool. The algorithm in Fig. 2 summarizes the therapy for colonic pseudo-obstruction in patients who initially respond to a first course of neostigmine therapy.

*Complications*

According to LaPlace's law, an increase in bowel diameter leads to increased wall tension, with a consequently increased risk of local ischemia

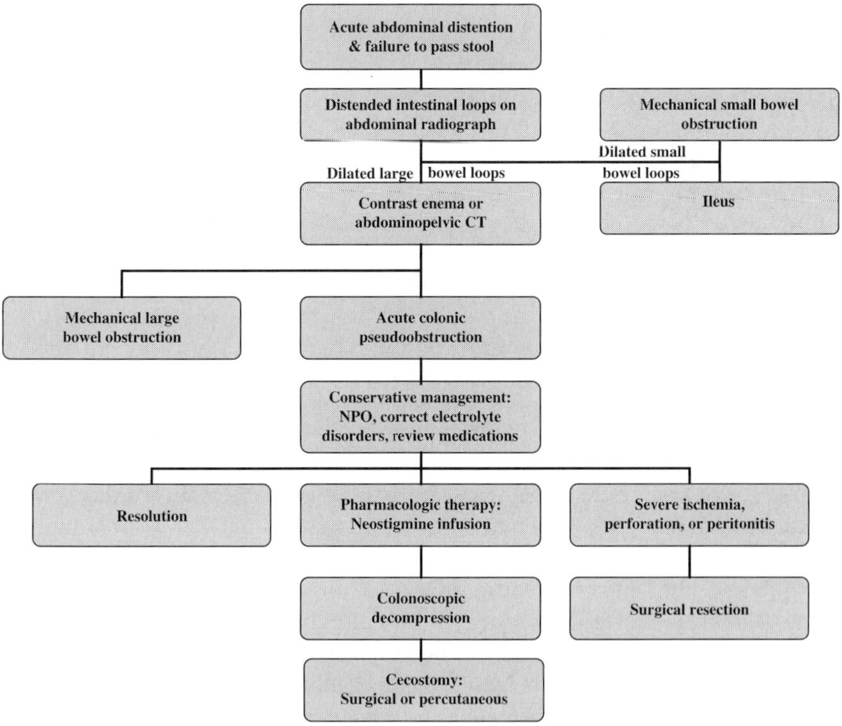


Fig. 1. Algorithm for management of colonic pseudo-obstruction presenting with acute abdominal distention and failure to pass stools. NPO, nothing per os.

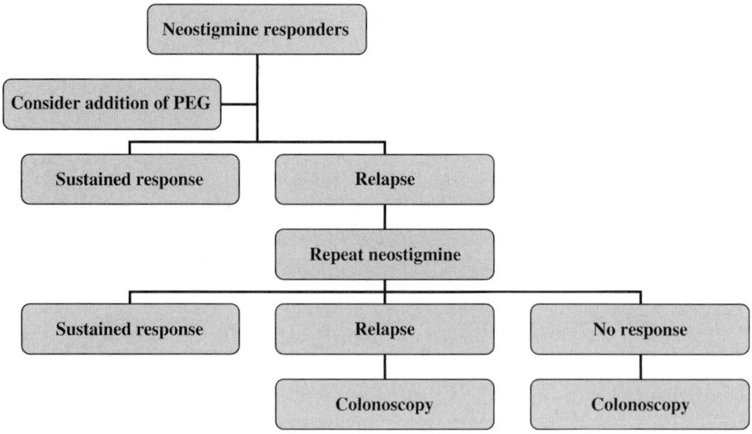


Fig. 2. Algorithm of clinical management in patients who initially respond to neostigmine therapy for acute colonic pseudo-obstruction. PEG, polyethylene glycol electrolyte.

and perforation. The analogous mechanical effect occurs when a balloon bursts or "perforates," as the balloon wall becomes progressively thinner and intramural tension increases during balloon overinflation [110]. The tension is greatest in the cecum because it has the largest colonic diameter. Animal and retrospective clinical data suggest critical thresholds of 12 cm for the cecum and 9 cm for the transverse colon for an increased risk of ischemia and perforation. In a review of 400 cases, no colonic perforation occurred with a cecal diameter less than 12 cm [57], but perforation has occasionally been reported with a cecal diameter of less than 10 cm. The true incidence of spontaneous perforation is unknown because of therapeutic intervention, but is estimated at between 3% and 20%. It has a mortality of 40% to 50% [57,94]. Renal transplant patients with ACPO have a higher perforation rate (22%) and a higher perforation-associated mortality (53%). A lower threshold for operative intervention is warranted in these patients if the initial colonoscopy is unsuccessful [111].

### *Outcome*

With appropriate treatment, ACPO usually resolves in 3 to 6 days, with a mean of 5.2 days [57]. The overall mortality of ACPO is about 15% [61,111,112]. The mortality in patients treated conservatively is about 12%, while the mortality in patients requiring surgery is about 30% [57,60,111,112]. Mortality is higher in the elderly and in patients with multiple comorbidities. Most deaths are caused by the underlying medical conditions [113]. Other factors increasing mortality include delayed colonic decompression, ischemic bowel, and increasing cecal diameter. Mortality increases fivefold when decompression is delayed 7 days or more versus 4 days or less after the diagnosis [57]. Surgical mortality is doubled in patients with ischemic or perforated bowel versus intact, viable bowel [57]. The mortality doubles when the cecal diameter becomes greater than 14 cm.

*Summary*

ACPO presents as massive colonic dilatation without a mechanical cause, usually in critically ill patients. It is believed to result from increased thoracic sympathetic stimulation or decreased sacral parasympathetic activity. The initial therapeutic approach is conservative, with supportive measures and correction of potential contributory metabolic, infectious, or pharmacologic factors. Mechanical obstruction should be excluded on plain abdominal radiographs or abdominal computed tomography by detecting air throughout the colonic segments, including the rectosigmoid. If air is not detected in the left colon, mechanical obstruction should be excluded by a contrast enema.

If the cecal diameter remains more than 9 cm after 72 hours of supportive measures, neostigmine, 2 mg should be administered during continuous electrocardiographic monitoring. The dose can be repeated 4 hours later if no response occurred or if colonic dilatation recurred. Patients who fail to respond to this therapy should undergo decompressive colonoscopy. Surgery is reserved for patients with clinical deterioration or with evidence of colonic ischemia or perforation.

## References


[1] Prasad M, Matthews JB. Deflating postoperative ileus. Gastroenterology 1999;117(2):489–92.

[2] Saunders MD, Kimmey MB. Systematic review: acute colonic pseudo-obstruction. Aliment Pharmacol Ther 2005;22:917–25.

[3] Loftus CG, Harewood GC, Baron TH. Assessment of predictors of response to neostigmine for acute colonic pseudo-obstruction. Am J Gastroenterol 2002;97(12):3118–22.

[4] Sϕreide O, Bjerkeset T, Fossdal JE. Pseudo-obstruction of the colon (Ogilvie's syndrome), a genuine clinical condition? Review of the literature (1948–1975) and report of five cases. Dis Colon Rectum 1977;20(6):487–91.

[5] Turnage RH, Heldmann M, Cole P, et al. Intestinal obstruction and ileus. In: Feldman M, Friedman LS, Brandt LJ, editors. Sleisenger and Fordtran's gastrointestinal and liver disease: pathophysiology, diagnosis, and management. 8th edition. Philadelphia: Elsevier Saunders; 2006. p. 2653–78.

[6] De Winter BY, Boeckxstaens GE, De Man JG, et al. Effect of adrenergic and nitrergic blockade on experimental ileus in rats. Br J Pharmacol 1997;120(3):464–8.

[7] Bauer AJ, Schwartz NT, Moore BA. Ileus in critical illness: mechanisms and management. Curr Opin Crit Care 2002;8(2):152–7.

[8] Wehner S, Behrendt FF, Lyutenski BN, et al. Inhibition of macrophage function prevents intestinal inflammation and postoperative ileus in rodents. Gut 2007;56(2):176–85.

[9] Schwarz NT, Kalff JC, Turler A, et al. Selective jejunal manipulation causes postoperative pan-enteric inflammation and dysmotility. Gastroenterology 2004;126(1):159–69.

[10] De Winter BY, Boeckxstaens GE, De Man JG, et al. Effects of mu- and kappa-opioid receptors on postoperative ileus in rats. Eur J Pharmacol 1997;339(1):63–7.

[11] Tache Y, Bonaz B. Corticotropin-releasing factor receptors and stress-related alterations of gut motor function. J Clin Invest 2007;117(1):33–40.
[12] Holte K, Kehlet H. Postoperative ileus: a preventable event. Br J Surg 2000;87(11):1480–93.
[13] Condon RE, Cowles VE, Ferraz AA, et al. Human colonic smooth muscle electrical activity during and after recovery from postoperative ileus. Am J Physiol 1995;269(3 Pt 1):G408–17.
[14] Livingston EH, Passaro EP Jr. Postoperative ileus. Dig Dis Sci 1990;35(1):121–32.
[15] Kurz A, Sessler DI. Opioid-induced bowel-dysfunction: pathophysiology and potential new therapies. Drugs 2003;63(7):649–71.
[16] Fallon MT, Hanks GW. Morphine, constipation and performance status in advanced cancer patients. Palliat Med 1999;13(2):159–60.
[17] Evers BM. Small intestine. In: Townsend CM, Beauchamp RD, Evers BM, Mattox KL, editors. Sabiston textbook of surgery: the biologic basis of modern surgical practice. 17th edition. Philadelphia: Elsevier Saunders; 2004. p. 1323–80.
[18] Pickleman J, Lee RM. The management of patients with suspected early postoperative small bowel obstruction. Ann Surg 1989;210(2):216–9.
[19] Moore FA, Feliciano DV, Andrassy RJ, et al. Early enteral feeding, compared with parenteral, reduces postoperative septic complications: the results of a meta-analysis. Ann Surg 1992;216(2):172–83.
[20] Binderow SR, Cohen SM, Wexner SD, et al. Must early postoperative oral intake be limited to laparoscopy? Dis Col Rectum 1994;37(6):584–9.
[21] Carr CS, Ling KD, Boulos P, et al. Randomized trial of safety and efficacy of immediate postoperative enteral feeding in patients undergoing gastrointestinal resection. Br Med J 1996;312(7035):869–71.
[22] Koretz RL, Avenell A, Lipman TO, et al. Does enteral nutrition affect clinical outcome? A systematic review of the randomized trials. Am J Gastroenterol 2007;102(2):412–29.
[23] Schilder JM, Hurteau JA, Look KY, et al. A prospective controlled trial of early postoperative oral intake following major abdominal gynecologic surgery. Gynecol Oncol 1997; 67(3):235–40.
[24] Asao T, Kuwano H, Nakamura J, et al. Gum chewing enhances early recovery from postoperative ileus after laparoscopic colectomy. J Am Coll Surg 2002;195(1):30–2.
[25] Matros E, Rocha F, Zinner M, et al. Does gum chewing ameliorate postoperative ileus? Results of a prospective, randomized, placebo-controlled trial. J Am Coll Surg 2006; 202(5):773–8.
[26] Quah HM, Samad A, Neathey AJ, et al. Does gum chewing reduce postoperative ileus following open colectomy for left-sided colon and rectal cancer? A prospective randomized controlled trial. Colorect Dis 2006;8(1):64–70.
[27] Schuster R, Grewal N, Greaney GC, et al. Gum chewing reduces ileus after elective open sigmoid colectomy. Arch Surg 2006;141(2):174–6.
[28] Waldhausen JH, Schirmer BD. The effect of ambulation on the recovery from postoperative ileus. Ann Surg 1990;212(6):671–7.
[29] Cheatham ML, Chapman WC, Key SP, et al. A meta-analysis of selective versus routine nasogastric decompression after elective laparotomy. Ann Surg 1995;221(5):469–76.
[30] Reasbeck PG, Rice ML, Herbison GP. Nasogastric intubation after intestinal resection. Surg Gynecol Obstet 1984;158(4):354–8.
[31] Behm B, Stollman N. Postoperative ileus: etiologies and intervention. Clin Gastroenterol Hepatol 2003;1(2):71–80.
[32] Bonacini M, Quiason S, Reynolds M, et al. Effect of intravenous erythromycin on postoperative ileus. Am J Gastroenterol 1993;88(2):208–11.
[33] Lightfoot AJ, Eno M, Kreder KJ, et al. Treatment of postoperative ileus after bowel surgery with low-dose intravenous erythromycin. Urology 2007;69(4):611–5.
[34] Smith AJ, Nissan A, Lanouette NM, et al. Prokinetic effect of erythromycin after colorectal surgery: randomized, placebo-controlled, double-blinded study. Dis Col Rectum 2000; 43(3):333–7.

[35] Hallerback B, Carlsen E, Carlsson K, et al. Beta-adrenoreceptor blockade in the treatment of postoperative adynamic ileus. Scand J Gastroenterol 1987;22(2):149–55.
[36] Cheape JD, Wexner SD, James K, et al. Does metoclopramide reduce the length of ileus after colorectal surgery? A prospective randomized trial. Dis Colon Rectum 1991;34(6): 437–41.
[37] Orlando E, Finelli F, Colla M, et al. (A double-blinded study of neostigmine versus placebo in paralytic ileus as a result of surgical interventions). Minerva Chir 1994;49(5):451–5 [in Italian].
[38] Kraus K, Fanning J. Prospective trial of early feeding and bowel stimulation after radical hysterectomy. Am J Obstet Gynecol 2000;182(5):996–8.
[39] Hansen CT, Sorensen M, Moller C, et al. Effect of laxatives on gastrointestinal function recovery in fast-track hysterectomy: a double-blind, placebo-controlled randomized study. Am J Obstet Gynecol 2007;196(4):311.e1–311.e7.
[40] Barnes J, Resch KL, Ernst E. Homeopathy for postoperative ileus? A meta-analysis. J Clin Gastroenterol 1997;25(4):628–33.
[41] Linde K, Clausius N, Ramirez G, et al. Are the clinical effects of homeopathy placebo effects? A meta-analysis of placebo-controlled trials. Lancet 1997;350(9081):834–43.
[42] Leslie JB. Alvimopan for the management of postoperative ileus. Ann Pharmacother 2005; 39(9):1502–10.
[43] Tan EK, Cornish J, Darzi AW, et al. Meta-analysis: alvimopan vs. placebo in the treatment of post-operative ileus. Aliment Pharmacol Ther 2007;25(1):47–57.
[44] Holzer P. Treatment of opioid-induced gut dysfunction. Expert Opin Investig Drugs 2007; 16(2):181–94.
[45] Aziz O, Athanasiou T, Tekkis PP, et al. Laparoscopic versus open appendectomy in children: a meta-analysis. Ann Surg 2006;243(1):17–27.
[46] Garcia-Caballero M, Vara-Thorbeck C. The evolution of postoperative ileus after laparoscopic cholecystectomy: a comparative study with conventional cholecystectomy and sympathetic blockade treatment. Surg Endosc 1993;7(5):416–9.
[47] LeBlanc-Louvry I, Coquerel A, Koning E, et al. Operative stress response is reduced after laparoscopic compared to open cholecystectomy: the relationship with postoperative pain and ileus. Dig Dis Sci 2000;45(9):1703–13.
[48] Ferraz AA, Cowles VE, Condon RE, et al. Nonopioid analgesics shorten the duration of postoperative ileus. Am Surg 1995;61(12):1079–83.
[49] Pairet M, Ruckenbusch Y. On the relevance of non-steroidal anti-inflammatory drugs in the prevention of paralytic ileus in rodents. J Pharm Pharmacol 1989;41(11):757–61.
[50] Ruoff G, Lema M. Strategies in pain management: new and potential indications for COX-2 inhibitors. J Pain Symptom Manage 2003;25(2 Suppl):S21–31.
[51] Sim R, Cheong DM, Wong KS, et al. Prospective randomized, double-blind, placebo-controlled study of pre- and postoperative administration of a COX-2-specific inhibitor as opioid-sparing analgesia in major colorectal surgery. Colorectal Dis 2007;9(1):52–60.
[52] Jorgensen H, Wetterslev J, Moiniche S, et al. Epidural local anaesthetics versus opioid-based analgesic regimens on postoperative gastrointestinal paralysis, PONV and pain after abdominal surgery. Cochrane Database Syst Rev 2000;(4) CD001893.
[53] Steinbrook RA. Epidural anesthesia and gastrointestinal motility. Anesth Analg 1998; 86(4):837–44.
[54] Ogilvie H. Large-intestine colic due to sympathetic deprivation: a new clinical syndrome. Br Med J 1948;2:671–3.
[55] Dudley HA, Sinclair IS, McLaren IF, et al. Intestinal pseudo-obstruction. J R Coll Surg Edinb 1958;3(3):206–17.
[56] Delgado-Aros S, Camilleri M. Pseudo-obstruction in the critically ill. Best Pract Res Clin Gastroenterol 2003;17(3):427–44.
[57] Vanek VW, Al-Salti M. Acute pseudo-obstruction of the colon (Ogilvie's syndrome): an analysis of 400 cases. Dis Colon Rectum 1986;29(3):203–10.

[58] Catchpole BN. Ileus: use of sympathetic blocking agents in its treatment. Surgery 1969; 66(5):811–20.
[59] Romeo DP, Solomon GD, Hover AR. Acute colonic pseudo-obstruction: a possible role for the colocolonic reflex. J Clin Gastroenterol 1985;7(3):256–60.
[60] Wegener M, Börsch G. Acute colonic pseudo-obstruction (Ogilvie's syndrome): presentation of 14 of our own cases and analysis of 1027 cases reported in the literature. Surg Endosc 1987;1(3):169–74.
[61] Nanni G, Garbini A, Luchetti P, et al. Ogilvie's syndrome (acute colonic pseudo-obstruction): review of the literature (October 1948 to March 1980) and report of four additional cases. Dis Colon Rectum 1982;25(2):157–66.
[62] Johnston G, Vitikainen K, Knight R, et al. Changing perspective on gastrointestinal complications in patients undergoing cardiac surgery. Am J Surg 1992;163(5):525–9.
[63] Kadesky K, Purdue GF, Hunt JL. Acute pseudo-obstruction in critically ill patients with burns. J Burn Care Rehabil 1995;16(2 Pt 1):132–5.
[64] Kahi CJ, Rex DK. Bowel obstruction and pseudo-obstruction. Gastroenterol Clin North Am 2003;32(4):1229–47.
[65] Adams JT. Adynamic ileus of the colon: an indication for cecostomy. Arch Surg 1974; 109(4):503–7.
[66] Chapman AH, McNamara M, Porter G. The acute contrast enema in suspected large bowel obstruction: value and technique. Clin Radiol 1992;46(4):273–8.
[67] Frager D. Intestinal obstruction: role of CT. Gastroenterol Clin North Am 2002;31(3): 777–99.
[68] Beattie GC, Peters RT, Guy S, et al. Computed tomography in the assessment of suspected large bowel obstruction. ANZ J Surg 2007;77(3):160–5.
[69] Sloyer AF, Panella VS, Demas BE, et al. Ogilvie's syndrome: successful management without colonoscopy. Dig Dis Sci 1988;33(11):1391–6.
[70] Abeyta BJ, Albrecht RM, Schermer CR. Retrospective study of neostigmine for the treatment of acute colonic pseudo-obstruction. Am Surg 2001;67(3):265–9.
[71] Mehta R, John A, Nair P, et al. Factors predicting successful outcome following neostigmine therapy in acute colonic pseudo-obstruction. A prospective study. J Gastroenterol Hepatol 2006;21(2):459–61.
[72] Paran H, Silverberg D, Mayo A, et al. Treatment of acute colonic pseudo-obstruction with neostigmine. J Am Coll Surg 2000;190(3):315–8.
[73] Ponec RJ, Saunders MD, Kimmey MB. Neostigmine for the treatment of acute colonic pseudo-obstruction. N Engl J Med 1999;341(3):137–41.
[74] Sgouros SN, Vlachogiannakos J, Vassiliadis K, et al. Effect of polyethylene glycol electrolyte balanced solution on patients with acute colonic pseudo obstruction after resolution of colonic dilation: a prospective, randomised, placebo-controlled trial. Gut 2006;55(5): 638–42.
[75] Stephenson BM, Morgan AR, Salaman JR, et al. Ogilvie's syndrome: a new approach to an old problem. Dis Colon Rectum 1995;38(4):424–7.
[76] Trevisani GT, Hyman NH, Church JM. Neostigmine: safe and effective treatment for acute colonic pseudo-obstruction. Dis Colon Rectum 2000;43(5):599–603.
[77] Turegano-Fuentes F, Munoz-Jimenez F, Del Valle-Hernandez E, et al. Early resolution of Ogilvie's syndrome with intravenous neostigmine: a simple, effective treatment. Dis Colon Rectum 1997;40(11):1353–7.
[78] Van Der Spoel JI, Oudemans-Van Straaten HM, Stoutenbeek CP, et al. Neostigmine resolves critical illness-related colonic ileus in intensive care patients with multiple organ failure: a prospective, double-blind, placebo-controlled trial. Intensive Care Med 2001; 27(5):822–7.
[79] Korsten MA, Rosman AS, Ng A, et al. Infusion of neostigmine-glycopyrrolate for bowel evacuation in persons with spinal cord injury. Am J Gastroenterol 2005;100(7): 1560–5.

[80] Briggs JC, Dobson-Smyth WE, Livingston A. Death due to a combination of treatment and disease. Br Med J 1969;4(5679):344.
[81] Marchand WE. An unusual case of neostigmine bromide poisoning. Gastroenterology 1959;36(6):877–80.
[82] Mazloum BW, Barnes JB, Lee M. Cisapride as successful treatment for acute intestinal pseudo-obstruction. South Med J 1996;89(8):828–30.
[83] Pelckmans PA, Michielsen PP, Jorens PG, et al. Cisapride in Ogilvie's syndrome. Gastroenterology 1990;99(4):1194–5.
[84] Mashour GA, Peterfreund RA. Spinal anesthesia and Ogilvie's syndrome. J Clin Anesth 2005;17(2):122–3.
[85] Armstrong DN, Ballantyne GH, Modlin IM. Erythromycin for reflex ileus in Ogilvie's syndrome. Lancet 1991;337(8737):378.
[86] Rovira A, Lopez A, Cambray C, et al. Acute colonic pseudo-obstruction (Ogilvie's syndrome) treated with erythromycin. Intensive Care Med 1997;23(7):798.
[87] Bonacini M, Smith OJ, Pritchard T. Erythromycin as therapy for acute colonic pseudo-obstruction (Ogilvie's syndrome). J Clin Gastroenterol 1991;13(4):475–6.
[88] Goodman AJ, Le Bourdonnec B, Dolle RE. Mu opioid receptor antagonists: recent developments. Chem Med Chem 2007;2(11):1552–70.
[89] Lembo A. Peripheral opioids for functional GI disease: a reappraisal. Dig Dis 2006;24(1–2): 91–8.
[90] Schmidt WK. Alvimopan (ADL 8-2698) is a novel peripheral opioid antagonist. Am J Surg 2001;182(5A Suppl):27S–38S.
[91] Simini B. Spinal anaesthesia in acute colonic pseudo-obstruction. Anaesthesia 1995;50(12): 1103.
[92] Lee JT, Taylor BM, Singleton BC. Epidural anesthesia for acute pseudo-obstruction of the colon (Ogilvie's syndrome). Dis Colon Rectum 1988;31(9):686–91.
[93] Jetmore AB, Timmcke AE, Gathright JB Jr, et al. Ogilvie's syndrome: colonoscopic decompression and analysis of predisposing factors. Dis Colon Rectum 1992;35(12):1135–42.
[94] Rex DK. Colonoscopy and acute colonic pseudo-obstruction. Gastrointest Endosc Clin N Am 1997;7(3):499–508.
[95] Bode WE, Beart RW Jr, Spencer RJ, et al. Colonoscopic decompression for acute pseudoobstruction of the colon (Ogilvie's syndrome). Report of 22 cases and review of the literature. Am J Surg 1984;147(2):243–5.
[96] Strodel WE, Nostrant TT, Eckhauser FE, et al. Therapeutic and diagnostic endoscopy in nonobstructive colonic dilatation. Ann Surg 1983;197(4):416–21.
[97] Pham TN, Cosman BC, Chu P, et al. Radiographic changes after colonoscopic decompression for acute pseudo-obstruction. Dis Colon Rectum 1999;42(12):1586–91.
[98] Harig JM, Fumo DE, Loo FD, et al. Treatment of acute nontoxic megacolon during colonoscopy: tube placement versus simple decompression. Gastrointest Endosc 1988; 34(1):23–7.
[99] Lavignolle A, Jutel P, Bonhomme J, et al. Ogilvie's syndrome: results of endoscopic exsufflation in a series of 29 cases. Gastroenterol Clin Biol 1986;10(2):147–51.
[100] Shishido SM, de Oliveira MG. Polyethylene glycol matrix reduces the rates of photochemical and thermal release of nitric oxide from S-niroso-N-acetylcysteine. Photochem Photobiol 2000;71(3):273–80.
[101] Duh QY, Way LW. Diagnostic laparoscopy and laparoscopic cecostomy for colonic pseudo-obstruction. Dis Colon Rectum 1993;36(1):65–70.
[102] Rivera MT, Kugathasan S, Berger W, et al. Percutaneous colonoscopic cecostomy for management of chronic constipation in children. Gastrointest Endosc 2001;53(2):225–8.
[103] Ramage JI, Baron TH. Percutaneous endoscopic cecostomy: a case series. Gastrointest Endosc 2003;57(6):752–5.
[104] Van Sonnenberg E, Varney RR, Casola G, et al. Percutaneous cecostomy for Ogilvie syndrome: laboratory observations and clinical experience. Radiology 1990;175(3):679–82.

[105] Chevallier P, Marcy PY, Francois E, et al. Controlled transperitoneal percutaneous cecostomy as a therapeutic alternative to the endoscopic decompression for Ogilvie's syndrome. Am J Gastroenterol 2002;97(2):471–4.
[106] Crass JR, Simmons RL, Frick MP, et al. Percutaneous decompression of the colon using CT guidance in Ogilvie syndrome. AJR Am J Roentgenol 1985;144(3):475–6.
[107] Maginot TJ, Cascade PN. Abdominal wall cellulitis and sepsis secondary to percutaneous cecostomy. Cardiovasc Intervent Radiol 1993;16(5):328–31.
[108] Ponsky JL, Aszodi A, Perse D. Percutaneous endoscopic cecostomy: a new approach to nonobstructive colonic dilation. Gastrointest Endosc 1986;32(2):108–11.
[109] Lynch CR, Jones RG, Hilden K, et al. Percutaneous endoscopic cecostomy in adults: a case series. Gastrointest Endosc 2006;64(2):279–82.
[110] Saunders MD, Cappell MS. Endoscopic management of acute colonic pseudo-obstruction. Endoscopy 2005;37(8):760–3.
[111] O'Malley KJ, Flechner SM, Kapoor A, et al. Acute colonic pseudo-obstruction (Ogilvie's syndrome) after renal transplantation. Am J Surg 1999;177(6):492–6.
[112] Ponzano C, Nardi S, Carrieri P, et al. (Diagnostic problems, pathogenetic hypothesis and therapeutic proposals in Ogilvie's syndrome. Review of 470 observations from the literature and presentation of 5 new cases). Minerva Chir 1997;52(11):1311–20 [in Italian].
[113] Kukora JS, Dent TL. Colonoscopic decompression of massive nonobstructive cecal dilatation. Arch Surg 1977;122(4):512–7.

ELSEVIER
SAUNDERS

Med Clin N Am 92 (2008) 671–686

THE MEDICAL
CLINICS
OF NORTH AMERICA

# Severe Complications of Inflammatory Bowel Disease

Francisco Marrero, MD, Mohammed A. Qadeer, MD,
Bret A. Lashner, MD*

*Department of Gastroenterology and Hepatology, Cleveland Clinic,
9500 Euclid Avenue/A30, Cleveland, OH 44195, USA*

Patients who have inflammatory bowel disease (IBD) occasionally have severe complications or emergency situations that require expedited, expert medical care, including toxic colitis, fistulas, abdominal abscesses, malignancy, primary sclerosing cholangitis, and pouchitis. Morbidity and mortality rates of Crohn's disease and ulcerative colitis (UC) are increased over the expected rates in the unaffected population. Knowledge of the presenting features, natural history, and treatment of these complications can lead to early and effective therapy and better outcomes.

## Epidemiology of severe or complicated inflammatory bowel disease

Patients who have IBD have an increased risk of mortality from several severe disease complications. In a meta-analysis of 10 population-based cohort studies of patients who had UC, the standardized mortality ratio (SMR) was 1.1 (95% confidence interval [CI], 0.9–1.2) [1]. The fact that patients who have ulcerative colitis are significantly less likely to smoke cigarettes than the unaffected population lowers the expected baseline SMR for these patients by as much as 40% [2,3]. Therefore, an SMR of 1.1 likely represents a substantially elevated risk of death. Approximately 17% of the mortality is directly related to UC [1], from colorectal cancer, postsurgical complications, and, to a lesser extent, primary sclerosing cholangitis (PSC).

In a European inception cohort of patients who had Crohn's disease, mortality was increased by 85% (SMR, 1.85; 95% CI, 1.30–2.55) [4]. Gastrointestinal complications, particularly abdominal sepsis, intestinal ischemia, and intestinal hemorrhage, accounted for most of the excess

* Corresponding author.
*E-mail address:* lashneb@ccf.org (B.A. Lashner).


doi:10.1016/j.mcna.2007.12.002 **medical.theclinics.com**

mortality. In a United States inception cohort of patients who had IBD, the SMR for Crohn's disease was 1.2 (95% CI, 0.9–1.6), and the SMR for UC was 0.8 (95% CI, 0.6–1.0) [5]. For Crohn's disease, the principal causes of death were gastrointestinal disease and chronic obstructive pulmonary disease, whereas in UC, the risk of cardiovascular death was significantly reduced. The large difference in mortality between Crohn's disease and UC is due to different rates of cigarette smoking. A manufacturer-maintained database of 6,290 patients who had Crohn's disease found that the risk of death was 0.53/100 patient-years in infliximab-treated patients and 0.43/100 patient-years in non-infliximab–treated patients (relative risk 1.24; 95% CI, 0.73–2.10) [6]. Mortality was related to older age and prednisone use and not necessarly to infliximab use.

Although the incidence of IBD is rising, the rate of IBD surgery is declining [6,7]. In Copenhagen County, 35% of patients who had Crohn's disease diagnosed between 1962 and 1987 had surgery within the first year of diagnosis, compared with 12% diagnosed between 2003 and 2005 ($P<.001$). In patients who have UC, surgery within the first year of disease was performed in 9% in the earlier cohort and 6% in the later cohort ($P = .09$). Lower surgery rates should translate into less surgically related mortality.

In theory, cardiovascular disease mortality should be increased in patients who have IBD because these patients have an elevated serum level of C-reactive protein, a risk factor for cardiovascular mortality. A meta-analysis of 11 studies showed no overall increased risk of cardiovascular mortality [8].

Mortality can apparently be minimized by performing surgery only for severe complications, performing effective cancer surveillance in high-risk patients, encouraging cancer chemoprevention, and strongly emphasizing the benefits of cigarette smoking cessation.

## Toxic megacolon and colonic perforation in the setting of severe acute colitis from inflammatory bowel disease

Toxic megacolon is a severe life-threatening emergency associated with IBD. It represents the most severe end of the broad spectrum of disease activity that ranges from mild disease to severe disease to toxic colitis to toxic magacolon. Toxic megacolon can occur with UC or Crohn's colitis.

### *Epidemiology*

In a review of 1,236 patients admitted with IBD between 1960 and 1979, 75 patients (6%) had toxic megacolon [9]. Of these cases, 10% had UC, and 2.3% had Crohn's disease. Seventy-nine percent of the patients underwent surgery during their hospitalization. Eleven of the 12 patients who died had suffered colonic perforation [10]. Although the lifetime incidence of toxic megacolon in patients who have UC is approximately 2.5%, the incidence among hospitalized patients ranges from 6% to 17% [11]. In a series of 500 patients who underwent surgery for Crohn's colitis, toxic megacolon was the major indication in 23% of cases [12].

*Etiology*

The etiology of toxic megacolon is incompletely understood. Defective colonic smooth muscle contractions, lowered basal pressure in the colonic lumen, or an inhibited gastro-colic reflex are thought to be key contributors [13,14]. The net result is bowel paralysis and dilation [15]. Hypokalemia and hypomagnesemia have also been implicated. Many biochemical mediators have been associated with toxic megacolon, particularly nitric oxide. It is unclear whether these electrolyte abnormalities and biochemical mediators reflect the toxic state, directly contribute to toxic megacolon, or both. Proximate triggers of megacolon include barium enema, rapid discontinuation of steroids or 5-aminosalicylic acid medications, administration of narcotics or anticholinergics, administration of chemotherapy, and colonoscopy [9,10,14]. Intense transmural vascular congestion and muscle disintegration commonly occur in toxic megacolon, whether from UC or Crohn's disease. Deep colonic ulceration occurs in toxic megacolon more frequently than in acute or chronic colitis [9].

*Diagnosis*

Toxic megacolon is diagnosed by a combination of clinical signs and symptoms. The diagnosis requires the presence of toxic colitis, defined by Truelove and Witts in 1955, as at least six bloody bowel movements daily, a hemoglobin of less than 10.5 g/dL, an erythrocyte sedimentation rate of at least 30 mm per hour, and a heart rate of 90 per beats minute or greater [16]. Jalen and colleagues described the clinical features of toxic megacolon in a series of 55 patients [17]. In addition to radiographic evidence of colonic dilation, at least three of the following needed to be present: temperature above 38°C, pulse rate above 90 beats per minute, leukocyte count greater than 10,500/mm$^3$ (with a left shift), and anemia with a hematocrit of less than 60% of normal. The patient must also have had one of the following signs or symptoms of systemic toxicity: dehydration, mental status changes, electrolyte abnormalities, or hypotension. Toxic megacolon is identified radiographically by plain abdominal roentgenograms. There should be thickening or loss of the haustral pattern, usually first affecting the inferior margin of the transverse colon (Fig. 1) [9]. Linear serrations, representing penetrating colonic wall ulceration, may occur from extensive, deep colonic ulceration. Toxic megacolon is radiographically defined as segmental or total colonic dilation, of at least 5 cm in diameter, in the setting of toxic colitis [9,10]. In one series, the mean maximal diameter of the dilated colon

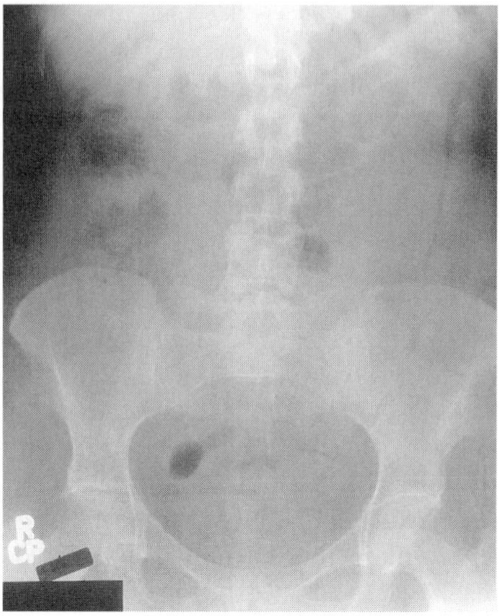

Fig. 1. Abdominal radiograph of a patient who has toxic megacolon. There are edematous haustral folds (thumbprinting) and a dilated transverse colon.

was 9.2 cm (range, 5–16 cm). Small intestinal or gastric distention may predict progression to toxic megacolon [18,19].

*Management*

Vigorous resuscitation with intravenous fluids is essential. Antibiotics are sometimes efficacious in severe Crohn's flares but are not effective in UC flares [20–22]. Broad-spectrum antibiotics to cover enteric organisms are recommended in the setting of toxic megacolon due to the risk of colonic perforation. Bowel rest with total parenteral nutrition may be an adjunctive therapy, but this intervention does not necessarily reduce the rate of surgical intervention or mortality. The use of 5-aminosalicylic acid agents is of little benefit in the setting of toxic megacolon. Although infliximab and cyclosporine are effective in some patients who have severely active colitis not responding to corticosteroids [23,24], these therapies have not been specifically studied in toxic megacolon.

Surgery is the best treatment option, but the timing of the surgery is debated. The patient can occasionally be managed conservatively with steroids, frequent abdominal imaging and laboratory studies, and close clinical monitoring. Surgery is indicated if the patient does not clinically improve within 7 days or if the patient clinically deteriorates. Another approach calls for surgery immediately at the diagnosis of toxic megacolon due to the high risk of perforation. Absolute indications for surgery in patients who have toxic megacolon include perforation, uncontrollable bleeding, and progressive dilation.

## Fistulizing Crohn's disease and intra-abdominal abscess

### *Fistulizing Crohn's disease*

Fistulizing disease is one of the three principal clinical phenotypes of Crohn's disease, the other two being inflammatory or stricturing behavior. Fistulas can occur in any part of the bowel. Fistulas may be external or internal. Internal fistulas may be enteroenteric or between the intestines and an adjacent structure. External fistulas arise from the intestine and communicate with the skin. The distribution of fistulas in patients in Olmsted County, Minnesota from 1970 to 1995 was 54% perianal, 24% enteroenteric, 9% rectovaginal, and 13% other [25]. The cumulative risk for developing a fistula was 50% at 20 years. There are no known specific risk factors for the development of fistulas in patients who have Crohn's disease.

### *Clinical presentation*

Patients present with variable symptoms depending on fistula location. Enteroenteric fistulas may be asymptomatic or otherwise present like an inflammatory Crohn's disease flare, and there may be a palpable mass on physical examination. Passage of air or feces from the vagina indicates an enterovaginal fistula. Recurrent polymicrobial urinary tract infections with enteric bacteria or pneumaturia suggest a fistula to the urinary bladder (enterovesicular). Fistulae to intra-abdominal compartments may present with an intra-abdominal abscess, such as a psoas abscess, or may lead to obstructive symptoms of the bowel or other intra-abdominal structures, such as the ureters. Observation of bowel contents leaking from a cutaneous site is consistent with an enterocutaneous fistula.

### *Diagnosis and treatment*

The diagnosis of these fistulas depends on the location. Generally, barium studies, small-bowel follow-through with fluoroscopy and manual manipulation, and CT or magnetic resonance (MR) enterography are helpful in the diagnosis (Fig. 2) [26]. Rectal endoscopic ultrasound, pelvic MRI, and an examination under anesthesia are helpful in assessing perianal fistulae [27].

The treatment is targeted at eradicating the fistulas or significantly reducing their symptoms. Treatment is typically medical and surgical, and the treatment plan is best decided by a surgeon and a gastroenterologist working together. The current literature regarding the medical management of fistulizing Crohn's disease is heavily weighted toward the treatment of enterocutaneous and enterovaginal fistulas; therefore, little is known about the medical therapy of other fistulas. Bowel rest, with total parenteral nutrition, often closes fistulas, but they recur soon after enteral feeding resumes.

Once a surgeon has drained a septic collection emanating from a fistula, the traditional first line of therapy for active fistulization is antibiotics. Metronidazole has been the most extensively studied antibiotic. Response

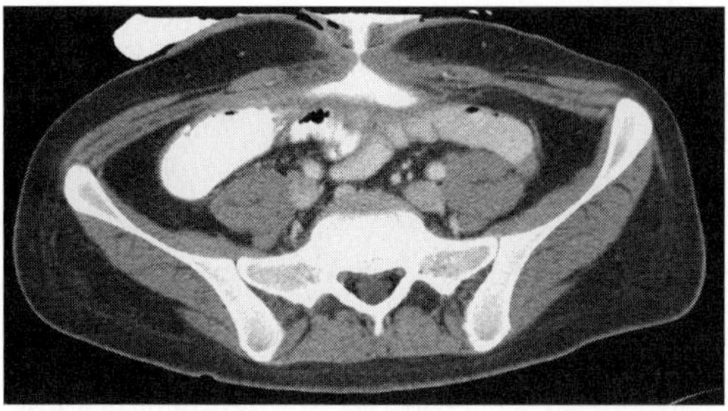

Fig. 2. Extravasation of barium through an enterocutanous fistula in the ventral abdominal wall.

to therapy, defined as healing or decreased discharge, approaches 50%. Although metronidazole alone is often effective, the fistulas typically recur upon metronidazole discontinuation. Ciprofloxacin, alone or in combination with metronidazole, is similarly effective as long as the medication is continued [28–30]. Side effects and loss of efficacy limit the usefulness of long-term antibiotic therapy. Antibiotics may be beneficial as a bridge to a more effective long-term therapy, such as infliximab or azathioprine [31].

Infliximab with 6-mercaptopurine is often effective for the management of enterocutaneous fistulas, with a better tolerated long-term side effect profile than antibiotics. A meta-analysis showed a 54% response rate to 6-mercaptopurine or azathioprine [32]. The ACCENT II trial showed a significantly higher response rate with long-term infliximab administration compared with infliximab induction followed by placebo [33]. A subanalysis of the CHARM trial showed that adalimumab was effective in treating fistulizing Crohn's disease [34].

Calcineurin inhibitors (cyclosporine and tacrolimus) are effective in inducing remission in fistulizing Crohn's disease. These medications should be used only as a bridge to immunosuppressives or TNF inhibitors due to their toxicity [35].

### *Intra-abdominal abscesses*

Intra-abdominal abscesses in patients who have IBD are usually related to fistulas into the mesentery or retroperitoneum with Crohn's disease. The diagnosis should be suspected in a patient who has Crohn's disease who presents with abdominal pain, fever, and leukocytosis, but all of these findings need not be present. An abscess is usually diagnosed by abdominopelvic CT or MRI.

The treatment is centered on abscess drainage. The management of an abscess should include input from a gastroenterologist, a surgeon, and, possibly, an interventional radiologist. If amenable to percutaneous drainage, the abscess should be drained. If not, the abscess can be surgically drained. Broad-spectrum antibiotics with coverage for enteric organisms should be administered. Closure of the fistula usually requires immunosuppressive and biologic therapy. In the setting of an intra-abdominal abscess, corticosteroids are avoided. Surgical resection is not always necessary after adequate drainage.

## Colorectal dysplasia and cancer

Colorectal dysplasia and cancer (CRC) have a much higher incidence in patients who have IBD than in the general population [36]. UC and Crohn's colitis have almost equivalent incremental risk for dysplasia and CRC when an equivalent length of large bowel is affected [37–39].

### *Types of dysplasia*

Dysplasia is classified according to the degree of stratification of the nuclei into low-grade dysplasia (LGD), high-grade dysplasia (HGD), and indefinite dysplasia. In LGD and HGD, the nuclei lose their orientation without extension into the lamina propria. Indefinite dysplasia has equivocal findings that may be mistaken for inflammatory changes [40]. Although interobserver agreement in the diagnosis of no dysplasia or HGD is excellent, agreement in the diagnosis of indefinite dysplasia or LGD is poor even among expert pathologists [39,41]. The finding of dysplasia is important because of the presence of synchronous cancers and development of metachronous cancers. At colectomy, the risk of having a synchronous cancer is 19% with LGD and 42% with HGD [42].

### *Risk factors for colorectal dysplasia and cancer*

Increased duration of disease, increased extent of disease, and the presence of primary sclerosing cholangitis are the most important risk factors for CRC in patients who have IBD. A meta-analysis demonstrated that the overall risk of CRC in any patient who has UC is 3.7% and increases to 5.4% with pancolitis [43]. The risk is 2% at 10 years, 8% at 20 years, and 18% at 30 years for any patient who has UC [43]. Another study found that that the relative risk for CRC was 14 with pancolitis and 1.7 with left-sided colitis as compared with the general population [44]. About 50% of CRC occur in the recto-sigmoid colon. Primary sclerosing cholangitis in patients who have IBD confers a synergistic effect with other risk factors for cancer or dysplasia and increases the risk by at least threefold [45].

### *Endoscopic findings*

The endoscopic appearance of dysplastic colonic mucosa varies from apparently normal to a granular, pebbly, or velvety pattern [40]. Advanced dysplasia may be associated with plaques, nodules, or overt polyps. Because patients who have UC can have sporadic adenomas (adenoma-like mass

[ALM]), it is critical to differentiate this lesion from a dysplasia-associated lesion or mass (DALM) due to a different prognosis and therapy. DALM is an irregularly shaped, dysplastic lesion within a background of active colitis, whereas an ALM is a dysplastic lesion that appears like a sporadic adenoma without dysplastic mucosa in the surrounding epithelium. DALM is significant due to a high risk of carcinoma development [46,47]. ALMs have a much lower risk of cancer development.

*Management*

The first step in management is confirmation of the dysplasia by a second gastrointestinal pathologist [48]. Patients who have unequivocal HGD or DALM should undergo total proctocolectomy in the absence of contraindications for surgery [41]. Patients who have sporadic adenoma (eg, ALM) should undergo colonoscopy with polypectomy and then undergo surveillance colonoscopies. The management of LGD in flat mucosa is controversial, but current evidence suggests that these patients should be offered total proctocolectomy [42,49,50]. Patients who have indefinite dysplasia should undergo repeat colonoscopy after anti-inflammatory treatment of the colitis.

*Natural history*

The risk of cancer in dysplasia detected on an initial colonoscopy is higher than that for dysplasia diagnosed on a subsequent surveillance colonoscopy (higher risk of synchronous cancers) [51]. The duration of transformation of dysplasia into cancer is unknown, but it may last for approximately 3 years [52].

*Surveillance for dysplasia*

The recommendations for surveillance are based on duration and extent of disease. The Crohn's and Colitis Foundation of America Concensus Conference recommends that screening should begin 8 years after the diagnosis of pancolitis (inflammation proximal to the splenic flexure) and 12 to 15 years after the diagnosis of left-sided colitis [53]. Colonoscopy is the best screening test because many flat lesions that commonly occur in patients who have IBD are missed by radiologic tests. Colonoscopy with 33 biopsies yields a 90% confidence for detecting dysplasia when it is present [54]. Four-quadrant biopsies are recommended every 10 cm of the normal-appearing mucosa in addition to extensive biopsies on and around abnormal mucosa or apparent strictures [55].

## Primary sclerosing cholangitis

PSC is a fibroinflammatory disorder of the bile ducts characterized by strictures and beading of the bile ducts, together with chronic cholestasis.

There is a strong but incompletely understood association between PSC and IBD, more so with UC than with Crohn's disease. The proportion of patients who have PSC who have coexisting UC varies from 70% in Northern Europeans to 35% in Southern Europeans and 20% in Japanese [56–58]. About 3% to 7% of patients who have UC have PSC [59]. PSC is predominantly a disease of young men, with a male/female ratio of 2:1.

### *Etiology*

The etiology of PSC is unknown, but different hypotheses have been proposed. The preponderance of HLA-B8, DR3, and DR52A haplotypes in patients who have PSC suggests that these haplotypes might play a significant role in pathogenesis [60,61]. Current evidence suggests that hepatic macrophages respond abnormally to the intestinal bacteria, resulting in disordered secretion of interleukins and TNF-$\alpha$ that causes chronic inflammation of the bile ducts.

### *Clinical features*

PSC has a variable presentation with fatigue, intermittent jaundice, weight loss, right upper quadrant abdominal pain, and pruritus [57,61], but patients are most commonly asymptomatic, and the diagnosis is suspected by finding an abnormally elevated serum alkaline phosphatase with otherwise normal liver function tests. Acute cholangitis does not commonly occur, except after instrumentation of the biliary system. Some patients have cirrhosis and portal hypertension at presentation.

### *Laboratory findings*

The laboratory findings vary among patients and within the same patient at different times. The most common abnormality is an elevated serum alkaline phosphatase with occasional serum transaminase elevations. The diagnostic role of serologic markers, such as p-ANCA, is yet to be proven [56]. The hallmark histologic feature of PSC is the "onion-ring appearance" of the bile duct due to mural inflammation and fibrosis.

### *Radiologic findings*

Endoscopic retrograde cholangiography is the diagnostic test of choice because forceful contrast injection can image ductal strictures to demonstrate intra- and extrahepatic ductal anatomy (Fig. 3) [56]. The bile ducts usually have a normal diameter, but the wall thickness is increased three- to fourfold due to fibrosis, which results in luminal narrowing. The patchy nature of the inflammation gives the bile ducts a "beaded" appearance due to intervening narrowing and dilation [56]. Percutaneous transhepatic cholangiography can be technically challenging when the disease is

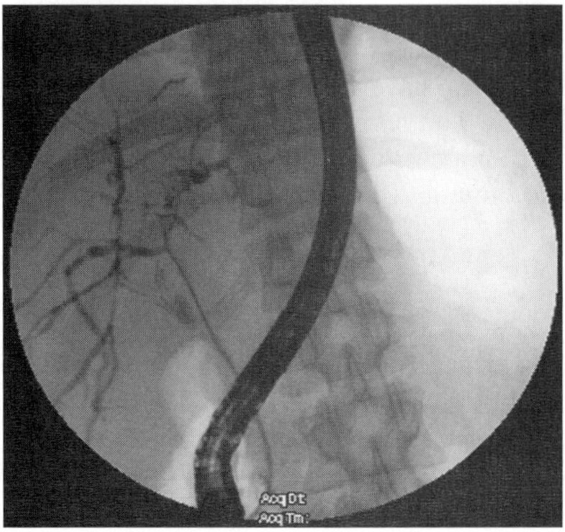


Fig. 3. Endoscopic retrograde cholangiopancreatography of a patient with PSC showing an attenuated biliary tree with a chain-of-lakes appearance, a dominant stricture in the left hepatic duct, and a stent across the stricture.

predominantly intrahepatic. MR cholangiography has a sensitivity of 85% and a specificity of 92% compared with endoscopic retrograde cholangiography [62]. Further refinements in MR technology are expected to improve its diagnostic accuracy.

*Therapy*

PSC is incurable, but different modes of palliation are successfully used. Pruritus is treated by cholestyramine, rifampicin, or naltrexone. Dilation and stenting of biliary strictures can produce significant symptom relief [59]. Steroids, immunosuppressives, and ursodeoxycholic acid have not been demonstrated to improve symptoms or mortality. Liver transplant is the definitive therapy, with an 85% to 90% 5-year survival [63]. PSC recurs in about 20% of patients after transplantation [64]. PSC can affect the outcome of surgery for UC. Ileostomy after total proctocolectomy in patients who have PSC is frequently complicated by recalcitrant peristomal varices with a high risk of bleeding due to portal hypertension [65], whereas ileal pouch creation has twice the cumulative risk of pouchitis compared with patients who do not have PSC. Ileal pouch–anal anastomosis is the preferred surgery for patients who have UC and PSC due to the risk of severe bleeding from peristomal varices.

*Natural history*

The onset of PSC may be unrelated to the onset of UC symptoms. Although colitis symptoms usually precede the diagnosis of PSC, some patients develop PSC symptoms up to 4 years before colitis symptoms [66]. The outcome of PSC is unrelated to the activity of the UC. Coexistent PSC significantly increases the cumulative risk of colon cancer, particularly proximal colon cancer, in patients who have UC. The median time of survival from the diagnosis of PSC is 12 years [57] in symptomatic patients, but about 75% of asymptomatic patients survive for 15 years or more. Cholangiocarcinoma is a complication of PSC that develops in 10% to 20% of patients. Median survival after the diagnosis of cholangiocarcinoma is about 9 months.

## Pouchitis

In 1977, Kock and colleagues [67] coined the term "pouchitis" to describe a nonspecific inflammatory disorder of the continent ileal reservoir (ileal pouch–anal anastomosis) after proctocolectomy performed for UC or familial adenomatous polyposis (FAP). Pouchitis is the most frequent long-term complication of ileal pouch-anal anastomosis in patients who have UC [68].

### *Etiologic factors*

The precise etiology of pouchitis is unknown, but implicated factors include bacterial overgrowth, fecal stasis, fecal bile acids, nutritional deficiencies, ischemic complications from surgery, recurrent UC, missed diagnosis of Crohn's disease, and a new form of IBD [69]. Pouchitis more frequently occurs in patients who have underlying UC than in patients who have FAP. Among patients who have UC, pouchitis is more common in those who have extraintestinal manifestations and in nonsmokers [70].

### *Diagnosis*

Pouchitis is diagnosed by a combination of clinical, endoscopic, and histologic features. The most common presentation of pouchitis is increased stool frequency. The diarrhea is predominantly watery, although bloody diarrhea can occur in patients who have cuffitis (inflammation of the rectal cuff, which likely represents recurrent UC). Fecal urgency and incontinence can sometimes be distressing and can severely affect the patient's quality of life [71]. Other symptoms include abdominal cramps, fever, and malaise. Pouchitis is defined as "acute" if the duration of symptoms is less than 4 weeks and as "chronic" if the duration is more than 4 weeks. Endoscopic characteristics include mucosal edema, granularity, friability, blunting of the vascular pattern, mucus exudates, and ulceration. Inflammation typically involves the entire pouch or only the distal pouch [72]. Histologic features include neutrophilic infiltration, crypt abscesses, and ulceration. Several classification schemes of pouchitis have been described to decrease the diagnostic variability among clinicians and researchers. The most commonly used classification is the Pouchitis Disease Activity Index, which incorporates clinical, endoscopic, and histologic parameters [73]. A score of 7 or greater is used to diagnose pouchitis (score range 0–26).

With complicated, atypical, or refractory pouchitis, other diagnostic tests can be performed to evaluate alternate causes. A pouchogram is an intraluminal contrast study that can demonstrate pouch fistulas, anastomotic strictures, and ileo-anal anastomotic dehiscence. CT enterography can assess the small bowel if Crohn's disease of the pouch is suspected. Anorectal manomtery is used to evaluate pelvic floor dysfunction, and pouch scintigraphy is used to evaluate pouch emptying.

### *Therapy*

The treatment is predominantly empiric, which reflects a poor understanding of the pathophysiology and the paucity of randomized controlled trials [74]. Several options are available for the successful treatment of pouchitis (Table 1). Antibiotics are the first line of therapy. Metronidazole 250 mg thrice daily for 7 to 10 days is the standard antibiotic. Response should occur within 2 to 3 days. Chronic pouchitis usually requires long-term antibiotic therapy with immunosuppressive therapy. Patients who have uncomplicated pouchitis that is unresponsive to antibiotics should be considered for other agents, such as 5-ASA suppositories (for cuffitis), steroids, immunosuppresives, or biologic agents (for Crohn's disease of the pouch or chronic pouchitis), and probiotics such as VSL#3 (for chronic pouchitis) [75]. Rarely, surgical pouch revision or excision is required for refractory or complicated pouchitis.

### *Natural history*

The cumulative risk of pouchitis during a 15-year period varies from 15% to 45% in patients who have FAP and UC, respectively [76]. The risk

Table 1
Medical treatment options for pouchitis

| | |
|---|---|
| Antibiotics | Metronidazole, ciprfloxacin, amoxicillin/clavulinic acid, erythromycin, tetracycline, rifaximin |
| Probiotics | Lactobacillus, bifidobacter, *Streptococcus salivarius* |
| 5-Aminosalicylates | Mesalamine, sulfasalazine |
| Steroids | Oral, enema |
| Nutritional agents | Short-chain fatty acids enemas, glutamine suppositories |
| Immunomodulators | Azathioprine, cyclosporine |
| Oxygen-free radical inhibitor | Allopurinol |
| Anti-diarrheals | Bismuth subsalicylate |
| Nicotine | Nicotine patch |

*Data from* Mahadevan U, Sandborn W. Pouchitis: clinical characteristics and management. In: Targan SR, Shanahan F, Karp LC, editors. Inflammatory bowel disease. From bench to bedside. 2nd edition. New York: Springer Scientific; 2003. p. 643–58.

increases to 80% if patients who have UC have concomitant PSC [69]. Recurrent pouchitis occurs in 20% of patients, whereas chronic pouchitis occurs in 5% of patients. Severe intractable pouchitis requiring surgical revision or excision occurs in 1% to 2% of pouch operations [74].

## References


[1] Jess T, Gambour M, Munkholm P, et al. Overall and cause-specific mortality in ulcerative colitis: Meta-analysis of population-based inception cohort studies. Am J Gastroenterol 2007;102:609–17.

[2] Palli D, Trallori G, Saieva C, et al. General and cancer specific mortality of a population based cohort of patients with inflammatory bowel disease: the Florence Study. Gut 1998;42:175–9.

[3] Bernstein CN, Wajda A, Svenson LW, et al. The epidemiology of inflammatory bowel disease in Canada: a population-based study. Am J Gastroenterol 2006;101:1559–68.

[4] Wolters FL, Russel MG, Sigbrandij J, et al. Crohn's disease: increased mortality 10 years after diagnosis in a Europe-wide population based cohort. Gut 2006;55:510–8.

[5] Jess T, Loftus EV, Harmsen WS, et al. Survival and cause specific mortality in patients with inflammatory bowel disease: a long term outcome study in Olmsted County, Minnesota, 1940–2004. Gut 2006;55:1248–54.

[6] Lichtenstein GR, Feagan BG, Cohen RD, et al. Serious infections and mortality in association with therapies for Crohn's disease: TREAT registry. Clin Gastroenterol Hepatol 2006;4:621–30.

[7] Vind I, Riis L, Jess T, et al. Increasing incidences of inflammatory bowel disease and decreasing surgery rates in Copenhagen City and County, 2003–2005: a population-based study from the Danish Crohn Colitis Database. Am J Gastroenterol 2006;101:1274–82.

[8] Dorn SD, Sandler RS. Inflammatory bowel disease is not a risk factor for cardiovascular disease mortality: results from a systemic review and meta-analysis. Am J Gastroenterol 2007; 102:662–7.

[9] Fazio VW. Toxic megacolon in ulcerative colitis and Crohn's colitis. Clin Gastroenterol 1980;9:389–407.

[10] Greenstein AJ, Sachar DB, Gibus A, et al. Outcome of toxic dilatation in ulcerative and Crohn's colitis. J Clin Gastroenterol 1985;7:137–43.

[11] Gan SI, Beck PL. A new look at toxic megacolon: an update and review of incidence, etiology, pathogenesis, and management. Am J Gastroenterol 2003;98:2363–71.

[12] Farmer RG, Hawk WA, Turnbull RB, et al. Indications for surgery in Crohn's disease: analysis of 500 cases. Gastroenterology 1976;71:245–50.

[13] Latella G, Vernia P, Viscido A, et al. GI distension in severe ulcerative colitis. Am J Gastroenterol 2002;97:1169–75.

[14] Berg DF, Bahadursingh AM, Kaminski DL, et al. Acute surgical emergencies in inflammatory bowel disease. Am J Surg 2002;184:45–51.

[15] Cheung O, Reguiero MD. Inflammatory bowel disease emergencies. Gastroenterol Clin North Am 2003;32:1269–88.

[16] Truelove SC, Witts LJ. Cortisone in ulcerative colitis: final report on a therapeutic trial. Br Med J 1955;2:1041–8.

[17] Jalan KN, Sircus W, Card WI, et al. An experience with ulcerative colitis: toxic dilation in 55 cases. Gastroenterology 1969;57:68–82.

[18] Caprilli R, Vernia P, Latella G, et al. Early recognition of toxic megacolon. J Clin Gastroenterol 1987;9:160–4.

[19] Chew CN, Nolan DJ, Jewell DP, et al. Small bowel gas in severe ulcerative colitis. Gut 1991; 32:1535–7.

[20] Chapman RW, Selby WS, Jewell DP, et al. Controlled trial of intravenous metronidazole as an adjunct to corticosteroids in severe ulcerative colitis. Gut 1986;27:1201–2.

[21] Mantzaris GJ, Petraki K, Archavlis E, et al. A prospective randomized controlled trial of intravenous ciprofloxacin as an adjunct to intravenous corticosteroids in severe ulcerative colitis. Scand J Gastroenterol 2001;36:971–4.
[22] Rahimi R, Nikfar S, Abdollahi M, et al. A meta-analysis of broad-spectrum antibiotic therapy in patients with active Crohn's disease. Clin Ther 2006;28(12):1983–8.
[23] Jarnerot G, Hertervig E, Friis-Liby I. Infliximab as rescue therapy in severe to moderately severe ulcerative colitis: a randomized, placebo controlled study. Gastroenterology 2005; 129:1358–9.
[24] Lichtiger S, Present DH, Kornbluth A, et al. Cyclosporine in severe ulcerative colitis refractory to steroid therapy. N Engl J Med 1994;330:1841–5.
[25] Schwartz DA, Loftus EV, Tremaine WJ, et al. The natural history of fistulizing Crohn's disease in Olmsted County, Minnesota. Gastroenterology 2002;122:875–80.
[26] MacKalski BA, Bernstein CN. New diagnostic imaging tools for inflammatory bowel disease. Gut 2006;55:733–41.
[27] Schwartz DA, Wiersema MJ, Dudiak KM, et al. A comparison of endoscopic ultrasound, magnetic resonance imaging, and exam under anesthesia for evaluation of Crohn's perianal fistulas. Gastroenterology 2001;121:1064–72.
[28] Bernstein LH, Frank MS, Brandt LJ, et al. Healing of perineal Crohn's disease with metronidazole. Gastroenterology 1980;79:357–65.
[29] Rubin DT, Kornbluth A. Role of antibiotics in the management of inflammatory bowel disease. Rev Gastroenterol Disord 2005;5:S10–5.
[30] Griggs L, Schwartz DA. Medical options for treating perianal Crohn's disease. Dig Liver Dis 2007;39:979–87.
[31] Dejaco C, Harrer M, Waldhoef T, et al. Antibiotics and azathioprine for the treatment of perianal fistulas in Crohn's disease. Aliment Pharmacol Ther 2003;18:1113–20.
[32] Pearson DC, May GR, Fick GH, et al. Azathioprine and 6-mercaptopurine in Crohn's disease: a meta-analysis. Ann Intern Med 1995;123:132–42.
[33] Sands BE, Anderson FH, Bernstein CN, et al. Infliximab maintenance therapy for fistulizing Crohn's disease. N Engl J Med 2004;350:876–85.
[34] Colombel JF, Sandborn WJ, Rutgeerts P, et al. Adalimumab for maintenance of clinical response and remission in patients with Crohn's disease: the CHARM trial. Gastroenterology 2007;132:52–65.
[35] Bressler B, Sands BE. Medical therapy for fistulizing Crohn's disease. Aliment Pharmacol Ther 2006;24:1283–93.
[36] Ekbom A, Helmick C, Zack M, et al. Ulcerative colitis and colorectal cancer: a population-based study. N Engl J Med 1990;323:1228–33.
[37] Gillen CD, Walmsley RS, Prior P, et al. Ulcerative colitis and Crohn's disease: a comparison of the colorectal cancer risk in extensive colitis. Gut 1994;35:1590–602.
[38] Greenstein AJ, Sachar DB, Smith H, et al. A comparison of cancer risk in Crohn's disease and ulcerative colitis. Cancer 1981;48:2741–5.
[39] Morson BC, Pang LSC. Rectal biopsy as an aid to cancer control in ulcerative colitis. Gut 1994;35:1590–2.
[40] Streutker CJ, Haggit RC, Riddell RH. Dysplasia in inflammatory bowel disease: clinical pathology and current surveillance methods. In: Targan SR, Shanahan F, Karp LC, editors. Inflammatory bowel disease. From bench to bedside. 2nd edition. New York: Springer Science; 2003. p. 719–29.
[41] Riddell RH, Goldman H, Ransohoff DF, et al. Dysplasia in inflammatory bowel disease: standardized classification with provisional clinical applications. Hum Pathol 1983;14: 931–68.
[42] Bernstein CN, Shanahan F, Weinstein WM. Are we telling patients the truth about surveillance colonoscopy in ulcerative colitis? Lancet 1994;343:71–4.
[43] Eaden JA, Abrams KR, Mayberry JF. The risk of colorectal cancer in ulcerative colitis: a meta-analysis. Gut 2001;48:526–35.

[44] Geboes K. Ulcerative colitis and malignancy. Acta Gastroenterol Belg 2000;63:279–83.
[45] Shetty K, Rybicki L, Brzezinski A, et al. The risk for cancer or dysplasia in ulcerative colitis patients with primary sclerosing cholangitis. Am J Gastroenterol 1999;94:1643–9.
[46] Blackstone MO, Riddell RH, Rogers BH, et al. Dysplasia associated lesion or mass (DALM) detected by colonoscopy in long-standing ulcerative colitis: an indication for colectomy. Gastroenterology 1981;80:366–74.
[47] Engelsgjerd M, Farraye FA, Odze RD. Polypectomy may be adequate treatment for adenoma-like dysplastic lesions in chronic ulcerative colitis. Gastroenterology 1999;117:1288–94.
[48] Dixon MF, Brown LJR, Gilmour HM, et al. Observer variation in the assessment of dysplasia in ulcerative colitis. Histopathology 1988;13:385–97.
[49] Gorfine SR, Bauer JJ, Harris MT, et al. Dysplasia complicating chronic ulcerative colitis: is immediate colectomy warranted? Dis Colon Rectum 2000;43:1575–81.
[50] Ullman T, Croog V, Harpaz N, et al. Progression of flat low-grade dysplasia to advanced neoplasia in patients with ulcerative colitis. Gastroenterology 2003;125:1311–9.
[51] Nugent FW, Haggitt RC, Gilpin PA. Cancer surveillance in ulcerative colitis. Gastroenterology 1991;100:1241–8.
[52] Lashner BA, Hanauer SB, Silverstein MD. Optimal timing of colonoscopy to screen for cancer in ulcerative colitis. Ann Intern Med 1988;108:274–8.
[53] Itzkowitz SH, Present DH. Consensus conference on colorectal cancer screening and surveillance in inflammatory bowel disease. Inflamm Bowel Dis 2005;11:314–21.
[54] Weinstein WM. Mucosal biopsy techniques and interaction with the pathologist. In: Weinstein WM, editor. Gastrointestinal endoscopy clinics of North America, 10Philadelphia: Elsevier Health Sciences; 2000. p. 555–71.
[55] Lashner BA, Turner BC, Bostwick DG, et al. Dysplasia and cancer complicating strictures in ulcerative colitis. Dig Dis Sci 1990;35:349–52.
[56] Chapman RW, Arborgh BA, Rhodes JM, et al. Primary sclerosing cholangitis: a review of its clinical features, cholangiography and hepatic histology. Gut 1980;21:870–7.
[57] Escorsell A, Pares A, Rodes J, et al. Epidemiology of primary sclerosing cholangitis in Spain. J Hepatol 1994;21:787–91.
[58] Takikawa H. Recent status of primary sclerosing cholangitis in Japan. J Hepatobiliary Pancreat Surg 1999;6:352–5.
[59] Olsson R, Danielson A, Jarnerot G, et al. Prevalence of primary sclerosing cholangitis in patients with ulcerative colitis. Gastroenterology 1991;100:1319–23.
[60] Chapman RW, Varghese Z, Gaul R, et al. Association of primary sclerosing cholangitis with HLA-B8. Gut 1983;24:38–41.
[61] Tobias R, Wright J, Kottler R. Primary sclerosing cholangitis associated with inflammatory bowel disease in Cape Town, 1975–1981. S Afr Med J 1983;63:229–35.
[62] Fulcher AS, Turner MA, Franklin KJ, et al. Primary sclerosing cholangitis: evaluation with MR cholangiography: a case control study. Radiology 2000;215:71–80.
[63] Gow PJ, Chapman RW. Liver transplantation for primary sclerosing cholangitis. Liver 2000;20:97–103.
[64] Graziadei IW, Wiesner RH, Batts KP, et al. Recurrence of primary sclerosing cholangitis following liver transplantation. Hepatology 1999;29:1050–6.
[65] Wiesner RH, La Russo NF, Dozois RR, et al. Peristomal varices after proctocolectomy in patients with primary sclerosing cholangitis. Gastroenterology 1986;90:316–22.
[66] Nemeth A, Ejderhamn J, Glaumann H, et al. Liver damage in juvenile inflammatory bowel disease. Liver 1990;10:239–48.
[67] Kock NG, Darle N, Hulten L, et al. Ileostomy. Curr Probl Surg 1977;14:1–52.
[68] Pemberton JH, Kelly KA, Beart RW, et al. Ileal pouch-anal anasotomosis for chronic ulcerative colitis: long term results. Ann Surg 1987;206:504–13.
[69] Mahadevan U, Sandborn W. Pouchitis: clinical characteristics and management. In: Targan SR, Shanahan F, Karp LC, editors. Inflammatory bowel disease. From bench to bedside. 2nd edition. New York: Springer Scientific; 2003. p. 643–58.

[70] Penna C, Dozois R, Tremaine W, et al. Pouchitis after ileal pouch-anal anastomosis for ulcerative colitis occurs with increased frequency in patients with associated primary sclerosing cholangitis. Gut 1996;38:234–9.
[71] Tiainen J, Matikainen M. Health-related quality of life after ileal pouch-anal anastomosis for ulcerative colitis: long term results. Scand J Gastroenterol 1999;34:601–5.
[72] Setti Carraro PG, Talbot IC, Nicholls JR. Patterns of distribution of endoscopic and histologic changes in the ileal reservoir after restorative proctocolectomy with ileoanal ileal reservoir: a long-term follow up study. Int J Colorectal Dis 1998;13:103–7.
[73] Sandborn W, Tremaine WJ, Batts KP, et al. Pouchitis following ileal pouch-anal anastomosis: a pouchitis disease activity index. Mayo Clin Proc 1994;69:409–15.
[74] Shen B, Fazio VW, Remzin FH, et al. Risk factors for diseases of the ileal pouch-anal anastomosis after restorative proctocolectomy for ulcerative colitis. Clin Gastroenterol Hepatol 2006;4:81–9.
[75] Shen B, Fazio VW, Remzi FH, et al. Clinical approach to diseases of ileal pouch-anal anastomosis. Am J Gastroenterol 2005;100:2796–807.
[76] Hurst RD, Molinari M, Chung TP, et al. Prospective study of the incidence, timing, and treatment of pouchitis in 104 consecutive patients after restorative procto-colectomy. Arch Surg 1996;131:497–500.

ELSEVIER
SAUNDERS

Med Clin N Am 92 (2008) 687–705

THE MEDICAL
CLINICS
OF NORTH AMERICA

# Endoscopic Mucosal Resection of Colonic Lesions: Current Applications and Future Prospects

David M. Poppers, MD, PhD,
Gregory B. Haber, MD, FRCPC*

*Division of Gastroenterology, Center for Advanced Therapeutic Endoscopy, Lenox Hill Hospital, 6 Black Hall, 100 East 77th Street, New York, NY 10021, USA*

## Conventional colonoscopic polypectomy

Adenomatous polyps within the colon represent dysplastic growths that can progress through successive stages of cellular atypia to localized intramucosal carcinoma, and then, if unchecked, breach the basement membrane, invade local structures, and eventually metastasize. Because colon cancer is the most common gastrointestinal malignancy in the United States and also common worldwide, much attention has been focused on detection and removal of its precursor lesions. Whereas conventional hyperplastic polyps are believed to have no premalignant potential, adenomas, whether tubular, tubulovillous, or villous, lie along the adenoma–carcinoma sequence with a progressively increasing likelihood of malignant transformation. Colonic polyps had been traditionally managed surgically, and are still so managed if a polyp contains invasive carcinoma [1]. Indeed, laparoscopic approaches have been refined to remove challenging polyps that cannot be safely removed endoscopically [2–4].

Pedunculated and sessile polyps have been managed during the past 3 decades by way of polypectomy under direct colonoscopic visualization. Pedunculated polyps have a stalk of mucosa and submucosa formed by the action of peristalsis. Most colonic polyps are sessile, however [5]. Polyps are removed either by grasping them with a forceps (either with or without electrocautery) for small lesions, or by using various polypectomy snares for large lesions. Coagulation and blended currents have been used safely. A Japanese review of 9555 procedures reported a bleeding incidence of

* Corresponding author.
*E-mail address:* ghaber@lenoxhill.net (G.B. Haber).

0025-7125/08/$ - see front matter 
doi:10.1016/j.mcna.2008.01.006 ***medical.theclinics.com***

only 1.1%, including 0.9% for standard snare polypectomy and 1.6% for electrocautery-assisted biopsy [6]. Colonoscopic therapy is safe and effective for various colorectal polyps, including adenomas, advanced adenomas, and benign inflammatory polyps, as demonstrated in a series of more than 11,000 procedures in a study from Taiwan [7]. Refinements of these colonoscopic techniques include the use of hemoclips, endoloops, or rubber band ligation for hemostasis, and the use of argon plasma coagulation (APC) to fulgurate residual adenomatous tissue at the polyp base following removal of most of the polyp (Fig. 1, A–D) [8]. With a piecemeal approach, large polyps can be resected by sequential application of the snare to remaining polyp tissue. The polyp is commonly raised or lifted by submucosal injection to form a submucosal fluid cushion to decrease the risk of tear or perforation for very large polyps or for moderately large polyps located in thin-walled sections of the colon, such as the cecum (Fig. 2, A–C) [9]. Large

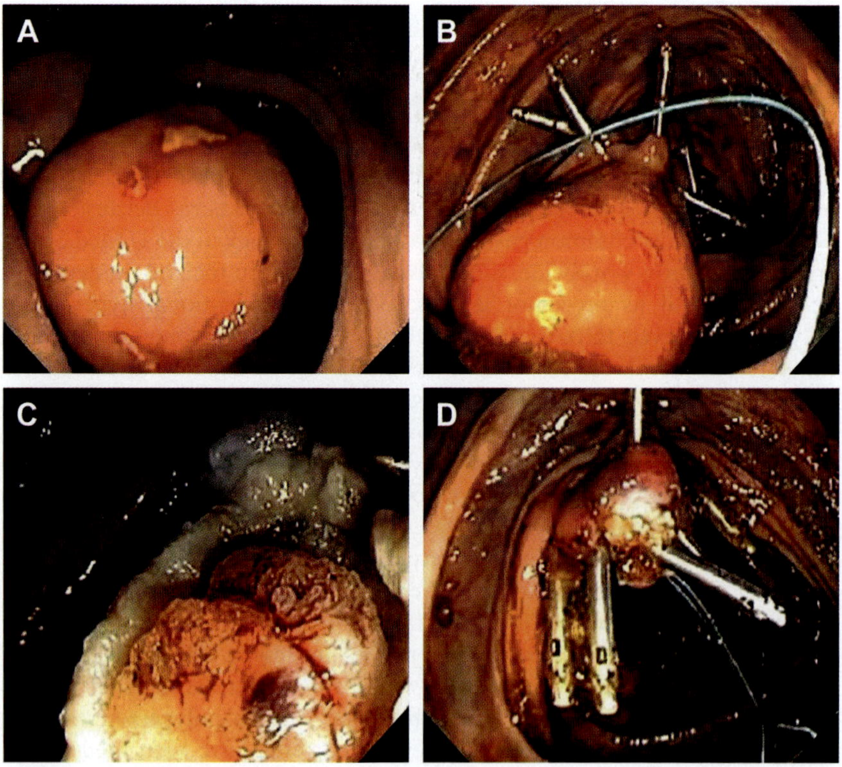


Fig. 1. (*A*) Large lipomatous polyp with superficial ulceration filling about 80% of the colonic lumen. (*B*) Securing the polyp base before snare polypectomy. Multiple endoclips have been deployed at the polyp base. A detachable nylon endoloop snare is about to be placed around the polyp base. (*C*) Polyp partially removed by piecemeal resection. Note the lipomatous nature of the polyp. (*D*) Residual polyp stalk after piecemeal snare resection. Note the presence of multiple endoclips and a single detachable snare on the polyp base.

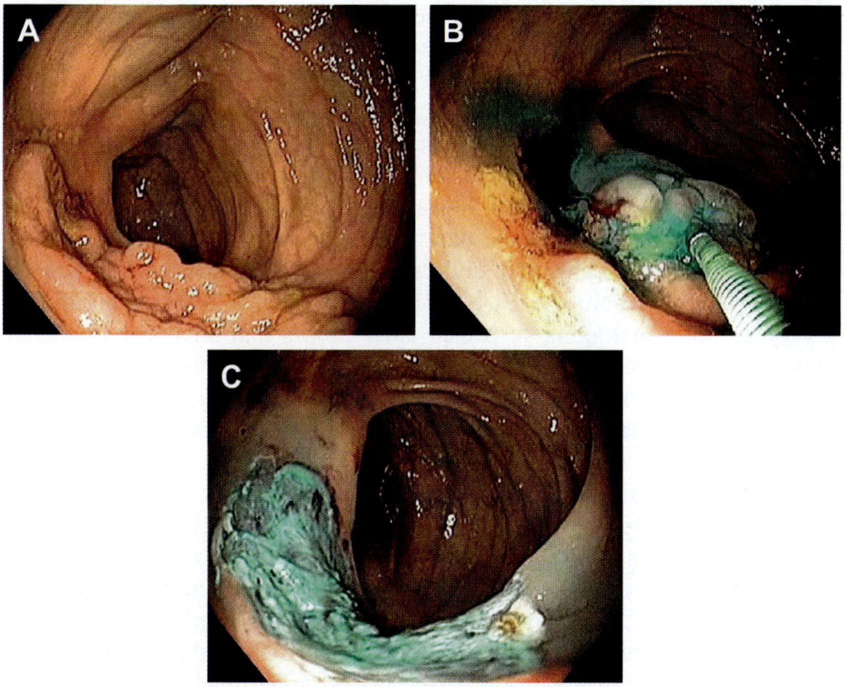


Fig. 2. (*A*) Flat, laterally extending (carpetlike) polyp in the ascending colon. (*B*) Submucosal injection with solution of dilute epinephrine and methylene blue in saline before polyp resection. Note the adequate lifting of the entire polyp. (*C*) Resection site after polyp removal. Note the residual methylene blue at the base of the lesion.

sessile or flat colorectal lesions pose a unique challenge. Approximately 0.8% to 5.2% of colonic polyps are greater than 2 cm in diameter. This size increases the likelihood of an associated malignancy. There is often a discrepancy between the endoscopic estimation and the actual pathologic size of the lesion, however, because of endoscopic magnification and polyp retraction after resection [10]. Large lesions without clear malignant features, and without evidence of invasion or lymphovascular involvement, are usually managed like moderately sized polyps, typically by piecemeal resection. For polyps that cannot be entirely removed at colonoscopy or that require surgical removal because of an invasive or lymphovascular component, submucosal injection of India ink at colonoscopy helps locate the polyp site at surgery [11].

## Staging of colonic lesions

Accurate staging is required to optimally treat benign colonic polyps or localized malignant polyps. The colonic lesion is typically identified by optical colonoscopy, despite increasing use of colorectal screening by CT colonography (CTC), or virtual colonoscopy, an endoluminal electronic reconstruction of CT scan slices of the purged colon [12]. Colorectal cancer is staged by the tumor node metastasis (TNM) system [13], which correlates with the classic Duke staging system. Staging is initially performed to exclude diffuse metastases, often by way of abdominal, pelvic, and chest CT, positron emission tomography scans, or bone scans to detect osseous metastases [14]. Endoscopic ultrasound (EUS) has become the gold standard for staging the depth of invasion of gastrointestinal lesions. It is highly accurate in assessing the depth of invasion of early gastric cancer, with rates of overstaging and understaging of 7.4% and 14.2%, respectively [15]. High-resolution EUS (HR-EUS) using a 20-MHz miniprobe is very accurate in staging suspected early esophageal adenocarcinoma or squamous cell carcinoma [16,17], with sensitivity of approximately 91% for mucosal tumors, but with lower sensitivity for submucosal lesions [18]. EUS also has a high negative predictive value for the absence of lymphadenopathy, which correlates well with superficial esophageal adenocarcinoma [19]. This observation is consistent with other studies, in which predictors of lymph node metastases include larger (>3 cm) tumors, poorer degrees of histologic differentiation, greater depth of invasion (especially as the level of m3/sm1 is reached), and the presence of angiolymphatic disease [20,21]. Staging by EUS may thus predict the level of invasion; for patients who have deeper lesions, EUS findings may predict angiolymphatic involvement and likely lymph node involvement that suggest a decreased likelihood of durable response to endoscopic techniques, such as endoscopic mucosal resection (discussed later in this article). EUS is also used to stage colorectal adenocarcinoma. In a prospective English study of 131 patients who had either colonic adenocarcinoma or broad-based colorectal polyps, staging with EUS at 12.5 MHz, by way of a through-the-scope miniprobe, was compared with histopathologic staging. Lymph node involvement at EUS was determined by the presence of round, clearly defined hypoechoic lymph nodes at least 1 cm in diameter [22]. The overall accuracy of EUS for nodal staging was 87%, with a sensitivity of 95%, specificity of 71%, positive predictive value of 87%, and negative predictive value of 88%. Only 4% (n = 5) of lesions were overstaged (EUS stage T3 versus pathologic T2 stage), and only 3 lesions were understaged (EUS stage T3 versus pathologic stage T4). The absence of lymphadenopathy at EUS may help to decide whether patients should undergo lower-morbidity interventions, such as endoscopic resection or ablation, rather than surgery.

### Optimal lesion visualization

Large pedunculated polyps tend to be easily detectable on standard optical colonoscopic evaluation, whereas flat and sessile lesions can be missed. Several chemical and electronic techniques, including chromoendoscopy, magnification endoscopy, narrow-band imaging, optical coherence tomography, and autofluorescence, help detect such lesions [23–25]. Contrast dyes, including indigo carmine, methylene blue, and cresyl violet, have been used to highlight polyps or tumors from the surrounding normal mucosa. Chromoendoscopy has been particularly useful in inflammatory conditions, such as ulcerative colitis and Crohn's disease, in which chronic inflammatory injury and repair of colonic mucosa may produce subtle lesions that represent adenomas or dysplasia [26]. Chromoendoscopy is useful to detect standard adenomatous and nonadenomatous colonic lesions [27,28]. Chromoendoscopy and high-pressure dye-spray techniques have been coupled with double balloon enteroscopy to screen for small intestinal polyps in patients who have hereditary polyposis syndromes, such as familial adenomatous polyposis. In these studies, flat lesions that were otherwise missed were identified and confirmed as adenomas on biopsy [29,30]. In a recent Italian study, patients underwent standard colonoscopy and, if a suspicious mucosal lesion was identified, the suspicious area was sprayed with 0.2% indigo carmine. This technique successfully identified an additional 244 neoplasms in 212 patients, including large, ulcerated, and advanced cancers, and nonadvanced lesions [31]. Small, depressed colonic lesions with varying degrees of cellular atypia were detected using an indigo carmine capsule followed by magnification chromoendoscopy [32].

High-magnification colonoscopy can also examine colonic mucosa more carefully. Kudo and colleagues [33] categorized difficult-to-identify nonpolypoid colorectal neoplasms as slightly elevated, laterally spreading, or depressed. Magnification enables detection of subtle color changes, abnormal capillary networks, colonic wall deformation, and grooves or bleeding spots in the colonic wall. Huang and colleagues [34] classified colonic pit patterns as types I and II, considered nonneoplastic, and types IIIL, IIIS, IV, and V, considered to represent varying degrees of neoplastic change. The type I pattern is characterized by round pits with a diameter of $0.07 \pm 0.02$ mm that are seen in normal colonic mucosa. The pits of type II are somewhat large (approximately $0.09 \pm 0.02$ mm) and have radial symmetry. Type IIIL are nonbranched elongated pits, roughly $0.22 \pm 0.09$ mm. Type IIIS pits are smaller round pits ($0.03 \pm 0.01$ mm). Type IV refers to branched pits ($0.93 \pm 0.32$ mm), whereas type V pits are irregularly arranged and often associated with dysplastic and neoplastic mucosa. Type I/II polyps are usually nonadenomatous and are located in the distal colon, whereas types III–IV polyps tend to be adenomatous and more proximal [35]. In experienced hands, magnification endoscopy, in combination with chromoendoscopy, is used to identify pit pattern subtypes that correlate with the pathologic findings of adenoma versus nonadenoma, with a sensitivity of 90%, negative predictive value of 73.6%, and accuracy of 86% [36]. There is good interobserver and intraobserver agreement in the assessment of colonic pit patterns [34]. Indigo carmine–based chromoendoscopy may provide much less incremental value, if the baseline endoscopy is performed with high magnification [37], but this combined approach may still be useful [38–41].

Narrow-band imaging (NBI) uses a narrow-range blue-wavelength light to enhance visualization of the topography and microvasculature of gastrointestinal mucosa [42,43], to improve detection of abnormal mucosa and polypoid lesions [44]. NBI is superior to conventional colonoscopy in distinguishing between adenomatous versus nonadenomatous polyps. NBI scores similarly to chromoendoscopy; both techniques are improved by concurrent use of high magnification [45]. In another study, chromoendoscopy and NBI had comparable sensitivities (approximately 95.7%), specificities (87.5%), and overall diagnostic accuracy (92.7%) [46].

Confocal laser microscopy allows for real-time in vivo diagnosis of dysplastic, metaplastic, and cancerous gastrointestinal mucosa [47,48]. Detection of altered tissue microarchitecture may permit targeted biopsies that provide a higher yield than random biopsies.

## Candidate colonic lesions for endoscopic mucosal resection

The increasing data on mucosal surveillance may enhance EMR-based management [49,50]. In the colon, EMR is indicated for carpetlike adenomatous polyps or for moderately well– or well-differentiated adenocarcinoma confined to the mucosa (layers m1, m2, or m3) or extending into the superficial submucosa (sm1a/sm1b) but with specific surface morphology. EMR is considered for sessile (type Is), flat elevated (IIa), and lateral spreading tumors (LST) no greater than 2.5 cm in diameter and for flat adenomatous lesions (IIb) that are moderately well- or well-differentiated and no greater than 10 mm in diameter. Mixed-type lesions (type IIc + IIa and type IIa + IIc) that are less than 10 mm in size may also be treated with EMR, but larger lesions have a higher rate of submucosal invasion and are less likely to be successfully managed with EMR [51]. The role of endoscopic submucosal dissection (ESD) is not yet established for larger lesions or for tumors with deeper invasion.

## Lifting the lesion in endoscopic mucosal resection

Once a candidate lesion is identified, the initial step is to lift the lesion with an injection of fluid to provide a submucosal cushion, to highlight the target lesion, and to decrease the risk for iatrogenic perforation. Failure to lift with injection, the "non-lift" sign, suggests deep invasion of the lesion that tethers the lesion to deep mural tissue and prevents mucosal separation [52].

Saline is the most common submucosal injection solution. Higher-viscosity solutions produce a more durable and consistent submucosal cushion. For example, sodium hyaluronate reliably produces a submucosal cushion for en bloc resections of large colonic or upper gastrointestinal lesions [53–55]. There is some experience with other solutions, including hypertonic dextrose with epinephrine, for colonic resections [56]. Normal saline, 5% and 10% dextrose, glycerol, and hyaluronan are safe, but hypertonic (3.75%) saline and higher (>20%) dextrose solutions may injure tissue [57]. The novel injection agent of autologous blood, for "blood patch" EMR is safe, cost effective, and efficacious, with a 97% lift success rate [58].

## Endoscopic mucosal resection—selected techniques

After successfully lifting the lesion, various techniques are used to remove it. Small (<2 cm) lesions can potentially be removed en bloc, whereas large lesions are typically removed piecemeal. The two major techniques are non-suction (lift-and-cut) and suction (suck-and-cut). With lift-and-cut, the lesion is lifted with submucosal injection. With suck-and-cut, snare resection is performed after aspiration of the tissue into a plastic cap fitted to the end of the endoscope [59–62]. Removal of the aspirated fragment of mucosa leaves a mucosal defect [63]. The cap-based EMR (EMR-C) was first developed for lesions in the esophagus, but has been applied to the colon [64]. These two techniques have multiple variations. A modified variceal ligator has been used for piecemeal resection of large lesions, especially of Barrett esophagus. In this technique, the lesion is suctioned into the cap, a rubber band is placed around the lesion and adjacent submucosa, and a hexagon-shaped snare is used to resect the lesion. Use of a reusable snare and a band ligator with six rubber bands permits six sequential piecemeal resections of a lesion during one esophageal intubation [65]. Band ligation has also been used for EMR of flat colorectal adenomas and adenocarcinomas [66].

Japanese physicians have used EMR for more than a decade to resect flat, sessile, and large colonic polyps, including adenomas, superficial mucosal and submucosally invasive adenocarcinoma, inflammatory and hyperplastic polyps, and carcinoid [67]. The rate of success is related to lesion size, morphology, and location, with flat lesions successfully removed in 87% of cases, whereas large lesions have a lower success rate. In a prospective study of 58 patients who had laterally spreading colonic tumors, patients underwent chromoendoscopy with indigo carmine to delineate the colon cancer, and with crystal violet to enhance the pit patterns. High-frequency (20 MHz) EUS was performed to exclude T2 disease. The patients were followed up to 24 months after EMR [68]. F-type lesions are laterally spreading colonic tumors that tend to have a smooth surface contour, whereas G-type lesions are an aggregate of nodules that form a broad-based lesion with an uneven and granular surface. In this study, F-type flat colonic lesions were more common in the proximal colon and were more often associated with T2/invasive disease. Twenty-one (36%) of 58 patients who had F-type lesions and 37 (64%) of 58 patients who had G-type lesions were treated with EMR. The lesion recurred within 6 months of EMR in

10 patients. G-type morphology and the need for piecemeal resection were risk factors for recurrence. After retreatment, patients who had these tumors had a 96% disease-free rate after 24 months. This study suggested that EMR is a safe and effective alternative to surgery for superficial resection in selected patients.

Bories and colleagues [69] described successful EMR for 52 sessile polyps and cancers (mean diameter = 27.5 mm, range 10–60 mm) by way of the lift-and-cut method. Pathologic examination of the resected lesions demonstrated 38 adenomas with high-grade dysplasia (HGD), 4 carcinomas, and 7 lesions extending to the deep or lateral margins. Of these patients, 98% had endoscopically determined complete resection, but 21.6% of the cases required APC to treat suspicious residual tissue at the base of the mucosal defect. Among 36 patients who had follow-up, 2 died, and 5 (15%) of the remaining 34 patients had recurrent disease [69]. Early colonic neoplasms seem to be candidates for EMR. Predictors of difficult EMR and a potential need for surgery include large tumors, sessile or flat/depressed morphology, and submucosal invasion [70].

## Large colonic neoplasms

Colonic polyps larger than 2 cm in diameter are detected in up to 5% of colonoscopies, and are more likely to contain foci of malignancy (estimates range from 5%–22%). Nonetheless, most large colonic lesions can be successfully removed with EMR [71]. EMR is becoming a first-line therapy for flat and sessile colorectal lesions, even for lesions larger than 2 cm in diameter [71]. In a review of 311 colonic polyps greater than 2 cm in diameter removed from 1989 to 2002 in 252 patients, 263 were removed by EMR (Table 1) [72]. Eighteen of these EMR-treated polyps required surgery for adenomatous recurrence, with the recurrence rate decreasing over time from 22% to 7%. EMR is a reasonably safe and effective technique to resect large colonic polyps and superficial cancers [73]. Tanaka and colleagues [74] showed that in 120 patients who had laterally spreading superficial colon cancers (including F-type in 33 and G-type in 87), F-type lesions were more likely associated with invasive disease (27.2% versus 10.3%, $P<.05$). G-type lesions were larger than F-type ($35.3 \pm 11.4$ mm versus $26 \pm 7.2$ mm, $P<.01$). Eighty-one (67.5%) of the colonic lesions were treated with EMR. Recurrences occurred in 7.4% of patients after a mean follow-up of 60.8 months. All recurrences were managed endoscopically with no detected metastasis, again demonstrating the efficacy of this technique for large colonic lesions. In another study of 136 patients who had a total of 139 sessile polyps (averaging 20 mm in the proximal colon and 30 mm elsewhere), the local recurrence rate was 21.9% at 12.3 months [75]. In a large study in which 40% of the lesions were flat/depressed, complete resection was confirmed in 576 (96%) of 599 lesions [76].

Table 1
Representative colonic endoscopic mucosal resection outcomes

| N | Size (mm) | Residual or recurrent disease | Adenocarcinoma (%) | Follow-up (mo) | Reference |
|---|---|---|---|---|---|
| 252 | 30.9–42.5 | 22% initially, then 7% | 11.5 | 156 | Church [72] |
| 120 | 31.2 | 7.7% | 10.3 (F-type), 27.2 (G-type) | 60.8 | Tanaka et al [74] |
| 136 | 20 (right) 30 (remainder) | 21.9% | 12.2 | 12.3 | Conio et al [75] |
| 599 | 6.5–6.8 | 2.5% | 5.4 | — | Hurlstone et al [76] |
| 161 | 32.5 | 4.6% | 2.5 | 9.2 | Arebi et al [77] |
| 33 | 20 | 0% | 23.3 | 21 | Jameel et al [78] |
| 30 | — | 0% | 43.3 | 45.2 | Kume et al [79] |
| 21 | 23.9–26.5 | 10% (APC), 63.6% (control) | NA | 3 | Brooker et al [80] |
| 176 | >30 | 16% (benign), 28.6% (malignant) | 12 | 20 | Binmoeller et al [81] |

*Abbreviation:* NA, not applicable.

A retrospective analysis of 161 large sessile and flat colorectal polyps (mean diameter = 32.5 mm) demonstrated a 95.4% success rate for EMR [77]. Smaller lesions had higher rates of resection and lower recurrence rates [77]. Sixty percent of the tumors were successfully managed with one EMR session, and only 2% required more than three sessions. Seven patients (4.6%) required surgery for residual or recurrent tumor. Jameel and colleagues [78] reported successful use of EMR for 33 colorectal adenomas or early carcinomas (size ranging from 10–50 mm), 22 of which were resected en bloc and 8 in piecemeal fashion. In this study, there was no recurrent disease at 21 months, no perforations, and only 2 cases of minor bleeding controlled with local epinephrine injection. Other studies, such as a study by Kume and colleagues [79], likewise show the usefulness of en bloc and piecemeal resection of large sessile colorectal tumors, with low rates of bleeding (1 patient, 3.3%), successfully managed endoscopically by clip placement, and with no evident disease recurrence for an average follow-up of 45 (range 3–104) months.

There is interest in methods to decrease the likelihood of recurrent dysplasia and malignancy. Large colonic lesions have an increased risk for recurrence. Larger polyps (> 1.5 cm) managed with piecemeal EMR were less likely to be associated with recurrent disease when potential residual adenomatous tissue, or the base of the post-EMR mucosal defect, is treated with APC. In one study only 1 of 10 APC-treated patients had recurrence at 1 year follow-up versus 7 of 10 recurrences in the control group ($P = .02$)

[80]. Large polyps greater than 3 cm in diameter, sometimes termed "giant polyps," have also been successfully treated with EMR [81]. Some 176 benign-appearing large polyps in 170 patients were removed either in toto (for pedunculated lesions) or piecemeal (for flat or sessile lesions), with the detection of malignancy in 12% of these patients. Eight of these patients underwent surgery for malignancy. Of the 124 of these patients (117 who had benign polyps, and 7 who had malignant change but who met "favorable" criteria) who were followed, 19 developed recurrent disease (18 adenomatous, 1 malignant), all of whom were successfully treated by either repeat EMR or surgical excision [81]. This finding supports use of EMR for large benign adenomas or low-risk adenocarcinomas.

### New colorectal endoscopic mucosal resection applications

Rectal lesions can be managed safely and effectively by EMR as well. In 83 patients who had rectal neoplasms, EUS was used for staging and for surgical referral for patients who had T2 or nodal disease [82]. Sixty-two patients underwent EMR, including patients who had laterally spreading tumors (mean diameter = 30 mm) or sessile tumors (mean diameter = 38 mm). The EMRs were generally performed in an ambulatory setting. Five patients (8%) who experienced bleeding achieved hemostasis with endoscopic clip placement. There were no perforations. In this series, 98% of patients had no neoplastic recurrence at a median follow-up of 16 months. EMR is thus likely a useful and safe treatment of large rectal adenomas.

EMR will likely be increasingly applied to other clinical scenarios. A British study examined EMR therapy for flat colonic lesions in 169 patients who had chronic ulcerative colitis [83]. The patients had 170 adenoma-like masses (ALMs), 18 dysplasia-associated lesions or masses (DALM), and 16 cancers. DALM lesions are usually flat or sessile, irregularly shaped, and arise from dysplastic mucosa. DALM often reflects underlying neoplasia. In contrast, ALMs represent typical sessile or pedunculated polyps, without dysplasia in the surrounding mucosa. Flat DALM and certain ALM were managed safely by EMR in these patients. These results could lead to increased EMR of flat dysplasia in selected patients, rather than automatic referral for colectomy. Complex techniques are being developed for colonic adenomas and early colorectal cancers that cannot be treated with standard EMR techniques, to avoid surgery. A new technique is EMR performed in a retroflexed position using a gastroscope as salvage therapy for Paris type I/II adenomas and superficial colonic adenocarcinomas, with a reported 98% recurrence-free rate at 24 months of follow-up [84].

### Endoscopic submucosal dissection

Adenomas and carcinomas with superficial submucosal invasion may sometimes be candidates for endoscopic therapy. Endoscopic submucosal dissection (ESD) permits submucosal dissection to separate target mucosa from the surrounding normal mucosa, or dissection to remove target submucosa from the underlying muscularis propria [65]. ESD is technically difficult and time consuming, requires meticulous dissection, and is associated with higher rates of bleeding and perforation than EMR. ESD permits en bloc resection of lesions larger than 5 cm in diameter [65]. Like EMR, ESR involves submucosal injection of a viscous submucosal fluid cushion, such as glycerin, hyaluronan, or lubricant jelly. ESD uses various distinct techniques depending on the type of electrosurgical knife used for submucosal dissection. The standard needle knife provides a rapid and sharp incision, but its naked monofilament wire and strong current are associated with a relatively high risk for bleeding and perforation. The insulated tip needle knife provides more controlled cutting that decreases the risk for inadvertent perforation because of a ceramic sphere that insulates the tip and permits only a peripheral cut. This knife is useful to dissect along tissue planes, but entails a risk for perforation because the dissection is performed partially blinded to the cutting plane. The hook knife has a bent monofilament blade approximately 1 to 1.3 mm in length. The rotatable hook blade is used to hook into and pull submucosal tissue before incision. This knife may be combined with a transparent hood to further decrease the risk for complications. Because of the short hook blade length, dissection with this device is painstaking, but it has a relatively low risk for perforation. It is useful for colonic or esophageal dissection in areas of preexistent ulcer or scar that are at higher risk for perforation. The flex knife possesses a short bent filament at the tip, which can be controlled to vary the cutting depth [85]. It is often combined with a transparent hood to improve visualization. Flex-knife ESD has a relatively low risk for perforation. The triangle-tip knife (with a triangular metal plate of 1.8 mm) may improve peri-tip coagulation. It can be used for dissection using the edge as a hook cut or with a safer but weaker cut using the tip. After complete lesion resection, additional fluid is injected to lift the resected area, and residual abnormal tissue can be removed by snare electrocautery. Because the colonic wall is thin, and the submucosal fluid leaks during the procedure, repeated submucosal fluid injections are important to reduce the perforation risk. ESD has been successfully used in a series of 200 colonic neoplasms in 18 patients, with lesions including adenomas, superficial carcinomas, and invasive carcinomas [86]. In this series, 183 (91.5%) of the lesions were treated with en bloc resection, with tumor-free margins in 70.5% of these. Eleven (5.5%) perforations were treated conservatively, with 1 (0.5%) delayed perforation that required surgery; 1.8% of the tumors had local recurrence, with no lymphadenopathy or metastasis detected at a median follow-up of 24 months. A recent Japanese study highlighted the success and safety of ESD for large colonic lesions. In a study of 71 colorectal neoplasms in 70 patients treated with ESD versus a group of 32 lesions managed by EMR, the ESD group (average lesion size = 32.7 mm) consisted primarily of laterally spreading tumors, with low-grade adenoma, HGD, and several cases of submucosal invasive cancer, with depths of invasion ranging from sm1 to sm3 [87]. For the ESD group, 98.6% of the lesions were removed by en bloc resection, with no tumor recurrence at a mean follow-up of 12.2 months, although some of these patients required repeated endoscopic resection. In contrast, the EMR group had a 6.3% recurrence rate, possibly because of the relatively high proportion of submucosal invasion.

## Complications of endoscopic mucosal resection

Although relatively safe, EMR is associated with complications (Table 2). The risk for bleeding ranges from 1.5% to 24% and seems to be higher than that for classical polypectomy. The bleeding rate depends on the type of lesion and the threshold for reporting the bleeding [88]. Bleeding is either immediate or delayed. It occurred in 22 instances, including 16 early and 6 delayed episodes, among 101 gastrointestinal lesions removed by EMR in 92 patients, including adenomas, areas of high-grade dysplasia, carcinoma, carcinoid, and others [89]. In one study, periprocedural bleeding occurred in 10.8% of EMRs for large sessile colonic polyps (n = 15), without delayed bleeding, and the postpolypectomy syndrome occurred in 3.7% (n = 5) [75]. An early study of 337 lesions, ranging from benign to submucosal invasive adenoma, demonstrated only one case (0.4%) of bleeding, and two cases (0.7%) of perforation [67]. Bleeding is usually controlled endoscopically, usually by endoscopic clips, which may have a decreased perforation rate compared with other modalities. ESD-related bleeding is usually controlled by endoscopic coaptive coagulation with an open biopsy forceps. Delayed bleeding may be reduced by administration of high-dose proton pump inhibitors and sucralfate. Complications, including bleeding and perforation, are associated with right-sided colonic location because of a relatively thin regional colonic wall, flat/sessile lesions, and large polyps (>3 cm in size). Large polyps are more advanced histologically and may require piecemeal resection with subsequent ablation to decrease the risk for recurrence [72]. Perforation is the most feared complication, with rates of 4% to 6% for ESD but lower rates for EMR. Small iatrogenic colonoscopic perforations that are promptly identified can be treated by closure

Table 2
Complications of colonic endoscopic mucosal resection

| N | Complication | Complication rate (%) | Reference |
|---|---|---|---|
| 50 | Bleeding | 10.8 | Conio et al [75] |
| | Postpolypectomy syndrome | 3.7 | |
| 337 | Bleeding | 0.4 | Yokota et al [67] |
| | Perforation | 0.7 | |
| 101 | Bleeding | 15.8 (early)<br>5.9 (delayed) | Ahmad et al [89] |

with endoscopically placed clips (Fig. 3, A–D) [90]. Extensive colonic perforations usually require urgent surgery. Post-EMR bacteremia rarely occurs. Two (5.3%) of 38 patients undergoing upper gastrointestinal EMR demonstrated transiently positive blood cultures with *Corynebacterium* or *Streptococcal* species, without signs or symptoms of systemic infection [91]. Stricture is associated with deep thermal injury from EMR or ESD during colonoscopy, but is more frequently associated with esophageal wall procedures. New techniques and modalities may reduce the risk for these complications [92].

## Current practice for endoscopic mucosal resection of the colon

There is little evidence that ESD provides a better patient outcome than EMR for either en bloc or piecemeal resection. The current management at our center is freehand en bloc or piecemeal resection of lesions after

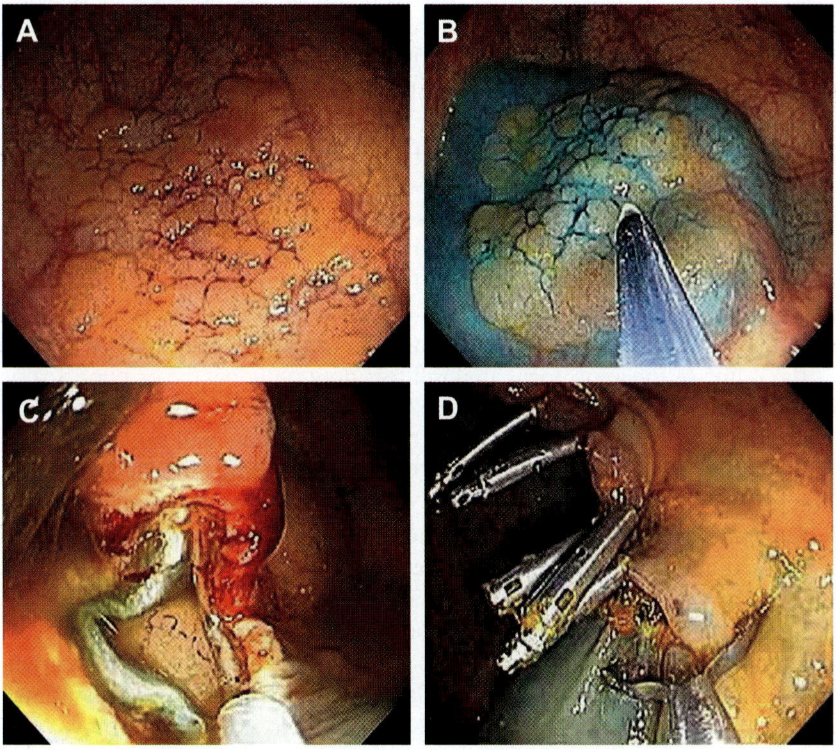


Fig. 3. (*A*) Flat, laterally spreading (carpetlike) polyp of the right colon. (*B*) Submucosal injection with a solution of dilute epinephrine and methylene blue in saline. Note the inadequate lifting of the left upper portion of the polyp. (*C*) Colonic perforation after snare resection of this polyp. (*D*) Successful closure of this colonic perforation with deployment of numerous endoclips. The patient experienced no adverse clinical sequelae.

submucosal fluid injection using a dilute solution of 1 of adrenaline to 150,000 of saline and a low concentration of methylene blue of 0.25 mL in 20 mL of saline. Highly viscous and hyperosmolar fluids are less important in snare resection because the time of resection is short and repeated injections before snare resection is adequate to lift the target tissue.

Very large polyps and polyps in the cecum, in the anal verge, near the appendiceal orifice, and on the ileocecal valve are difficult to remove. A large polyp requires more time for resection, rather than additional dexterity or instrumentation. Enough time should be scheduled to remove a large polyp at one session. Polyp removal in more than one session is counterproductive because scarring and retraction after the initial session impedes the subsequent lifting of the residual polyp.

At the detection of a polyp at an index endoscopy, suspicious areas, with retraction, ulceration, or rigidity, should be biopsied. If no suspicious areas are present, different parts of the polyp are sampled. The patient is then rescheduled at the same institution or referred to an outside expert for complete resection after the biopsy results confirm the absence of invasive cancer. For a long procedure to remove a giant polyp, the endoscopic field must be kept dry, and hemostasis with APC or electrocoagulation with hot biopsy forceps is often necessary to stem bleeding. For polyps that extend across two or more transverse folds, the upstream side of the polyp may be difficult to observe with a forward view and retroflexion may be necessary. Visualization is usually possible with a pediatric colonoscope but a gastroscope is a simple alternative in the left colon.

Polyps on the ileocecal valve or at the anal verge are challenging because of gathering and collapse of mucosal folds at these locations. A transparent friction cap is a useful device to splay open the area of concern and to provide an operating field with good illumination and visualization. For a polyp at the Z line of the anus, local anal infiltration with lidocaine or bupivacaine is necessary to prevent pain from the electrocautery.

Colonoscopic retroflexion is often necessary to view and treat polyps on the lower lip of the ileocecal valve and polyps extending into the anal verge. Polyps extending to the appendiceal orifice can be safely removed only if a clear margin is achievable. It is difficult to deploy even a small snare into a recessed area, such as the appendiceal orifice. After removing as much as possible by snare, the residual polyp is removed with multiple "flea bites" using a hot biopsy forceps. If a clear margin of resection cannot be achieved, combined laparoscopic and endoscopic removal can be attempted with intentional full-thickness snaring under laparoscopic control. This combined approach permits a modified wedge resection without hemicolectomy.

## Summary

The introduction of submucosal fluid injection has remarkably extended the range of endoscopically resectable polyps. The limiting factor for endoscopic resection is not polyp size, but polyp depth. Endoscopic ultrasound is a useful adjunctive diagnostic tool to assess the depth of invasion. The success of a resection ultimately depends on pathologic confirmation of benignity or of cancer limited to the mucosa. Selected well-differentiated cancers without lymphovascular invasion to the superficial submucosa can be successfully resected endoscopically.

## Acknowledgments

We thank Dr. Evin McCabe for his assistance in the preparation of the photographic images.

## References

[1] Hassan C, Zullo A, Winn S, et al. The colorectal malignant polyp: scoping a dilemma. Dig Liver Dis 2007;39(1):92–100.
[2] Beck DE, Margolin DA. Laparoscopic treatment of colonic polyps. Semin Laparosc Surg 2004;11(1):23–6.
[3] Baig MK, Wexner SD. Laparoscopic treatment of colonic polyps. A review. Minerva Chir 2003;58(4):447–57.
[4] Repici A, Tricerri R. Endoscopic polypectomy: techniques, complications and follow-up. Tech Coloproctol 2004;8(Suppl 2):s283–90.
[5] Waye JD. Advanced polypectomy. Gastrointest Endosc Clin N Am 2005;15(4):733–56.
[6] Parra-Blanco A, Kaminaga N, Kojima T, et al. Colonoscopic polypectomy with cutting current: is it safe? Gastrointest Endosc 2000;51(6):676–81.
[7] Su M-Y, Ho Y-P, Hsu C-M, et al. How can colorectal neoplasms be treated during colonoscopy? World J Gastroenterol 2005;11(18):2806–10.
[8] Waye JD. New methods of polypectomy. Gastrointest Endosc Clin N Am 1997;7(3):413–22.
[9] Waye JD. Endoscopic mucosal resection of colon polyps. Gastrointest Endosc Clin N Am 2001;11(3):537–48.
[10] Morales TG, Sampliner RE, Garewal HS, et al. The difference in colon polyp size before and after removal. Gastrointest Endosc 1996;43(1):25–8.
[11] Nizam R, Siddiqi N, Landas SK, et al. Colonic tattooing with India ink: benefits, risks, and alternatives. Am J Gastroenterol 1996;91(9):1804–8.
[12] Sosna J, Morrin MM, Copel L, et al. Computed tomography colonography (virtual colonoscopy): update on technique, applications, and future developments. Surg Technol Int 2003; 11:102–10.
[13] Compton CC, Greene FL. The staging of colorectal cancer: 2004 and beyond. CA Cancer J Clin 2004;54(6):295–308.
[14] Gollub MJ, Schwartz LH, Akhurst T. Update on colorectal cancer imaging. Radiol Clin North Am 2007;45(1):85–118.
[15] Yanai H, Matsumoto Y, Harada T, et al. Endoscopic ultrasonography and endoscopy for staging depth of invasion in early gastric cancer: a pilot study. Gastrointest Endosc 1997; 46(3):212–6.
[16] Gillard V. Evaluation of polyps by endoscopic ultrasonography (EUS): implication for endotherapy. Acta Gastroenterol Belg 1999;62(2):196–9.
[17] Waxman I, Saitoh Y. Clinical outcome of endoscopic mucosal resection for superficial GI lesions and the role of high-frequency US probe sonography in an American population. Gastrointest Endosc 2000;52(3):322–7.

[18] May A, Günter E, Roth F, et al. Accuracy of staging in early oesophageal cancer using high resolution endoscopy and high resolution endosonography: a comparative, prospective, and blinded trial. Gut 2004;53(5):634–40.
[19] Buskens CJ, Westerterp M, Lagarde SM, et al. Prediction of appropriateness of local endoscopic treatment for high-grade dysplasia and early adenocarcinoma by EUS and histopathologic features. Gastrointest Endosc 2004;60(5):703–10.
[20] Gotoda T, Yanagisawa A, Sasako M, et al. Incidence of lymph node metastasis from early gastric cancer: estimation with a large number of cases at two large centers. Gastric Cancer 2000;3(4):219–25.
[21] Eguchi T, Nakanishi Y, Shimoda T, et al. Histopathological criteria for additional treatment after endoscopic mucosal resection for esophageal cancer: analysis of 464 surgically resected cases. Mod Pathol 2006;19(3):475–80.
[22] Hurlstone DP, Brown S, Cross SS, et al. Endoscopic ultrasound miniprobe staging of colorectal cancer: can management be modified? Endoscopy 2005;37(8):710–4.
[23] Hurlstone DP, Sanders DS. Recent advances in chromoscopic colonoscopy and endomicroscopy. Curr Gastroenterol Rep 2006;8(5):409–15.
[24] DaCosta RS, Wilson BC, Marcon NE. Optical techniques for the endoscopic detection of dysplastic colonic lesions. Curr Opin Gastroenterol 2005;21(1):70–9.
[25] Bruno MJ. Magnification endoscopy, high resolution endoscopy, and chromoscopy: towards a better optical diagnosis. Gut 2003;52(Suppl 4):7–11.
[26] Thorlacius H, Toth E. Role of chromoendoscopy in colon cancer surveillance in inflammatory bowel disease. Inflamm Bowel Dis 2007;13(7):911–7.
[27] Axelrad AM, Fleischer DE, Geller AJ, et al. High-resolution chromoendoscopy for the diagnosis of diminutive colon polyps: implications for colon cancer screening. Gastroenterology 1996;110(4):1253–8.
[28] Kiesslich R, von Bergh M, Hahn M, et al. Chromoendoscopy with indigo carmine improves the detection of adenomatous and nonadenomatous lesions in the colon. Endoscopy 2001; 33(12):1001–6.
[29] Kanamori T, Itoh M, Yoshimi N. Pressure dye-spray: a simple and reliable method for differentiating adenomas from hyperplastic polyps in the colon. Gastrointest Endosc 2002; 55(6):695–700.
[30] Mönkemüller K, Fry LC, Ebert M, et al. Feasibility of double-balloon enteroscopy-assisted chromoendoscopy of the small bowel in patients with familial adenomatous polyposis. Endoscopy 2007;39(1):52–7.
[31] Trecca A, Gaj F, Di Lorenzo GP, et al. Improved detection of colorectal neoplasms with selective use of chromoendoscopy in 2005 consecutive patients. Tech Coloproctol 2006; 10(4):339–44.
[32] Mitooka H, Fujimori T, Maeda S, et al. Minute flat depressed neoplastic lesions of the colon detected by contrast chromoscopy using an indigo carmine capsule. Gastrointest Endosc 1995;41(5):453–9.
[33] Kudo S, Kashida H, Tamura T, et al. Colonoscopic diagnosis and management of nonpolypoid early colorectal cancer. World J Surg 2000;24(9):1081–90.
[34] Huang Q, Fukami N, Kashida H. Interobserver and intra-observer consistency in the endoscopic assessment of colonic pit patterns. Gastrointest Endosc 2004;60(4):520–6.
[35] Ince A, Bölükbas C, Peker O, et al. Pit pattern type analyses of colon polyps with high-resolution colonoscope. Hepatogastroenterology 2007;54(73):67–70.
[36] Liu HH, Kudo SE, Juch JP. Pit pattern analysis by magnifying chromoendoscopy for diagnosis of colorectal polyps. J Formos Med Assoc 2003;102(3):178–82.
[37] Apel D, Jakobs R, Schilling D, et al. Accuracy of high-resolution chromoendoscopy in prediction of histologic findings in diminutive lesions of the rectosigmoid. Gastrointest Endosc 2006;63(6):824–8.
[38] Hurlstone DP, Fujii T. Practical uses of chromoendoscopy and magnification at colonoscopy. Gastrointest Endosc Clin N Am 2005;15(4):687–702.

[39] Fu KI, Sano Y, Kato S, et al. Chromoendoscopy using indigo carmine dye spraying with magnifying observation is the most reliable method for differential diagnosis between non-neoplastic and neoplastic colorectal lesions: a prospective study. Endoscopy 2004;36(12): 1089–93.
[40] Eisen GM, Kim CY, Fleischer DE, et al. High-resolution chromoendoscopy for classifying colonic polyps: a multicenter study. Gastrointest Endosc 2002;55(6):687–94.
[41] De Palma GD, Rega M, Masone S, et al. Conventional colonoscopy and magnified chromoendoscopy for the endoscopic histological prediction of diminutive colorectal polyps: a single operator study. World J Gastroenterol 2006;12(15):2402–5.
[42] Gross SA, Wallace MB. Hold on Picasso, narrow band imaging is here. Am J Gastroenterol 2006;101(1):2717–8.
[43] Muto M, Katada C, Sano Y, et al. Narrow band imaging: a new diagnostic approach to visualize angiogenesis in superficial neoplasia. Clin Gastroenterol Hepatol 2005; 3(7 Suppl 1):S16–20.
[44] Kuznetsov K, Lambert R, Rey JF. Narrow-band imaging: potential and limitations. Endoscopy 2006;38(1):76–81.
[45] Chiu HM, Chang CY, Chen CC, et al. A prospective comparative study of narrow-band imaging, chromoendoscopy, and conventional colonoscopy in the diagnosis of colorectal neoplasia. Gut 2007;56(3):373–9.
[46] Su MY, Hsu CM, Ho YP, et al. Comparative study of conventional colonoscopy, chromoendoscopy, and narrow-band imaging systems in differential diagnosis of neoplastic and nonneoplastic colonic polyps. Am J Gastroenterol 2006;101(12):2711–6.
[47] Goetz M, Hoffman A, Galle PR, et al. Confocal laser endoscopy: new approach to the early diagnosis of tumors of the esophagus and stomach. Future Oncol 2006;2(4):469–76.
[48] Hoffman A, Goetz M, Vieth M, et al. Confocal laser endomicroscopy: technical status and current indications. Endoscopy 2006;38(12):1275–83.
[49] Rembacken BJ, Gotoda T, Fujii T, et al. Endoscopic mucosal resection. Endoscopy 2001; 33(8):709–18
[50] Larghi A, Waxman I. Endoscopic mucosal resection: treatment of neoplasia. Gastrointest Endosc Clin N Am 2005;15(3):431–54.
[51] Larghi A, Waxman I. State of the art on endoscopic mucosal resection and endoscopic submucosal dissection. Gastrointest Endosc Clin N Am 2007;17(3):441–69.
[52] Uno Y, Munakata A. The non-lifting sign of invasive colon cancer. Gastrointest Endosc 1994;40(4):485–9.
[53] Yamamoto H, Yube T, Isode N, et al. A novel method of endoscopic mucosal resection using sodium hyaluronate. Gastrointest Endosc 1999;50(2):251–6.
[54] Yamamoto H, Kawata H, Sunada K, et al. Success rate of curative endoscopic mucosal resection with circumferential mucosal incision assisted by submucosal injection of sodium hyaluronate. Gastrointest Endosc 2002;56(4):507–12.
[55] Yamamoto H, Kawata H, Sunada K, et al. Successful en-bloc resection of large superficial tumors in the stomach and colon using sodium hyaluronate and small-caliber-tip transparent hood. Endoscopy 2003;35(8):690–4.
[56] Katsinelos P, Kountouras J, Paroutoglou G, et al. Endoscopic mucosal resection of large sessile colorectal polyps with submucosal injection of hypertonic 50 percent dextrose-epinephrine solution. Dis Colon Rectum 2006;49(9):1384–92.
[57] Fijishiro M, Yahagi N, Kashimura K, et al. Tissue damage of different submucosal injection solutions for EMR. Gastrointest Endosc 2005;62(6):933–42.
[58] Sato T. A novel method of endoscopic mucosal resection assisted by submucosal injection of autologous blood (blood patch EMR). Dis Colon Rectum 2006;49(10):1636–41.
[59] Inoue H, Endo M. Endoscopic esophageal mucosal resection using a transparent tube. Surg Endosc 1990;4(4):198–201.
[60] Inoue H, Endo M, Takeshita K, et al. A new simplified technique of endoscopic esophageal mucosal resection using a cap-fitted panendoscope (EMRC). Surg Endosc 1992;6(5):264–5.

[61] Inoue H, Takeshita K, Hori H, et al. Endoscopic mucosal resection with a cap-fitted panendoscope for esophagus, stomach, and colon mucosal lesions. Gastrointest Endosc 1993; 39(1):58–62.
[62] Tada M, Inoue H, Yabata E, et al. Feasibility of the transparent cap-fitted colonoscope for screening and mucosal resection. Dis Colon Rectum 1997;40(5):618–21.
[63] Larghi A, Waxman I. State of the art on endoscopic mucosal resection and endoscopic submucosal dissection. Gastrointest Endosc Clin N Am 2007;17(3):445–8.
[64] Inoue H, Kawano T, Tani M, et al. Endoscopic mucosal resection using a cap: techniques for use and preventing perforation. Can J Gastroenterol 1999;13(6):477–80.
[65] Sumiyama K, Gostout CJ. Novel techniques and instrumentation for EMR, ESD, and full-thickness endoscopic luminal resection. Gastrointest Endosc Clin N Am 2007;17(3): 471–85.
[66] Van Os EC, Gostout CJ, Geller A, et al. Band ligation-assisted endoscopic resection of a flat rectal adenoma containing infiltrating adenocarcinoma. Gastrointest Endosc 1997;45(3):322–4.
[67] Yokota T, Sugihara K, Yoshida S. Endoscopic mucosal resection for colorectal neoplastic lesions. Dis Colon Rectum 1994;37(11):1108–11.
[68] Hurlstone DP, Sanders DS, Cross SS. Colonoscopic resection of lateral spreading tumours: a prospective analysis of endoscopic mucosal resection. Gut 2004;53(9):1334–9.
[69] Bories E, Pesenti C, Monges G, et al. Endoscopic mucosal resection for advanced sessile adenoma and early-stage colorectal carcinoma. Endoscopy 2006;38(3):231–5.
[70] Tung SY, Wu CS. Clinical outcome of endoscopically removed early colorectal cancer. J Gastroenterol Hepatol 2003;18(10):1175–9.
[71] Fukami N, Lee JH. Endoscopic treatment of large sessile and flat colorectal lesions. Curr Opin Gastroenterol 2006;22(1):54–9.
[72] Church JM. Experience in the endoscopic management of large colonic polyps. ANZ J Surg 2003;73(12):988–95.
[73] Hawes RH. Perspectives in endoscopic mucosal resection. Gastrointest Endosc Clin N Am 2001;11(3):549–52.
[74] Tanaka S, Haruma K, Oka S, et al. Clinicopathologic features and endoscopic treatment of superficially spreading colorectal neoplasms larger than 20mm. Gastrointest Endosc 2001; 54(1):62–6.
[75] Conio M, Repici A, Demarquay JF, et al. EMR of large sessile colorectal polyps. Gastrointest Endosc 2004;60(2):234–41.
[76] Hurlstone DP, Cross SS, Drew K, et al. An evaluation of colorectal endoscopic mucosal resection using high-magnification chromoscopic colonoscopy: a prospective study of 1000 colonoscopies. Endoscopy 2004;36(6):491–8.
[77] Arebi N, Swain D, Suzuki N, et al. Endoscopic mucosal resection of 161 cases of large sessile or flat colorectal polyps. Scand J Gastroenterol 2007;42(7):859–66.
[78] Jameel JK, Pillinger SH, Moncur P, et al. Endoscopic mucosal resection (EMR) in the management of large colorectal polyps. Colorectal Dis 2006;8(6):497–500.
[79] Kume K, Murata I, Yoshikawa I, et al. Endoscopic piecemeal mucosal resection of large colorectal tumors. Hepatogastroenterology 2005;52(62):429–32.
[80] Brooker JC, Saunders BP, Shah SG, et al. Treatment with argon plasma coagulation reduces recurrence after piecemeal resection of large sessile colonic polyps: a randomized trial and recommendations. Gastrointest Endosc 2002;55(3):371–5.
[81] Binmoeller KF, Bohnacker S, Seifert H, et al. Endoscopic snare excision of "giant" colorectal polyps. Gastrointest Endosc 1996;43(3):183–8.
[82] Hurlstone DP, Sanders DS, Cross SS, et al. A prospective analysis of extended endoscopic mucosal resection for large rectal villous adenomas: an alternative technique to transanal endoscopic microsurgery. Colorectal Dis 2005;7(4):339–44.
[83] Hurlstone DP, Sanders DS, Atkinson R, et al. Endoscopic mucosal resection for flat neoplasia in chronic ulcerative colitis: can we change the endoscopic management paradigm? Gut 2007;56(6):838–46.

[84] Hurlstone DP, Sanders DS, Thomson M, et al. "Salvage" endoscopic mucosal resection in the colon using a retroflexion gastroscope dissection technique: a prospective analysis. Endoscopy 2006;38(9):902–6.
[85] Kodashima S, Fujishiro M, Yahagi N, et al. Endoscopic submucosal dissection using flex-knife. J Clin Gastroenterol 2006;40(5):378–84.
[86] Fujishiro M, Yahagi N, Kakushima N, et al. Endoscopic submucosal dissection of esophageal squamous cell neoplasms. Clin Gastroenterol Hepatol 2006;4(6):688–94.
[87] Tamegai Y, Saito Y, Masaki N, et al. Endoscopic submucosal dissection: a safe technique for colorectal tumors. Endoscopy 2007;39(5):418–22.
[88] Larghi A, Waxman I. State of the art on endoscopic mucosal resection and endoscopic submucosal dissection. Gastrointest Endosc Clin N Am 2007;17(3):448–50.
[89] Ahmad NA, Kochman ML, Long WB, et al. Efficacy, safety, and clinical outcomes of endoscopic mucosal resection: a study of 101 cases. Gastrointest Endosc 2002;55(3):390–6.
[90] Yoshikane H, Hidano H, Sakakibara A, et al. Endoscopic repair by clipping of iatrogenic colonic perforation. Gastrointest Endosc 1997;46(5):464–6.
[91] Lee T-H, Hsueh P-R, Yeh W-C, et al. Low frequency of bacteremia after endoscopic mucosal resection. Gastrointest Endosc 2000;52(2):223–5.
[92] Fatima H, Rex DK. Minimizing endoscopic complications: colonoscopic polypectomy. Gastrointest Endosc Clin N Am 2007;17(1):145–56.

THE MEDICAL CLINICS OF NORTH AMERICA

ELSEVIER SAUNDERS

Med Clin N Am 92 (2008) 707–715

# Index

*Note:* Page numbers of article titles are in **boldface** type.



0025-7125/08/$ - see front matter 
doi:10.1016/S0025-7125(08)00039-4 